Plant-Derived Phenolic Compounds: From Molecular Mechanisms to Clinical Application

Plant-Derived Phenolic Compounds: From Molecular Mechanisms to Clinical Application

Editors

Stefano Castellani
Massimo Conese

MDPI • Basel • Beijing • Wuhan • Barcelona • Belgrade • Manchester • Tokyo • Cluj • Tianjin

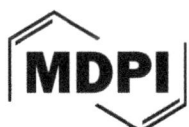

Editors

Stefano Castellani
Department of Precision and
Regenerative Medicine and
Ionian Area - (DiMePRe-J)
University Aldo Moro of Bari
Bari
Italy

Massimo Conese
Department of Clinical and
Experimental Medicine
University of Foggia
Foggia
Italy

Editorial Office
MDPI
St. Alban-Anlage 66
4052 Basel, Switzerland

This is a reprint of articles from the Special Issue published online in the open access journal *Molecules* (ISSN 1420-3049) (available at: www.mdpi.com/journal/molecules/special_issues/ Proanthocyanidins_Natural).

For citation purposes, cite each article independently as indicated on the article page online and as indicated below:

LastName, A.A.; LastName, B.B.; LastName, C.C. Article Title. *Journal Name* **Year**, *Volume Number*, Page Range.

ISBN 978-3-0365-7759-3 (Hbk)
ISBN 978-3-0365-7758-6 (PDF)

© 2023 by the authors. Articles in this book are Open Access and distributed under the Creative Commons Attribution (CC BY) license, which allows users to download, copy and build upon published articles, as long as the author and publisher are properly credited, which ensures maximum dissemination and a wider impact of our publications.

The book as a whole is distributed by MDPI under the terms and conditions of the Creative Commons license CC BY-NC-ND.

Contents

About the Editors vii

Preface to "Plant-Derived Phenolic Compounds: From Molecular Mechanisms to Clinical Application" ix

El Hadi Erbiai, Abdelfettah Maouni, Luís Pinto da Silva, Rabah Saidi, Mounir Legssyer and Zouhaire Lamrani et al.
Antioxidant Properties, Bioactive Compounds Contents, and Chemical Characterization of Two Wild Edible Mushroom Species from Morocco: *Paralepista flaccida* (Sowerby) Vizzini and *Lepista nuda* (Bull.) Cooke
Reprinted from: *Molecules* **2023**, *28*, 1123, doi:10.3390/molecules28031123 1

Katarzyna Ratajczak, Natalia Glatzel-Plucińska, Katarzyna Ratajczak-Wielgomas, Katarzyna Nowińska and Sylwia Borska
Effect of Resveratrol Treatment on Human Pancreatic Cancer Cells through Alterations of Bcl-2 Family Members
Reprinted from: *Molecules* **2021**, *26*, 6560, doi:10.3390/molecules26216560 15

Elisa Aranda, José A. Teruel, Antonio Ortiz, María Dolores Pérez-Cárceles, José N. Rodríguez-López and Francisco J. Aranda
Effects of a Semisynthetic Catechin on Phosphatidylglycerol Membranes: A Mixed Experimental and Simulation Study
Reprinted from: *Molecules* **2023**, *28*, 422, doi:10.3390/molecules28010422 37

Marta Oleszek, Iwona Kowalska, Terenzio Bertuzzi and Wiesław Oleszek
Phytochemicals Derived from Agricultural Residues and Their Valuable Properties and Applications
Reprinted from: *Molecules* **2023**, *28*, 342, doi:10.3390/molecules28010342 53

Nadia Naim, Marie-Laure Fauconnier, Nabil Ennahli, Abdessalem Tahiri, Mohammed Baala and Ilham Madani et al.
Chemical Composition Profiling and Antifungal Activity of Saffron Petal Extract
Reprinted from: *Molecules* **2022**, *27*, 8742, doi:10.3390/molecules27248742 103

Mongi Saoudi, Riadh Badraoui, Ahlem Chira, Mohd Saeed, Nouha Bouali and Salem Elkahoui et al.
The Role of *Allium subhirsutum* L. in the Attenuation of Dermal Wounds by Modulating Oxidative Stress and Inflammation in *Wistar* Albino Rats
Reprinted from: *Molecules* **2021**, *26*, 4875, doi:10.3390/molecules26164875 119

Mongi Saoudi, Riadh Badraoui, Ahlem Chira, Mohd Saeed, Nouha Bouali and Salem Elkahoui et al.
Correction: Saoudi et al. The Role of *Allium subhirsutum* L. in the Attenuation of Dermal Wounds by Modulating Oxidative Stress and Inflammation in *Wistar* Albino Rats. *Molecules* 2021, *26*, 4875
Reprinted from: *Molecules* **2022**, *27*, 5332, doi:10.3390/molecules27165332 135

Xiaoli Zhu and Khaled Athmouni
HPLC Analysis and the Antioxidant and Preventive Actions of *Opuntia stricta* Juice Extract against Hepato-Nephrotoxicity and Testicular Injury Induced by Cadmium Exposure
Reprinted from: *Molecules* **2022**, *27*, 4972, doi:10.3390/molecules27154972 137

Adriana Trapani, María Ángeles Esteban, Francesca Curci, Daniela Erminia Manno, Antonio Serra and Giuseppe Fracchiolla et al.
Solid Lipid Nanoparticles Administering Antioxidant Grape Seed-Derived Polyphenol Compounds: A Potential Application in Aquaculture †
Reprinted from: *Molecules* **2022**, *27*, 344, doi:10.3390/molecules27020344 . . . . **151**

Wei Gao, Tingting Yu, Guomeng Li, Wei Shu, Yongxun Jin and Mingjun Zhang et al.
Antioxidant Activity and Anti-Apoptotic Effect of the Small Molecule Procyanidin B1 in Early Mouse Embryonic Development Produced by Somatic Cell Nuclear Transfer
Reprinted from: *Molecules* **2021**, *26*, 6150, doi:10.3390/molecules26206150 . . . . **173**

Cristiane Okuda Torello, Marisa Claudia Alvarez and Sara T. Olalla Saad
Polyphenolic Flavonoid Compound Quercetin Effects in the Treatment of Acute Myeloid Leukemia and Myelodysplastic Syndromes
Reprinted from: *Molecules* **2021**, *26*, 5781, doi:10.3390/molecules26195781 . . . . **187**

Wedad S. Sarawi, Ahlam M. Alhusaini, Laila M. Fadda, Hatun A. Alomar, Awatif B. Albaker and Amjad S. Aljrboa et al.
Curcumin and Nano-Curcumin Mitigate Copper Neurotoxicity by Modulating Oxidative Stress, Inflammation, and Akt/GSK-3β Signaling
Reprinted from: *Molecules* **2021**, *26*, 5591, doi:10.3390/molecules26185591 . . . . **199**

Nellysha Namela Muhammad Abdul Kadar, Fairus Ahmad, Seong Lin Teoh and Mohamad Fairuz Yahaya
Caffeic Acid on Metabolic Syndrome: A Review
Reprinted from: *Molecules* **2021**, *26*, 5490, doi:10.3390/molecules26185490 . . . . **213**

About the Editors

Stefano Castellani

Stefano Castellani, Ph.D., is associate professor in General Pathology at the Department of Precision and Regenerative Medicine and Ionian Area (DiMePRe-J), Aldo Moro University of Bari, Bari, Italy. His research interests have concerned the pathophysiology of cystic fibrosis and gene- and drug-based delivery for its treatment. In recent years, he has been involved in in vitro studies of nanoparticle delivery for the treatment of pathologies, such as chronic airway inflammatory diseases and Parkinson's disease. In particular, from 2015 to 2018 he was project manager of the research project "Delivery of natural anti-oxidants to the lung using paramagnetic nanoparticles for the treatment of chronic respiratory diseases" and of the project "Nanotechnologies applied to the delivery of natural substances for the therapy of chronic respiratory diseases". As per Scopus, Dr. Castellani has currently published 59 peer-reviewed scientific articles with a h-index of 18.

Massimo Conese

Massimo Conese, M.D., Ph.D., is full professor in General Pathology and the Director of the Laboratory of Experimental and Regenerative Medicine at the University of Foggia, Foggia, Italy. His general interests are in the pathophysiology of cystic fibrosis, as well as in gene-, drug-, and stem cell-based treatments. He is presently working on nanoparticle-mediated drug delivery and plant-derived extracellular vesicles aimed at treating chronic airway inflammatory diseases, Parkinson's disease, and inflammatory bowel disease. He is also studying the role of human adipose-derived stem cells in the treatment of intractable wounds. He was appointed Coordinator in the European Community (EC) project (FP5) "Development and application of chromosome-based gene transfer vectors for cell therapy" (2003–2006) and was Partner in two EC projects (FP6) "Improved precision of nucleic acid based therapy of cystic fibrosis" (2005–2008) and "European Coordination Action for Research in Cystic Fibrosis" (2005–2009). As per Scopus, Dr. Conese has published 169 peer-reviewed scientific articles, with a h-index of 39.Dr. Conese is Editorial Board Member of *Open Medicine, Current Stem Cell Research & Therapy, Case Reports in Medicine, International Journal of Molecular Sciences, Cells, Journal of Respiration, Pathophysiology* and *Stem Cell Investigation*.

Preface to "Plant-Derived Phenolic Compounds: From Molecular Mechanisms to Clinical Application"

Plant-derived phenolic compounds have gained attention over time since they have proved effective antioxidant, anticarcinogenic, anti-inflammatory, neuroprotective and cardioprotective properties.This Special Issue entitled "Plant-Derived Phenolic Compounds: From Molecular Mechanisms to Clinical Application" collects the accumulative effort of several leading international scientists who have contributed to the research on these phenolic molecules derived from fruits, seeds, leaves, and flowers, focusing on their extraction, synthesis, characterization, and delivery for a wide variety of purposes, ranging from their use in prevention and therapy of several diseases, to the study their biological properties for different applications. The purpose of the Special Issue is to shed light on various aspects related to phenolic extracts, collecting reviews of recent avances relating to their use in various research fields, and novel research works aimed at obtaining new informations on the biological features of these molecules. This Special Issue, which provides an opportunity to both highlight the recent avances in the field of plant-derived phenolic compounds and elucidating previously unaddressed aspects, such as the mechanisms involved in their protective activity, is addressed to scientists who deal with this topic, encouraging new lines of research. A large audience should be interested in this Special Issue. In particular, in addition to the pharmacological interest in these compounds, their biological activities should be explored to benefit a range of applications, such as in the functional food, in the cosmetic, and in the packaging industries.

Stefano Castellani and Massimo Conese
Editors

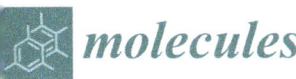

Article

Antioxidant Properties, Bioactive Compounds Contents, and Chemical Characterization of Two Wild Edible Mushroom Species from Morocco: *Paralepista flaccida* (Sowerby) Vizzini and *Lepista nuda* (Bull.) Cooke

El Hadi Erbiai [1,2], Abdelfettah Maouni [1], Luís Pinto da Silva [2], Rabah Saidi [1], Mounir Legssyer [1], Zouhaire Lamrani [1] and Joaquim C. G. Esteves da Silva [2,*]

[1] Biology, Environment, and Sustainable Development Laboratory, Higher School of Teachers (ENS), Abdelmalek Essaadi University, Tetouan 93000, Morocco
[2] Chemistry Research Unit (CIQUP), Institute of Molecular Sciences (IMS), Department of Geosciences, Environment and Territorial Planning, Faculty of Sciences, University of Porto, Rua do Campo Alegre s/n, 4169-007 Porto, Portugal
* Correspondence: jcsilva@fc.up.pt; Tel.: +351-220402569

Abstract: Mushrooms have been consumed for centuries and have recently gained more popularity as an important source of nutritional and pharmaceutical compounds. As part of the valorization of mushroom species in northern Morocco, the current study aimed to investigate the chemical compositions and antioxidant properties of two wild edible mushrooms, *Paralepista flaccida* and *Lepista nuda*. Herein, the bioactive compounds were determined using spectrophotometer methods, and results showed that the value of total phenolic content (TPC) was found to be higher in *P. flaccida* (32.86 ± 0.52 mg) than in *L. nuda* (25.52 ± 0.56 mg of gallic acid equivalents (GAEs)/mg of dry methanolic extract (dme)). On the other hand, the value of total flavonoid content (TFC) was greater in *L. nuda* than in *P. flaccida*, with values of 19.02 ± 0.80 and 10.34 ± 0.60 mg of (+)-catechin equivalents (CEs)/g dme, respectively. Moreover, the ascorbic acid, tannin, and carotenoids content was moderate, with a non-significant difference between the two samples. High-performance liquid chromatography–mass spectrometry (HPLC-MS) analysis allowed the identification and quantification of thirteen individual phenolic compounds in both *P. flaccida* and *L. nuda*, whereas *p*-Hydroxybenzoic acid was recognized as the major compound detected, with values of 138.50 ± 1.58 and 587.90 ± 4.89 µg/g of dry weight (dw), respectively. The gas chromatography–mass spectrometry (GC-MS) analysis of methanolic extracts of *P. flaccida* and *L. nuda* revealed the presence of sixty-one and sixty-six biomolecules, respectively. These biomolecules can mainly be divided into four main groups, namely sugars, amino acids, fatty acids, and organic acids. Moreover, glycerol (12.42%) and mannitol (10.39%) were observed to be the main chemical compositions of *P. flaccida*, while *L. nuda* was predominated by linolelaidic acid (21.13%) and leucine (9.05%). *L. nuda* showed a strong antioxidant property, evaluated by DPPH (half maximal effective concentration (EC_{50}) 1.18–0.98 mg/mL); β-carotene bleaching (EC_{50} 0.22–0.39 mg/mL); and reducing power methods (EC_{50} 0.63–0.48 mg/mL), respectively. These findings suggested that both mushrooms are potential sources of various biomolecules, many of which possess important biological activities which are interesting for the foods and pharmaceuticals industry.

Keywords: *Paralepista flaccida*; *Lepista nuda*; bioactive compounds; biomolecules; antioxidant activity; Moroccan mushroom; wild edible mushroom

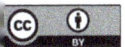

1. Introduction

Mushrooms have been consumed for centuries due to their nutritional and medicinal benefits. In terms of nutritional value, the fruiting bodies of mushrooms are known to be rich in high-quality protein, essential and non-essential amino acids, have a high proportion of unsaturated fatty acids, a good source of fiber, and a higher amount of carbohydrates, and are also full of micronutrients, such as vitamin B complex, and a high level of mineral elements that are essential for human health [1,2]. In medicinal terms, several studies have demonstrated that mushrooms contain a wide variety of bioactive compounds, such as alkaloids, carotenoids, enzymes, fats, glycosides, organic acids, phenolics, polysaccharides, proteins, terpenoids, tocopherols, vitamins, and volatile compounds in general. These compounds from mushrooms have shown a wide range of biological activities, including antioxidant, antibacterial, antifungal, antitumor, immunomodulating, cardiovascular-protective, antiviral, antiparasitic, antifibrotic, anti-inflammatory, antidiabetic, anti-atherosclerotic, hypoallergenic, antiatherogenic, hypoglycemic, hepatoprotective, and hypotensive properties [1,2]. Consequently, mushrooms have become more attractive as functional foods and as a source of nutraceuticals and pharmaceutical compounds.

Oxidative stress is involved in many diseases, as a trigger or associated with complications. Most of these diseases appear with age, which leads to serious pathologies such as cardiovascular and neurodegenerative diseases, cancer, diabetes, metabolic syndrome, and digestive disease [3]. Many important molecules with antioxidant properties can help the endogenous defense system against oxidative stress caused by the excess of reactive oxygen and nitrogen species (ROS and RNS) [4]. Wild mushrooms contain different antioxidants such as phenolic compounds, tocopherols, ascorbic acid, carotenoids and more other molecules which could be extracted to be used as functional ingredients, namely against chronic diseases related to oxidative stress [4,5].

Paralepista flaccida (Sowerby) Vizzini, (2012) is a wild edible basidiomycete mushroom belonging to the order *Agaricales* and the family *Tricholomataceae* [6]. It is known to form fairy rings [7]. *Paralepista* species were generally assigned either to the genus *Lepista* or *Clitocybe*, until 2012 when Alfredo Vizzini and Enrico Ercole published a paper that confirmed by molecular analysis that these mushrooms are a separate clade from other *Lepista* species (such as *Lepista nuda*) and also from *Clitocybe* species (such as *Clitocybe fragrans*) [8]. This genus is recognized by Species Fungorum [9], and the Global Biodiversity Information Facility [10].

The naming of this mushroom is complicated, and some references generally listed the *flaccida* and *inversa* forms as separate species, in which the case of *inversa* is distinguished because it grows under conifers rather than broad-leaved trees, has a shinier cap surface, and is more rigid (less flaccid), which is according to our collected samples. However, other mycologists are considering *inversa* as a variety of *flaccida*, and, finally, some modern authors merge the two into one [7,9–14].

P. flaccida is saprophytic species growing naturally on humus-rich soil and compost under deciduous trees, while the *inversa* form grows under conifer needles. It is frequently distributed in Europe [12] and has also been reported wildly in forests of *Quercus*, *Cedrus*, *Acacia*, and *Pinus* in diverse areas of Morocco including Chefchaouen, Ktama, Tangier, Lalla Mimouna, Middle Atlas and Rabat [15–20].

Lepista nuda (Bull.) Cooke, (1871) (also called *Clitocybe nuda*, commonly known as blewits) is an edible basidiomycete mushroom belonging to the same order and family as *P. flaccida*. It is a saprotrophic species found in both deciduous and mixed forest areas in Europe, North America, Asia and Australia [21,22]. Due to its special fragrance and delicate texture, *L. nuda* has been cultivated in several countries, including France, Holland, Britain, and Taiwan [21]. In Morocco, *L. nuda* has been found widely under *Quercus*, *Cedrus*, and *Pinus* trees in several sites, including Chefchaouen, Dardara, Oued Laou, Bouhachem, Gourougou, Ain Sferjla, Oued Cherrat, Lalla Mimouna, Mamora, Rabat and also in coastal plateau from Essaouira to Tangier [16,18–20,23–25].

Many studies on the chemical compositions and biological activities of mushrooms have been made in northern Mediterranean countries concerning the species growing in this region. However, as far as we know, there are few studies on mushrooms in southern countries, especially in Morocco, which is considered one of the richest Mediterranean countries in terms of biodiversity [25–27].

Several studies have been carried out on the chemical compositions and biological activities of *L. nuda* [2,22], while few data were reported about *P. flaccida* which were in the case of *inversa* form [2,28]. However, as we know no studies were reported on these two species growing in Morocco, except one study which was performed on the total phenolic and antioxidant activity of *L. nuda* collected from Natural Parc of Bouhachem [25].

The objective of the present study was to investigate the chemical compositions and antioxidant activity of two wild edible mushrooms, *Paralepista flaccida* and *Lepista nuda*, collected from northern Morocco. Herein, the contents of the bioactive compounds including total phenolic, total flavonoid, total ascorbic acid, total tannin, and total carotenoids contents (β-carotene and lycopene) were determined using a UV-Visible spectrophotometer, while high-performance liquid chromatography-mass spectrometry (HPLC-MS) was used for the identification and quantification of phenolic compounds, and gas chromatography-mass spectrometry (GC-MS) for biomolecules identification. Moreover, the antioxidant properties were evaluated by three different assays, including DPPH radical-scavenging, β-carotene bleaching inhibition, and reducing power assay.

2. Results and Discussion

2.1. Extraction Yield

As presented in Table 1, the extraction yields of methanolic extracts of *P. flaccida* (30.32 %) and *L. nuda* (31.69 %) were statistically similar to each other's, while lower than the previous yield in the Portuguese *Lepista inversa* (39%) which was reported by Heleno et al. [29].

Table 1. Extraction yield and bioactive compound contents in the dried fruiting body of mushroom studies [1].

Bioactive Compounds	*P. flaccida*	*L. nuda*	One-Way ANOVA *
Extraction yield (%)	30.32 ± 1.14	31.69 ± 2.04	0.4736
Total phenolic (mg GAE/g dme)	32.86 ± 0.52 [a]	25.52 ± 0.56 [b]	<0.0001
Total flavonoid (mg CE/g dme)	10.34 ± 0.06 [b]	19.02 ± 0.80 [a]	<0.0001
Ascorbic acid (mg AAE/g dw)	1.27 ± 0.06	1.31 ± 0.03	0.9048
Tannin (mg CE/g dw)	2.67 ± 0.04	2.26 ± 0.19	>0.9999
β-Carotene (µg/g dme)	0.30 ± 0.02	0.64 ± 0.01	0.9982
Lycopene (µg/g dme)	0.23 ± 0.01	0.38 ± 0.01	>0.9999

[1] Values are expressed as means ± SD of three independent measurements. * $p < 0.05$ indicates that the mean value of at least one component differs from the others. For each mushroom sample, means within a line with different letters differ significantly ($p < 0.05$).

2.2. Estimation of Bioactive Compounds

The bioactive compound contents in the studied mushroom samples were estimated using a UV-Visible spectrophotometer, and the results are presented in Table 1.

Total phenolic contents in the methanolic extract were observed to be significantly important in both tested species, although *P. flaccida* was shown to have a higher amount, with the value of 32.86 mg GAE/g of dme, which is higher than the previous studies by Heleno et al., (3.60 mg) [29] and Vaz et al., (10.8 mg in ethanolic extract) [30] in *Lepista inversa*. Similarly, *L. nuda* content (25.52 mg) was noted to be higher than several works from Morocco, Turkey, Portugal and Turkey, with values of 11.83, 7.7, 6.31, and 4.18 mg GAE/g of dme, respectively [25,31–33], which was close to the amount in the given results in the Argentinian (27.34 mg) [34] and the Indian mushrooms (23.77 mg) [35].

Concerning total flavonoid contents, the methanolic extract of *L. nuda* was given, statically, as a more important content than *P. flaccida*, with the values of 19.02 and 10.34 mg CE/g of dme, respectively. However, Barros et al. [32] (3.36 mg CE/g dme) and Sharma et al. [35] (2.47 mg quercetin equivalent/g dme) found lower flavonoid contents in *L. nuda* than in the present study.

Regarding ascorbic acid content, the fruiting body of samples presented a moderate result and there were no significant differences between *P. flaccida* (1.27 mg/g) and *L. nuda* (1.31 mg/g). The amount of ascorbic acid in *L. nuda* was observed to be higher than the values of 0.34 and 0.23 mg/g obtained in the previous studies [32,35], respectively. However, ascorbic acid was not detected in the work by Lkay Koca et al. [31].

The amount of tannin content in *P. flaccida* was found to be significantly similar to *L. nuda*, with the values of 2.67 and 2.26 mg CE/g of dw, respectively. To our knowledge, there were no previous studies on the tannin content of both samples.

As shown in Table 1, β-carotene and lycopene contents were observed to be present statistically in small quantities in comparison with the premier bioactive compounds. However, the values of β-carotene and lycopene from *L. nuda* were higher than the previous study from India [35] (0.39 and 0.20 µg/100 g), while smaller than the one reported in the Portuguese sample [32] (2.52 and 0.98 µg/g).

Overall, the content of bioactive compounds determined in the studied wild edible mushrooms from Morocco was very important, although these compounds have been previously estimated in many other mushrooms and are known for their strong antioxidant capacity [5].

2.3. Phenolic Compounds by HPLC–MS Analysis

The identification and quantification of individual phenolic compounds in fruiting body extracts of *P. flaccida* and *L. nuda* were performed using the HPLC–MS technique. The chromatogram illustrating the phenolic compounds peaks in *P. flaccida* and *L. nuda* is shown in Figure 1 and Figure S1, respectively, whereas Table 2 gives the amounts of the thirteen compounds identified and quantified by using standards and their mass spectra. The HPLC-MS results showed that *p*-hydroxybenzoic acid was recognized as the major phenolic compound identified and quantified in both mushrooms *P. flaccida* and *L. nuda*, with values of 138.50 and 587.90 µg/g dw, respectively. Chlorogenic acid (136.30 µg/g) was classified as the second main compound in *P. flaccida*, followed by gallic acid (132 µg/g) and cinnamic acid (124.20 µg/g), while catechin (400.20 µg/g), ellagic acid (362.60 µg/g) and chlorogenic acid (327.60 µg/g) were listed as the second, the third and the fourth main phenolic compounds detected in *L. nuda* extract, respectively. The lowest component that had been detected was syringic acid for both *P. flaccida* and *L. nuda*, with values of 11.25 and 8.57 µg/g dw, respectively. However, the phenolic compounds rutin, vanillin, rosmarinic acid, salicylic acid and quercetin were not detected in either sample. Statistically, and except gallic acid, all phenolic compounds characterized in the current work showed a significant difference in the comparison between the two tested mushrooms (Table 2).

There have been a few investigations on phenolic compounds of the studied mushrooms, whereas *P. flaccida* phenolics characterization was only reported by the study of Vaz et al. [36] under the name *Lepista inversa*, without detecting any compounds in their samples; however, *L. nuda* individual phenolic compounds were analyzed in three previous research works from two countries (Portugal and Argentina). Herein, from Portugal, Pinto et al. [37] identified two compounds, *p*-hydroxybenzoic (sample from wild pine forest: 100 µg/g dw and from the wild oak forest: 150 µg/g) and cinnamic acids (from wild pine forest: trace and from the wild oak forest: 10 µg/g), with their concentrations significantly lower than the present work, while the study by Barros at al. [38] detected three phenolic acids which are protocatechuic: *p*-hydroxybenzoic and *p*-coumaric acids, with the values of 33.57, 29.31 and 3.75 µg/g dw, respectively. Regarding Argentina, Toledo et al. [34] did not find any of the phenolic compounds analyzed (gallic, *p*-hydroxybenzoic and *p*-coumaric acids) in their *L. nuda*. The phenolic compounds from mushrooms have already been studied in several species, and it was reported that these compounds have been attributed to different biological activities such as antioxidant, antimicrobial and antitumor activities [5,39].

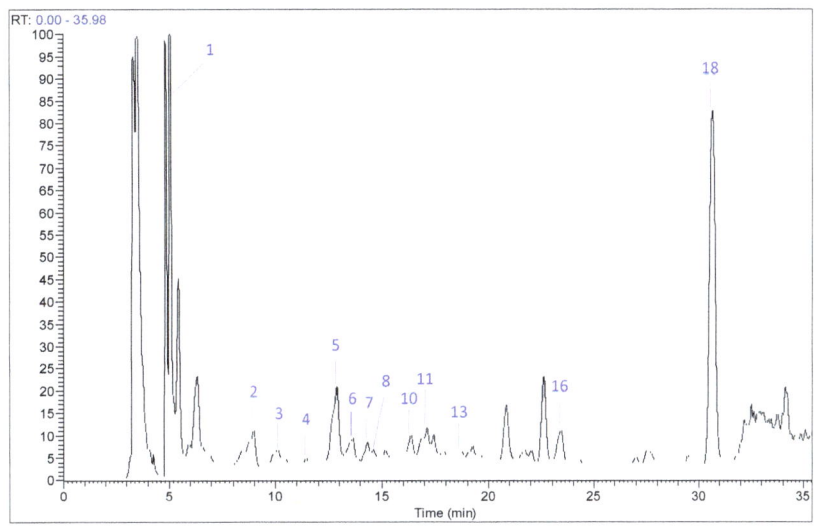

Figure 1. HPLC–MS chromatogram of phenolic compounds in *Paralepista flaccida* extract detected at 280 nm.

Table 2. Phenolic acids and related compounds characterized by HPLC–MS [1].

N°.	Phenolic Compounds	P. flaccida (µg/g dw)	L. nuda (µg/g dw)	One-Way ANOVA *
1	Gallic acid	132 ± 1.79 [a]	131.7 ± 1.11 [a]	0.9955
2	Protocatechuic acid	79.91 ± 2.02 [b]	97.28 ± 1.10 [a]	<0.0001
3	Chlorogenic acid	136.3 ± 1.27 [b]	327.6 ± 3.68 [a]	<0.0001
4	Catechin	102 ± 1.32 [b]	400.2 ± 6.13 [a]	<0.0001
5	p-Hydroxybenzoic acid	138.5 ± 1.58 [b]	587.9 ± 4.89 [a]	<0.0001
6	Caffeic acid	13.28 ± 0.60 [b]	77.37 ± 0.66 [a]	<0.0001
7	Vanillic acid	26.59 ± 0.81 [a]	23.53 ± 1.10 [b]	0.0114
8	Syringic acid	11.25 ± 0.72 [a]	8.57 ± 0.49 [b]	0.001
9	Rutin	nd	nd	-
10	Ellagic acid	100.5 ± 3.62 [b]	362.6 ± 2.80 [a]	<0.0001
11	p-Coumaric acid	35.9 ± 0.53 [b]	124.2 ± 2.73 [a]	<0.0001
12	Vanillin	nd	nd	-
13	Ferulic acid	11.61 ± 0.32 [b]	27.3 ± 0.53 [a]	<0.0001
14	Rosmarinic acid	nd	nd	-
15	Salicylic acid	nd	nd	-
16	Methylparaben	47.12 ± 1.04 [b]	271.6 ± 3.21 [a]	<0.0001
17	Quercetin	nd	nd	-
18	Cinnamic acid	124.2 ± 0.44 [b]	274.3 ± 1.00 [a]	<0.0001

[1] Each value is expressed as means ± SD of three independent measurements. * $p < 0.05$ indicates that the mean value of at least one component differs from the others. For each mushroom sample, means within a line with different letters differ significantly ($p < 0.05$). nd = not detected.

2.4. Biomolecules by GC–MS Analysis

The chemical compositions of the fruiting bodies' methanolic extracts after their derivatization were established by GC–MS, a powerful tool for qualitative and quantitative analysis of various compounds present in natural products and the technique widely used in medical, biological, and food research [40]; the summarized results of this analysis are represented in Tables S1–S5. The GC–MS chromatogram of *P. flaccida* (Figure S2) and *L. nuda* (Figure 2) revealed the presence of sixty-one and sixty-six biologically active compounds, respectively. The identified biomolecules can be mainly divided into five main groups of constituents of each sample, namely sugars, amino acids, fatty acids, organic acids, and the five composed of rest groups, whereas sugars (52.51%) and fatty acids (29.72%) were observed to be the main chemical group in *P. flaccida* and *L. nuda*, respectively (Table 3).

Glycerol (12.42%), mannitol (10.39%) and linoleic acid (9.67%) were recognized as major chemical compositions of *P. flaccida*, while *L. nuda* was predominated by linolelaidic acid (21.13%), leucine (9.05%) and mannitol (5.05%). The two main compounds detected in this study, mannitol and linoleic acid, were previously considered antioxidants [41,42]. Alongside nutritional values, the biomolecules identified in both mushrooms could be responsible for various pharmacological actions such as antioxidant, anti-inflammatory, antimicrobial, antiviral and antitumor activities.

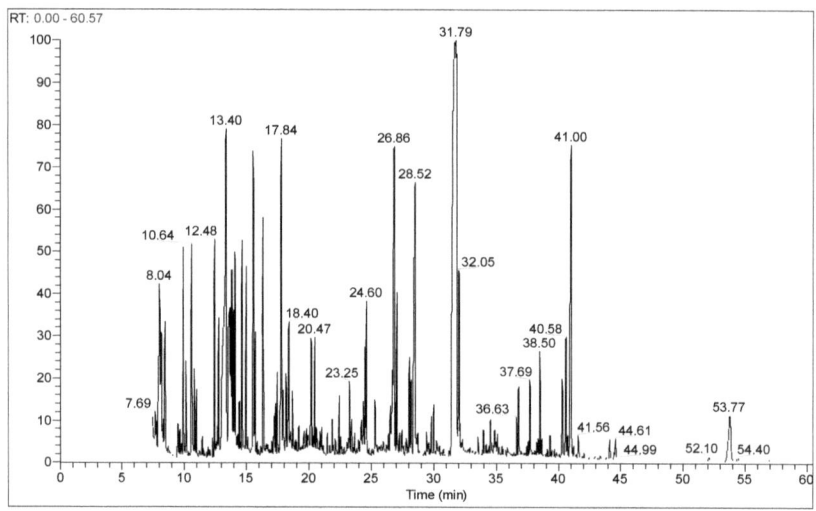

Figure 2. GC-MS chromatogram of *L. nuda* derivatized methanolic extract.

Table 3. Biomolecule groups of the derivatized methanolic extracts by GC–MS analysis.

Compound Names	*P. flaccida* (%)	*L. nuda* (%)
Sugar compositions	52.51	22.88
Fatty acids	11.71	29.72
Amino acids	16.03	18.29
Organic acids	10.53	11.11
Other groups	9.21	17.97
Total	99.99	99.97

As presented in Table S1, the contents of sugar compositions of methanolic extracts of the two analyzed mushrooms were strong and diverse. *P. flaccida* extract contained 21 compounds which were dominated by glycerol (12.42%), mannitol (10.39%) and trehalose (8.58%). Likewise, *L. nuda* methanolic extract was composed of 16 components, in which mannitol (5.16%), threitol (4.16%) and trehalose (4.13%) were the most abundant sugar compounds detected. Heleno et al. previously reported the presence of two sugar compounds, trehalose and mannitol, in *L. inversa* [43]. The presence of the two main sugars in *L. nuda*, mannitol and trehalose, were also observed in several previous studies [31,38,41]. Moreover, glucose, rhamnose, mannose, and xylose were the four monosaccharides quantified in *L. nuda* from India without detecting galactose and fructose [35]. Trehalose, a naturally occurring nontoxic disaccharide, functions as an antioxidant and may be useful to treat many chronic diseases, involving oxidative stress [44].

Concerning fatty acids, *L. nuda* methanolic extract contained the major diversity (11) of compounds, representing 29.72% of the total of compounds identified, whereas linolelaidic (21.13%), palmitic (4.49%) and stearic acids (1.78%) were the major fatty acids detected (Table S2). In contrast, only four fatty acids were detected in *P. flaccida*, which were predominated by linoleic (9.67%) and palmitic (1.63%) (Table S2). Several previous works studied the fatty acids of *L. nuda*, and all of them reported that linoleic acid was the main compound identified, which was not detected in our mushroom [34,35,37,45]. According to these previous studies on *L. nuda* and our *P. flaccida* result, two studies from Bulgaria and Portugal also found linoleic acid as the main fatty acid determined in the species' *inversa* form (*Lepista inversa*) [28,43].

Regarding amino acids, the major diversity of amino acids was observed in *P. flaccida* (15 amino acids), while there was less in *L. nuda*, with eight compounds (Table S3). Gamma-aminobutyric acid (3.04%), glutamine (1.99%) and threonine (1.42%) were classified as the main amino acids detected in *P. flaccida*. For *L. nuda*, leucine, threonine and alanine represented the majority of the amino acids identified, with percentages of 9.05%, 2.69% and 2.15%, respectively. To our knowledge, there have been no previous studies on the amino acids of *P. flaccida* or of *inversa* form; however, one study was performed on *L. nuda* from India with the identification of four amino acids, namely aspartic acid, arginine, tyrosine and proline [35].

For organic acids, GC–MS analysis of the derivatized methanolic extracts showed the presence of eight compounds in *P. flaccida* and eleven compounds in *L. nuda* (Table S4). The *P. flaccida* was predominated by 3,4-dihydroxybutanoic (2.59%), malic (2.26%), succinic (1.85%) and citric (1.83%) acids, while acetoacetic (2%), oxalic (1.66%), maleic (1.44%) and lactic (1.32%) acids were observed to be the highest presented organic acids in *L. nuda*. Three analyses were realized on organic acids in *L. nuda*, and the results demonstrated that quinic and oxalic acids were listed as the main compounds in the three studies [34,37,46]. Contrary to our work, quinic and fumaric acids were not detected in *L. nuda*; citric acid was not detected in a study from Portugal [46], and citric and malic acids were not identified in the previous work from Argentina [34]. Organic acids may have a protective role against various diseases due to their antioxidant activity (such as in the case of tartaric, malic, citric or succinic acids), being able to chelate metals or to delocalize the electronic charge coming from free radicals [46].

Alongside sugars, fatty acids, amino acids and organic acids, the GC–MS analyses of derivatized methanolic extracts of the studied mushrooms showed that the samples also contained many other biologically active compounds belonging to the group of alcohols, steroids, nucleic acids, lipids, glycerides, etc. (Table S5). Ergosterol was noted to represent 1.97% and 1.61% of total biomolecules in *P. flaccida* and *L. nuda*, respectively. This biomolecule is the most abundant sterol found in mushrooms, and it has several biological activities including antioxidant, anti-inflammatory, anti-hyperlipidemic, anti-tyrosinase and antimicrobial activities [47,48].

2.5. Antioxidant Activity

Natural antioxidants have become scientifically interesting compounds due to their many benefits for human health [49]. There are numerous methods available to determine the antioxidant capacity of extracts or pure compounds. Herein, the antioxidant activity of methanolic extracts of the two Moroccan mushrooms *P. flaccida* and *L. nuda* were evaluated spectrophotometrically using three different assays: DPPH radical scavenging, β-carotene/linoleate, and Ferricyanide/Prussian blue activity. The antioxidant results are expressed in EC_{50} values, as summarized in Table 4. In addition, the results have been graphically represented in Figures S3–S5. The methanolic extracts of *P. flaccida* and *L. nuda* showed a strong antioxidant capacity, which was in agreement with the important amount of phenolic compounds and other bioactive compounds found in both mushrooms. These important results were significantly different with Trolox, a standard that was used as a control. On the other hand, the strongest antioxidant capacity was observed in *P. flaccida* extract using a β-carotene bleaching inhibition assay with the value of 0.22 mg/mL (lower EC_{50} value), and in the same mushroom the lowest antioxidant activity by using DPPH radical-scavenging activity with the value of 1.18 mg/mL (higher EC_{50} value) was noted.

Table 4. EC_{50} (mg/mL) of antioxidant properties of the methanolic extracts from Northern Morocco and of the standard Trolox®.

Assays	P. flaccida (mg/mL)	L. nuda (mg/mL)	Trolox (mg/mL)	One-Way ANOVA *
DPPH radical-scavenging activity	1.18 ± 0.11 [a]	0.98 ± 0.01 [b]	0.020 ± 0.01 [c]	<0.0001
β-carotene/linoleate assay	0.22 ± 0.01 [b]	0.39 ± 0.02 [a]	0.006 ± 0.01 [c]	<0.0001
Ferricyanide/Prussian blue assay	0.63 ± 0.01 [a]	0.48 ± 0.00 [b]	0.080 ± 0.02 [c]	<0.0001

The results are presented as mean ± SD (n = 3). * $p < 0.05$ indicates that the mean value of at least one component differs from the others. For each mushroom sample, means within a line with different letters differ significantly ($p < 0.05$).

Concerning DPPH radical-scavenging activity (Figure S3), the results showed that the two studied samples exhibited significant free radical reducing capacity. Herein, the methanolic extract of L. nuda gave higher antioxidant capacity than P. flaccida extract, with EC_{50} values of 0.98 and 1.18 mg/mL, respectively. A previous study was released on L. nuda from Morocco, and the antioxidant activity was 10.60 mg of Trolox equivalent per gram of lyophilized mushroom. Moreover, several works from other countries, namely Portugal, Argentina, Turkey and India, evaluated the DPPH radical-scavenging activity of L. nuda extracts and the EC_{50} values ranged between 2.16 and 16.20 mg/mL, which were significantly higher than our values [31,32,34,35,37]. Another work from Portugal, by Heleno et al., noted that L. inversa gave the EC_{50} value of 10.57 mg/mL, which was highly different from our results [29]. This important radical-scavenging activity is due to the high content of total phenolic and flavonoids found in the studied mushrooms [5].

Regarding the β-carotene-linoleate bleaching assay (Figure S4), the biomolecules existing in the methanolic extract of the two mushrooms were able to inhibit the discoloration of β-carotene and have demonstrated strong antioxidant properties. The methanolic extract of P. flaccida revealed significantly higher antioxidant activity than the L. nuda extract, with values of 0.22 and 0.39 mg/mL, respectively, which were more effective than L. inversa (1.80 mg/mL) from Portugal reported previously by Heleno et al. [29]. Furthermore, recent studies have also demonstrated the antioxidant activity of L. nuda extract using β-carotene-linoleate bleaching assay and the results were observed to be lower than our samples, with higher EC_{50} values which were between 3.53 and 14.24 mg/mL [32,34,37]. These important β-carotene-linoleate bleaching results could be due to the high quantity of carotenoids and other major biomolecules found in the methanolic extract of P. flaccida and L. nuda.

For reducing power by Ferricyanide/Prussian blue assay (Figure S5), the natural antioxidant compounds exiting in methanolic extracts of the two edible Moroccan mushrooms were able to convert Fe^{3+} into Fe^{2+} and, therefore, exhibited high reducing power with EC50 values of 0.48 mg/mL for the L. nuda and 0.63 mg/mL for P. flaccida. Our extracts have given a strong reducing power in comparison with previous results by Heleno et al. in L. inversa (2.9 mg/mL) [29], and with the ones reported in various works on L. nuda extracts, in which their EC_{50} values ranged between 0.75 and 4.21 mg/mL [32,34,35,37]. This finding of reducing power could be related to the ability of biomolecules found in the samples to reduce Fe^{3+} [50].

Overall, the investigated edible mushrooms are sources of powerful antioxidants such as phenolic compounds, ascorbic acid, carotenoids, and other bioactive compounds, which could be used against diseases related to oxidative stress, dermatological applications, cosmetics, and as supplements in the food industry [29].

3. Materials and Methods

3.1. Standards and Reagents

N,O-Bis(trimethylsilyl)trifluoroacetamide (BSTFA), alkane standards (C_8-C_{20} and C_{21}-C_{40}), meta-Phosphoric acid, 2,6-Dichloroindophenol sodium salt hydrate, l-ascorbic acid, (+)-catechin, vanillin reagent, Folin–Ciocalteu's phenol reagent, (±)-6-Hydroxy-2,5,7,8-tetramethylchromane-2-carboxylic acid (Trolox), β-carotene, Tween 40, linoleic acid, iron (III) chloride, sodium hydroxide, sodium nitrite, and phenolic standards including, caffeic acid, catechin, chlorogenic acid, cinnamic acid, ellagic acid, ferulic acid, gallic acid, methylparaben, *p*-coumaric acid, *p*-hydroxybenzoic acid, protocatechuic acid, quercetin, rosmarinic acid, rutin, salicylic acid, syringic acid, vanillic acid, and vanillin were purchased from SIGMA-ALDRICH, Co., (St. Louis, MO, USA). Acetonitrile, ethyl acetate, hydrochloric acid fuming 37%, pyridine, aluminum chlorure, and sodium chloride were obtained from Merck KGaA (Darmstadt, Germany), and 2,2-diphenyl-l-picrylhydrazyl (DPPH) was from Alfa Aesar (Ward Hill, MA, USA). Acetone, n-hexane, and hexane were purchased from CABLO ERBA Reagent, S.A.S (Val de Reuil Cedex, France). Methanol and all other chemicals and solvents were of the highest commercial grade and obtained from Honeywell (St. Muskegon, MI, USA).

3.2. Mushroom Material

The edible mushrooms *P. flaccida* and *L. nuda* were harvested from Koudiat Taifour forest, a Biological and Ecological Interest Site (SIBE) (35°40′45.4″N 5°17′36.3″W 180 m of altitude) in northwestern Morocco during January 2018, under *Quercus suber*, *Pinus halepensis*, *Eucalyptus rostrata* and *Pistacia lentiscus* trees. The identifications of the harvested species were undertaken in the Biology, Environment, and Sustainable Development (BEDD) laboratory at the École Normale Supérieure (ENS) of Tetouan, Morocco, and were based on macroscopic and microscopic characterizations and ecological conditions. These identifications were made according to the two determination keys [51,52]. Voucher specimens were deposited at the herbarium of the BEDD laboratory, Department of Matter and Life Sciences, ENS of Tetouan, Morocco. The fruiting bodies were immediately cleaned, weighed, cut into small pieces, air-dried, and reduced to a fine powder (20 mesh).

3.3. Preparation of Crude Methanolic Extracts

The methanol extraction was carried out following the previous work by Barros et al. [32], with some modifications. A total of 1 g of fine-dried mushroom power (20 mesh) was extracted by stirring with 20 mL of methanol at 25 °C at 150 rpm for 24 h and filtered through Whatman N °4 paper. The residue from the filtration was extracted again, twice, using the procedure described earlier. The combined methanolic extracts were evaporated at 40 °C to dryness. Then, the dried extracts were weighed and stored at −81 °C for further use. The extraction yield was calculated for each studied species. This preparation and all the further works were carried out at the Faculty of Sciences of the University of Porto, Portugal.

3.4. Estimation of Bioactive Compounds

The contents of bioactive compounds, including total phenolic compound content (TPC), total flavonoid content (TFC), total ascorbic acid content (TAAC), total tannin content (TTC), and total carotenoids contents (β-carotene (Tβ-CC) and lycopene (TLC)), in fruiting bodies of *P. flaccida* and *L. nuda* were determined by spectrophotometry using the same conditions, equipment and procedures described previously by Erbiai et al. [26].

TPC was determined by Folin–Ciocalteu assay. Briefly, one ml of extract methanolic solution was mixed with 5 mL of Folin–Ciocalteu reagent and 4 mL of sodium carbonate solution (7.5%). The tubes were vortex mixed for 15 s and allowed to stand for 30 min at 40 °C in the dark. Then, the absorbance of the solution was measured at 765 nm against the blank. The results were expressed as milligrams of gallic acid equivalents (GAE) per gram of dry methanolic extract (dme).

TFC was determined by using an aluminum chloride colorimetric method, based on the formation of a complex between aluminum chloride and the C-4 keto group and either the C-3 or C-5 hydroxyl group of flavones and flavonols. The intensity of the pink color was measured at 510 nm using a UV-Visible spectrophotometer against the blank, which contained all reagents except extract samples. The results were expressed as mg of (+)-catechin equivalents (CEs) per gram of dme.

TAAC was determined using a method based on the reaction of ascorbic acid existing in the extract with the reagent 2,6 dichlorophenolindophenol. Meta-phosphoric acid (1%) was used for ascorbic acid extraction. The absorbance was measured at 515 nm against a blank. The results were expressed as mg of $_L$-ascorbic acid equivalents (AAEs) per gram of dw.

TTC of the sample powder was assayed by the Vanillin-HCL method, which is a method specific to dihydroxyphenols and particularly sensitive to molecules containing meta-substituted, di- and tri-hydroxybenzene. The absorbance of color developed was measured at 500 nm against the blank. The TTC was expressed as mg of (+)-catechin equivalents per gram (CEs/g) of dme.

Tβ-CC and TLC were determined following a method based on the mixture of methanol extract and acetone-hexane (4:6). The solution absorbance (A) was measured at 453, 505, 645, and 663 nm using a UV-Vis spectrophotometer. Tβ-CC and TLC were calculated according to the following equations: *Lycopene* (mg/100 mL) = $[(0.0458\ A_{663}) + (0.372\ A_{505}) - (0.0806\ A_{453})]$; *β-Carotene* (mg/100 mL) = $[(0.216\ A_{663}) - (0.304\ A_{505}) + (0.452\ A_{453})]$.

3.5. Phenolic Compounds Analysis by HPLC–MS

The extraction and analysis of individual phenolic compounds of *P. flaccida* and *L. nuda* were carried out following the same procedure, conditions and HPLC equipment used in our previous published work [26]. Briefly, the phenolic extract was analyzed by high-performance liquid chromatography-mass spectrometry (HPLC–MS). Chromatographic separation was accomplished using Acclaim™ 120 reverse phase C18 columns (3 μm 150 × 4.6 mm) thermostatted at 35 °C, and peaks were detected at 280 nm as the preferred wavelength. The mobile phase used was composed of 1% acetic acid and 100% acetonitrile. The identification of phenolic compounds in the samples was characterized according to their UV-Vis spectra and identified by their mass spectra and retention times in comparison with commercial standards. Quantification was made from the areas of the peaks recorded at 280 nm by comparison with calibration curves obtained from the standard of each compound. The results were expressed in μg per gram of dry weight (dw).

3.6. Biomolecules Analysis by GC–MS

Before GC–MS analysis, the crude methanolic extracts of each mushroom (10 mg) were derivatized by adding 100 μL of anhydrous pyridine and 100 μL BSTFA, and the mixture was heated at 80 °C for 25 min, then the mixture was diluted with 200 μL chloroform [53,54]. The derivatized solution was analyzed by using Gas Chromatography (GC) (Trace 1300 gas chromatography; Thermo Fisher Scientific, Waltham, MA, USA) linked to a mass spectrometry (MS) system (ISQ single quadrupole mass spectrometer; Thermo Fisher Scientific) and automatic injector. The GC separation was conducted with a TG5-MS capillary column (60 m × 0.25 mm i.d.; 0.25 μm film thickness) with a non-polar stationary phase (5% Phenyl 95% dimethylpolysiloxane). The injection and detector temperature were made at 300 °C using splitless injection mode (1:10). Helium was used as a carrier gas at a flow rate of 1.2 mL/min. The oven temperature was programmed from 40 °C (2 min) to 200 °C at a rate of 6 °C/min (2 min), and then at a rate of 6 °C/min (6 min) up to 300 °C. The total run time was 65 min. MS conditions were: electron ionization mass spectra were set at 70 eV, the mass ranged from 50 to 650 amu, and the ion source temperature was 300 °C. Retention indices were calculated for all components, using a homologous series of known standards of alkanes mixture (C_8–C_{20} and C_{21}–C_{40}) injected in conditions equal to sample ones. Identification of components of mushroom extracts was based on retention indices (RI) relative to alkanes, with those of authentic compounds and with the spectral data obtained from the databases of the National Institute Standard and Technology (NIST) and PubChem Libraries of the corresponding compounds. Data acquisition was operated by Software Thermo Xcalibur™ 2.2 SP1.48, and data analysis was performed using NIST MS Search 2.2 Library 2014.

3.7. Evaluation of Antioxidant Activity

The antioxidant activity of methanolic extracts from the two edible mushrooms *P. flaccida* and *L. nuda* was evaluated by three different assays, including DPPH radical-scavenging, reducing power, and β-carotene bleaching inhibition assay, and by following the same procedures, equipment and conditions used previously by Heleno et al. [29]. The extract concentration providing 50% of antioxidant capacity or 0.5 of absorbance (EC_{50}) was calculated from the graphs of antioxidant activity percentages (DPPH, and β-carotene/linoleate assays) or absorbance at 690 nm (ferricyanide/Prussian blue assay) against extract concentrations. Trolox was used as a reference standard.

DPPH radical-scavenging activity (RSA) of the samples was determined using the stable free radical DPPH (1.1-diphenyl-2-picrylhydrazyl). The absorbance was measured at 517 nm using a UV-Vis spectrophotometer against a blank. The RSA was calculated as a percentage of DPPH discoloration using the equation: RSA (%) = [($A_{DPPH} - A_{Sample}$)/A_{DPPH}] × 100, where A_{DPPH} is the absorbance of the DPPH solution and A_{Sample} is the absorbance of the test extract.

For the β-carotene-linoleate bleaching assay, the antioxidant activity of the methanolic extracts was carried out using the β-carotene linoleate model system, in which the presence of antioxidants in the extracts and their capacity to neutralize the linoleate free radicals avoids β-carotene bleaching. The absorbance was measured immediately at zero-time at 470 nm against a blank, and measured for the second time at 120 min. A control containing methanol instead of the extract was realized in parallel. β-carotene bleaching inhibition was calculated using the following formula: (%) = (β-carotene content after 2 h of the assay/initial β-carotene content) × 100.

Reducing power by Ferricyanide/Prussian blue assay, the methodology of which is based on the capacity to convert Fe^{3+} into Fe^{2+}, the absorbance of the solution was measured at 690 nm using a UV-Vis spectrophotometer against a blank containing the same solution mixture without mushroom extract.

3.8. Statistical Analysis

Three samples were used, and all assays were carried out in triplicate. Extraction yield, bioactive compounds, and antioxidant activity values were expressed as mean ± standard deviation (SD). The statistical significance of the data was made with a one-way analysis of variance (ANOVA), followed by post hoc Tukey's multiple comparison tests with $\alpha = 0.05$ using GraphPad Prism 8.0.1 software (San Diego, CA, USA).

4. Conclusions

This research work constitutes the first report on the chemical characterizations and antioxidant properties of the two wild edible mushrooms *P. flaccida* and *L. nuda* from southern Mediterranean countries and, in particular, from Morocco. The fruiting bodies of the studied samples demonstrated an important content of bioactive compounds, namely phenolic compounds (individual and total contents), ascorbic acid and carotenoids. In addition, the GC–MS analysis of *P. flaccida* and *L. nuda* extracts revealed the presence of more than sixty biologically active compounds for each. On the other hand, the two edible mushrooms showed strong antioxidant properties by using three assays: DPPH radical scavenging activity, inhibition of β-carotene bleaching, and ferric-reducing power. The highly considered antioxidant capacity of the samples could be related to their richness of bioactive compounds. In general, the findings may encourage more people from southern Mediterranean countries to consume edible mushrooms as food due to their benefits on human health. They may also allow researchers to make the valorization of mushrooms from these regions an interesting objective for their investigation to open up new perspectives in nutritional and pharmaceutical research, and to contribute to discovering novel antioxidant agents and medicaments which can be used for the treatment of many diseases.

Supplementary Materials: The following supporting information can be downloaded at: https://www.mdpi.com/article/10.3390/molecules28031123/s1, Figure S1: HPLC–MS chromatogram of phenolic compounds in *Lepista nuda* extract detected at 280 nm, Figure S2: GC–MS chromatogram of *P. flaccida* derivatized methanolic extract, Table S1: Sugar compositions of the derivatized methanolic extract by GC–MS analysis, Table S2: Fatty acids of the derivatized methanolic extract by GC–MS analysis, Table S3: Amino acids of the derivatized methanolic extract by GC–MS, Table S4: Organic acids of the derivatized methanolic extract by GC–MS analysis, Table S5: Rest of the biomolecule constituents of the derivatized methanolic extract by GC–MS analysis, Figure S3: Radical-scavenging activity on DPPH radicals. Each value is expressed as mean ± SD (n = 3), Figure S4: Lipid peroxidation inhibition measured by the β-carotene bleaching inhibition. Each value is expressed as mean ± SD (n = 3), Figure S5: Reducing power. Each value is expressed as mean ± SD (n = 3).

Author Contributions: Conceptualization, E.H.E. and A.M.; Data curation, E.H.E. and A.M.; Formal analysis, E.H.E.; Funding acquisition, J.C.G.E.d.S. and A.M.; Investigation, J.C.G.E.d.S. and A.M.; Methodology, E.H.E., L.P.d.S., A.M. and J.C.G.E.d.S.; Project administration, J.C.G.E.d.S. and A.M.; Resources, J.C.G.E.d.S. and A.M.; Software, E.H.E.; Supervision, J.C.G.E.d.S., L.P.d.S., and A.M.; Validation, Z.L., J.C.G.E.d.S. and A.M.; Visualization, R.S., Z.L. and M.L.; Writing—original draft, E.H.E.; Writing—review and editing, J.C.G.E.d.S. and L.P.d.S.; All authors have read and agreed to the published version of the manuscript.

Funding: Our research work is part of a Moroccan project supported by MESRSI and CNRST (PPR2-35/2016, titled "Biological control of crop diseases and cancer & Valorization of plants and superior fungi from Northern Morocco"). Secondly, this work was completed in the Faculty of Sciences of the University of Porto, within the framework of program Erasmus (Key Action 1, MOBILE+3), and within the framework of FCT ("Fundação para a Ciência e Tecnologia", Portugal)-funded projects PTDC/QEQ-QAN/5955/2014, PTDC/QUI-QFI/2870/2020, UIDB/00081/2020 (CIQUP), and LA/P/0056/2020 (IMS). Luís Pinto da Silva acknowledges funding from the FCT under the Scientific Employment Stimulus (CEECINST/00069/2021), while El Hadi Erbiai also acknowledges the FCT for funding his postdoctoral position (under project PTDC/QUI-QFI/2870/2020).

Institutional Review Board Statement: Not applicable.

Informed Consent Statement: Not applicable.

Data Availability Statement: Data is contained within the article or Supplementary Material.

Conflicts of Interest: The authors declare no conflict of interest.

Sample Availability: Samples of the compounds are not available from the authors.

References

1. Niego, A.G.; Rapior, S.; Thongklang, N.; Raspé, O.; Jaidee, W.; Lumyong, S.; Hyde, K.D. Macrofungi as a Nutraceutical Source: Promising Bioactive Compounds and Market Value. *J. Fungi* **2021**, *7*, 397. [CrossRef] [PubMed]
2. Ferreira, I.C.F.R.; Fernandes, Â.; Heleno, S.A. Chemical, Nutritional, and Bioactive Potential of Mushrooms. In *Edible and Medicinal Mushrooms*; Diego, C.Z., Pardo-Giménez, A., Eds.; John Wiley & Sons, Ltd.: Chichester, UK, 2017; pp. 455–501. ISBN 978-1-119-14944-6.
3. Benoutman, A.; Erbiai, E.H.; Edderdaki, F.Z.; Cherif, E.K.; Saidi, R.; Lamrani, Z.; Pintado, M.; Pinto, E.; Esteves da Silva, J.C.G.; Maouni, A. Phytochemical Composition, Antioxidant and Antifungal Activity of Thymus Capitatus, a Medicinal Plant Collected from Northern Morocco. *Antibiotics* **2022**, *11*, 681. [CrossRef] [PubMed]
4. Reis, F.S.; Pereira, E.; Barros, L.; Sousa, M.J.; Martins, A.; Ferreira, I.C.F.R. Biomolecule Profiles in Inedible Wild Mushrooms with Antioxidant Value. *Molecules* **2011**, *16*, 4328–4338. [CrossRef] [PubMed]
5. Ferreira, I.; Barros, L.; Abreu, R. Antioxidants in Wild Mushrooms. *Curr. Med. Chem.* **2009**, *16*, 1543–1560. [CrossRef] [PubMed]
6. Bon, M.; Wilkinson, J.; Ovenden, D. *The Mushrooms and Toadstools of Britain and North-Western Europe*, 1st ed.; Hodder & Stoughton General Division: London, UK, 1987; ISBN 978-0-340-39953-8.
7. Crevel, R. *van Funga Nordica: Agaricoid, Boletoid and Cyphelloid Genera*; CRC Press: Boca Raton, FL, USA, 1995; Volume 1, ISBN 978-90-5410-616-6.
8. Vizzini, A.; Ercole, E. Paralepistopsis Gen. Nov. and Paralepista (Basidiomycota, Agaricales). *Mycotaxon* **2012**, *120*, 253–267. [CrossRef]
9. Royal Botanic Gardens Kew Paralepista Flaccida—Species Fungorum. Available online: http://www.speciesfungorum.org/Names/NamesRecord.asp?RecordID=564347 (accessed on 21 October 2022).

10. GBIF Secretariat Paralepista Flaccida (Sowerby) Vizzini. Available online: https://www.gbif.org/species/7978027 (accessed on 21 October 2022).
11. Eyssartier, G.; Roux, P. *Le guide des champignons. France et Europe 3e édition—Guillaume Eyssartier, Pierre Roux; Les Guides des fous de Nature*; Belin: Paris, France, 2013; ISBN 978-2-7011-8289-6.
12. Courtecuisse, R.; Duhem, B. *Champignons de France et d'Europe - Régis Courtecuisse, Bernard Duhem; Guide Delachaux*.; Delachaux et Niestlé: Paris, France, 2012; ISBN 978-2-603-02038-8.
13. Bézivin, C.; Lohézic, F.; Sauleau, P.; Amoros, M.; Boustie, J. Cytotoxic Activity of Tricholomatales Determined with Murine and Human Cancer Cell Lines. *Pharm. Biol.* **2002**, *40*, 196–199. [CrossRef]
14. Işıloğlu, M.; Yılmaz, F.; Merdivan, M. Concentrations of Trace Elements in Wild Edible Mushrooms. *Food Chem.* **2001**, *73*, 169–175. [CrossRef]
15. El-Assfouri, A.; Ouazzani Touhami, A.; Zidane, L.; Fennane, M.; Douira, A. Inventaire Des Spécimens Fongiques de l'Herbier National de l'Institut Scientifique de Rabat. *Bull. Inst. Sci. Rabat Maroc Sect. Sci. Vie* **2003**, *25*, 1–23.
16. Outcoumit, A.; Kholfy, S.E.; Touhami, A.O.; Douira, A. Bibliographic Inventory of Tangier Fungi: Catalogue of the Basidiomycetes Fungal Flora. *IJPAES* **2014**, *4*, 52.
17. Kholfy, S.E.; El-Assfouri, A.; Ouazzani Touham, A.; Belahbib, N.; Douira, A. Bibliographic Catalog of Endemic or Rare Mushrooms of Morocco. *Int. J. Plant Anim. Environ. Sci.* **2014**, 103–116.
18. Haimed, M.; Nmichi, A.; Ouazzani Touhami, A.; Douira, A. Bibliographic Inventory of Moroccan Central Plateau Fungi. *J. Anim. Plant Sci.* **2013**, *18*, 2723–2749.
19. Ouabbou, A.; El-Assfouri, A.; Ouazzani, A.; Benkirane, R.; Douira, A. Bibliographic Catalog of the Forest of Mamora (Morocco) Fungal Flora. *J. Anim. Plant Sci.* **2012**, *15*, 2200–2242.
20. El kholfy, S.; Aït Aguil, F.; Ouazzani Touhami, A.; Benkirane, R.; Douira, A. Bibliographic Inventory of Moroccan Rif's Fungi: Catalog of Rifain Fungal Flora. *J. Anim. Plant Sci.* **2011**, *12*, 1493–1526.
21. Chen, M.-H.; Li, W.-S.; Lue, Y.-S.; Chu, C.-L.; Pan, I.-H.; Ko, C.-H.; Chen, D.-Y.; Lin, C.-H.; Lin, S.-H.; Chang, C.-P.; et al. Clitocybe Nuda Activates Dendritic Cells and Acts as a DNA Vaccine Adjuvant. *Evid. Based Complement. Alternat. Med.* **2013**, *2013*, e761454. [CrossRef]
22. De, J.; Nandi, S.; Acharya, K. A Review on Blewit Mushrooms (Lepista Sp.) Transition from Farm to Pharm. *J. Food Process. Preserv.* **2022**, *46*, e17028. [CrossRef]
23. Haimed, M.; Kholfy, S.E.; El-Assfouri, A.; Ouazzani-Touhami, A.; Benkirane, R.; Douira, A. Inventory of Basidiomycetes and Ascomycetes Harvested in the Moroccan Central Plateau. *Int J Pure Appl Bio* **2015**, *3*, 100–108.
24. Alcántara, D.M.; Ferrezuelo, T.I.; Díaz, C.M.; Bouziane, H. Estudio de La Micobiota Del Norte de Marruecos II. *Micobotánica-Jaén* **2018**, *XIII*, 1–44.
25. Aliaño-González, M.J.; Barea-Sepúlveda, M.; Espada-Bellido, E.; Ferreiro-González, M.; López-Castillo, J.G.; Palma, M.; Barbero, G.F.; Carrera, C. Ultrasound-Assisted Extraction of Total Phenolic Compounds and Antioxidant Activity in Mushrooms. *Agronomy* **2022**, *12*, 1812. [CrossRef]
26. Erbiai, E.H.; da Silva, L.P.; Saidi, R.; Lamrani, Z.; Esteves da Silva, J.C.G.; Maouni, A. Chemical Composition, Bioactive Compounds, and Antioxidant Activity of Two Wild Edible Mushrooms Armillaria Mellea and Macrolepiota Procera from Two Countries (Morocco and Portugal). *Biomolecules* **2021**, *11*, 575. [CrossRef]
27. Erbiai, E.H.; Bouchra, B.; da Silva, L.P.; Lamrani, Z.; Pinto, E.; da Silva, J.C.G.E.; Maouni, A. Chemical Composition and Antioxidant and Antimicrobial Activities of Lactarius Sanguifluus, a Wild Edible Mushroom from Northern Morocco. *Euro-Mediterr. J. Environ. Integr.* **2021**, *6*. [CrossRef]
28. Marekov, I.; Momchilova, S.; Grung, B.; Nikolova-Damyanova, B. Fatty Acid Composition of Wild Mushroom Species of Order Agaricales—Examination by Gas Chromatography–Mass Spectrometry and Chemometrics. *J. Chromatogr. B* **2012**, *910*, 54–60. [CrossRef] [PubMed]
29. Heleno, S.A.; Barros, L.; Sousa, M.J.; Martins, A.; Ferreira, I.C.F.R. Tocopherols Composition of Portuguese Wild Mushrooms with Antioxidant Capacity. *Food Chem.* **2010**, *119*, 1443–1450. [CrossRef]
30. Vaz, J.A.; Heleno, S.A.; Martins, A.; Almeida, G.M.; Vasconcelos, M.H.; Ferreira, I.C.F.R. Wild Mushrooms Clitocybe Alexandri and Lepista Inversa: In Vitro Antioxidant Activity and Growth Inhibition of Human Tumour Cell Lines. *Food Chem. Toxicol.* **2010**, *48*, 2881–2884. [CrossRef] [PubMed]
31. Keleş, A.; Koca, I.; Gençcelep, H. Antioxidant Properties of Wild Edible Mushrooms. *J. Food Process. Technol.* **2011**, *02*. [CrossRef]
32. Barros, L.; Venturini, B.A.; Baptista, P.; Estevinho, L.M.; Ferreira, I.C.F.R. Chemical Composition and Biological Properties of Portuguese Wild Mushrooms: A Comprehensive Study. *J. Agric. Food Chem.* **2008**, *56*, 3856–3862. [CrossRef]
33. Elmastas, M.; Isildak, O.; Turkekul, I.; Temur, N. Determination of Antioxidant Activity and Antioxidant Compounds in Wild Edible Mushrooms. *J. Food Compos. Anal.* **2007**, *20*, 337–345. [CrossRef]
34. Toledo, C.; Barroetaveña, C.; Fernandes, Â.; Barros, L.; Ferreira, I. Chemical and Antioxidant Properties of Wild Edible Mushrooms from Native Nothofagus Spp. Forest, Argentina. *Molecules* **2016**, *21*, 1201. [CrossRef]
35. Sharma, S.K.; Gautam, N. Chemical, Bioactive, and Antioxidant Potential of Twenty Wild Culinary Mushroom Species. *BioMed Res. Int.* **2015**, *2015*, 1–12. [CrossRef]
36. Vaz, J.A.; Barros, L.; Martins, A.; Morais, J.S.; Vasconcelos, M.H.; Ferreira, I.C.F.R. Phenolic Profile of Seventeen Portuguese Wild Mushrooms. *LWT - Food Sci. Technol.* **2011**, *44*, 343–346. [CrossRef]

37. Pinto, S.; Barros, L.; Sousa, M.J.; Ferreira, I.C.F.R. Chemical Characterization and Antioxidant Properties of Lepista Nuda Fruiting Bodies and Mycelia Obtained by in Vitro Culture: Effects of Collection Habitat and Culture Media. *Food Res. Int.* **2013**, *51*, 496–502. [CrossRef]
38. Barros, L.; Dueñas, M.; Ferreira, I.C.F.R.; Baptista, P.; Santos-Buelga, C. Phenolic Acids Determination by HPLC–DAD–ESI/MS in Sixteen Different Portuguese Wild Mushrooms Species. *Food Chem. Toxicol.* **2009**, *47*, 1076–1079. [CrossRef]
39. Heleno, S.A.; Martins, A.; Queiroz, M.J.R.P.; Ferreira, I.C.F.R. Bioactivity of Phenolic Acids: Metabolites versus Parent Compounds: A Review. *Food Chem.* **2015**, *173*, 501–513. [CrossRef]
40. Kałużna-Czaplińska, J. GC-MS Analysis of Biologically Active Compounds in Cosmopolitan Grasses. *Acta Chromatogr.* **2007**, 279–282.
41. André, P.; Villain, F. Free Radical Scavenging Properties of Mannitol and Its Role as a Constituent of Hyaluronic Acid Fillers: A Literature Review. *Int. J. Cosmet. Sci.* **2017**, *39*, 355–360. [CrossRef]
42. Chen, Z.Y.; Chan, P.T.; Kwan, K.Y.; Zhang, A. Reassessment of the Antioxidant Activity of Conjugated Linoleic Acids. *J. Am. Oil Chem. Soc.* **1997**, *74*, 749–753. [CrossRef]
43. Heleno, S.A.; Barros, L.; Sousa, M.J.; Martins, A.; Ferreira, I.C.F.R. Study and Characterization of Selected Nutrients in Wild Mushrooms from Portugal by Gas Chromatography and High Performance Liquid Chromatography. *Microchem. J.* **2009**, *93*, 195–199. [CrossRef]
44. Mizunoe, Y.; Kobayashi, M.; Sudo, Y.; Watanabe, S.; Yasukawa, H.; Natori, D.; Hoshino, A.; Negishi, A.; Okita, N.; Komatsu, M.; et al. Trehalose Protects against Oxidative Stress by Regulating the Keap1-Nrf2 and Autophagy Pathways. *Redox Biol.* **2018**, *15*, 115–124. [CrossRef] [PubMed]
45. Ayaz, F.A.; Chuang, L.T.; Torun, H.; Colak, A.; Sesli˙, E.; Presley, J.; Smith, B.R.; Glew, R.H. Fatty Acid and Amino Acid Compositions of Selected Wild-Edible Mushrooms Consumed in Turkey. *Int. J. Food Sci. Nutr.* **2011**, *62*, 328–335. [CrossRef]
46. Barros, L.; Pereira, C.; Ferreira, I.C.F.R. Optimized Analysis of Organic Acids in Edible Mushrooms from Portugal by Ultra Fast Liquid Chromatography and Photodiode Array Detection. *Food Anal. Methods* **2013**, *6*, 309–316. [CrossRef]
47. Barreira, J.C.M.; Oliveira, M.B.P.P.; Ferreira, I.C.F.R. Development of a Novel Methodology for the Analysis of Ergosterol in Mushrooms. *Food Anal. Methods* **2014**, *7*, 217–223. [CrossRef]
48. Taofiq, O.; Heleno, S.A.; Calhelha, R.C.; Fernandes, I.P.; Alves, M.J.; Barros, L.; González-Paramás, A.M.; Ferreira, I.C.F.R.; Barreiro, M.F. Phenolic Acids, Cinnamic Acid, and Ergosterol as Cosmeceutical Ingredients: Stabilization by Microencapsulation to Ensure Sustained Bioactivity. *Microchem. J.* **2019**, *147*, 469–477. [CrossRef]
49. Zehiroglu, C.; Ozturk Sarikaya, S.B. The Importance of Antioxidants and Place in Today's Scientific and Technological Studies. *J. Food Sci. Technol.* **2019**, *56*, 4757–4774. [CrossRef] [PubMed]
50. Ferreira, I.C.F.R.; Baptista, P.; Vilas-Boas, M.; Barros, L. Free-Radical Scavenging Capacity and Reducing Power of Wild Edible Mushrooms from Northeast Portugal: Individual Cap and Stipe Activity. *Food Chem.* **2007**, *100*, 1511–1516. [CrossRef]
51. Malençon, G.; Bertault, R. *Flore des champignons superieurs du Maroc: Tome I*; Travaux de l'Institut Scientifique Chérifien et de la Faculté des Sciences de Rabat. Série Botanique et Biologie Végétale; Institut Scientifique Chérifien: Rabat, Morocco, 1970; Volume 1.
52. Régis, C. *LES CHAMPIGNONS DE FRANCE—Guide encyclopédique*; Eclectis: Paris, France, 1994; Volume 1, ISBN 978-2-908975-19-2.
53. Çayan, F.; Tel, G.; Duru, M.E.; Öztürk, M.; Türkoğlu, A.; Harmandar, M. Application of GC, GC-MSD, ICP-MS and Spectrophotometric Methods for the Determination of Chemical Composition and In Vitro Bioactivities of Chroogomphus Rutilus: The Edible Mushroom Species. *Food Anal. Methods* **2014**, *7*, 449–458. [CrossRef]
54. Popova, M.; Silici, S.; Kaftanoglu, O.; Bankova, V. Antibacterial Activity of Turkish Propolis and Its Qualitative and Quantitative Chemical Composition. *Phytomedicine* **2005**, *12*, 221–228. [CrossRef] [PubMed]

Disclaimer/Publisher's Note: The statements, opinions and data contained in all publications are solely those of the individual author(s) and contributor(s) and not of MDPI and/or the editor(s). MDPI and/or the editor(s) disclaim responsibility for any injury to people or property resulting from any ideas, methods, instructions or products referred to in the content.

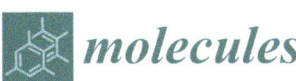

Article

Effect of Resveratrol Treatment on Human Pancreatic Cancer Cells through Alterations of Bcl-2 Family Members

Katarzyna Ratajczak *, Natalia Glatzel-Plucińska, Katarzyna Ratajczak-Wielgomas, Katarzyna Nowińska and Sylwia Borska

Division of Histology and Embryology, Department of Human Morphology and Embryology, Wroclaw Medical University, 50-368 Wroclaw, Poland; natalia.glatzel-plucinska@umed.wroc.pl (N.G.-P.); katarzyna.ratajczak-wielgomas@umed.wroc.pl (K.R.-W.); katarzyna.nowinska@umed.wroc.pl (K.N.); sylwia.borska@umed.wroc.pl (S.B.)
* Correspondence: katarzyna.ratajczak@umed.wroc.pl; Tel.: +48-71-784-1354

Abstract: Pancreatic cancers are among of the most lethal types of neoplasms, and are mostly detected at an advanced stage. Conventional treatment methods such as chemotherapy or radiotherapy often do not bring the desired therapeutic effects. For this reason, natural compounds are increasingly being used as adjuvants in cancer therapy. Polyphenolic compounds, including resveratrol, are of particular interest. The aim of this study is to analyze the antiproliferative and pro-apoptotic mechanisms of resveratrol on human pancreatic cells. The study was carried out on three human pancreatic cancer cell lines: EPP85-181P, EPP85-181RNOV (mitoxantrone-resistant cells) and AsPC-1, as well as the normal pancreatic cell line H6c7. The cytotoxicity of resveratrol in the tested cell lines was assessed by the colorimetric method (MTT) and the flow cytometry method. Three selected concentrations of the compound (25, 50 and 100 μM) were tested in the experiments during a 48-h incubation. TUNEL and Comet assays, flow cytometry, immunocytochemistry, confocal microscopy, real-time PCR and Western Blot analyses were used to evaluate the pleiotropic effect of resveratrol. The results indicate that resveratrol is likely to be anticarcinogenic by inhibiting human pancreatic cancer cell proliferation. In addition, it affects the levels of Bcl-2 pro- and anti-apoptotic proteins. However, it should be emphasized that the activity of resveratrol was specific for each of the tested cell lines, and the most statistically significant changes were observed in the mitoxantrone-resistant cells.

Keywords: resveratrol; Bax; Bcl-2; Caspase-3; apoptosis; multidrug resistance; pancreatic cancer

Citation: Ratajczak, K.; Glatzel-Plucińska, N.; Ratajczak-Wielgomas, K.; Nowińska, K.; Borska, S. Effect of Resveratrol Treatment on Human Pancreatic Cancer Cells through Alterations of Bcl-2 Family Members. *Molecules* **2021**, *26*, 6560. https://doi.org/10.3390/molecules26216560

Academic Editors: Stefano Castellani, Massimo Conese and Diego Muñoz-Torrero

Received: 31 August 2021
Accepted: 27 October 2021
Published: 29 October 2021

Publisher's Note: MDPI stays neutral with regard to jurisdictional claims in published maps and institutional affiliations.

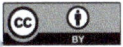

Copyright: © 2021 by the authors. Licensee MDPI, Basel, Switzerland. This article is an open access article distributed under the terms and conditions of the Creative Commons Attribution (CC BY) license (https://creativecommons.org/licenses/by/4.0/).

1. Introduction

Despite developments in the field of early cancer detection, the number of new cases is increasing at an alarming rate [1]. Pancreatic cancers, classified as one of the most aggressive malignant neoplasms in humans, pose a particular problem [2–4].

Cancer treatment focuses mainly on surgery, radiotherapy, and chemotherapy, depending on the type and severity of the disease at the time of diagnosis. In the case of pancreatic cancer, surgery is the most effective treatment [5]. However, due to the diagnosis of this disease in its late stage of development, only 15–20% of patients qualify for surgical removal of the tumor [6]. At the time of diagnosis, the vast majority of patients have numerous metastases, disqualifying them from surgery [5,6]. In turn, the use of chemotherapeutic agents has led to the development of acquired multidrug resistance [7,8].

The abovementioned methods of treatment often turn out to be ineffective, especially if the cancer is diagnosed at an advanced stage. For this reason, chemoprevention and the search for alternative treatment methods showing no or minimal side effects are becoming more and more important [8]. High hopes are placed on compounds of natural origin, including polyphenols, which are characterized by a wide range of biological activities. Many plant-derived compounds participate in the neoplastic process by affecting cell survival, inhibiting angiogenesis or inducing apoptosis [9]. Apoptosis, as a complex physiological process following a specific pattern, has a significant effect on the proper functioning of the body, leading to the removal of unnecessary and damaged cells that could pose a threat to the body over time (e.g., cancer cells). Proteins from the Bcl-2 family are involved in the process of apoptosis. Within them, we can distinguish two functional groups: one which has an inhibitory effect on apoptosis (e.g., Bcl-2) and one which influences the promotion of the apoptosis process (e.g., Bax). Maintaining the balance between pro- and anti-apoptotic proteins is essential for cell survival [10].

An example of a compound exhibiting anticancer properties is resveratrol. Resveratrol (3,5,4′-trihydroxystilbene) is a polyphenol belonging to the stilbene group, found in many plant foods such as grapes, blueberries, peanuts, tea and dark chocolate [11,12]. However, its main source is red wine, due to the fact that its highest concentration can be found in the skin of red grapes (50–100 µg/g) [13]. Resveratrol exists in the form of cis and trans isomers (Figure 1). The *trans* isomer is used for research due to its greater activity compared to the *cis* one [14–16].

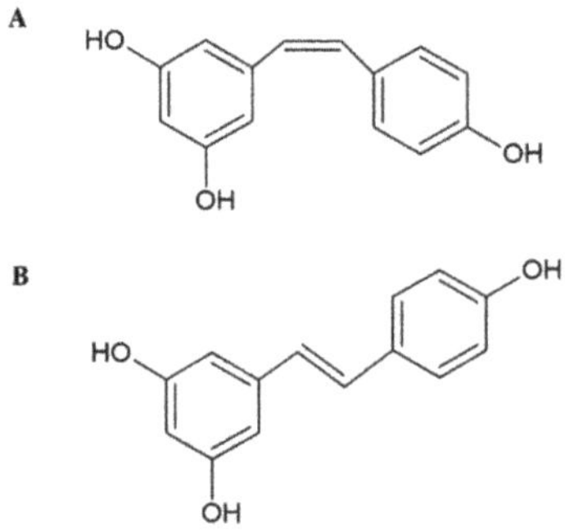

Figure 1. Chemical structures of resveratrol isomers: (**A**) *cis*-resveratrol, (**B**) *trans*-resveratrol.

Resveratrol is a phytoalexin that is produced in very small amounts by plants in response to the harmful effects of environmental factors, such as excessive UV radiation, exposure to heavy metals or fungal infections [11,17–19]. This compound is characterized by a wide range of biological activities, including antitumor activity [20]. Numerous scientific studies have shown that resveratrol exhibits antitumor activity at all stages of the carcinogenesis process in various types of neoplasms, including pancreatic neoplasm [3,21–23]. In addition, it also participates in overcoming the phenomenon of multidrug resistance (MDR), which has been demonstrated in research on cell models of gastric and pancreatic cancer [24,25].

The aim of our research is to demonstrate the potential antiproliferative and pro-apoptotic effects of *trans*-resveratrol on normal cells and various types of pancreatic cancer cells in vitro. So far, in vitro studies on the effects of resveratrol on members of the Bcl-2 family in pancreatic cancer cells have not been compared with studies on normal cells. It was also important to include cells resistant to cytostatics in the presented comparative studies in this field.

2. Results
2.1. Assessment of the Effect of Resveratrol on Cell Viability

Cell viability was analyzed with the MTT colorimetric assay. For this purpose, the cells of the tested lines were treated with increasing concentrations of resveratrol (0, 5, 10, 25, 50, 100, 150, 200 µM) for 24 h, 48 h and 72 h (37 °C, 5% CO_2). It was observed that the exposure of pancreatic cell lines to resveratrol inhibited proliferation in a concentration- and time-dependent manner compared to untreated cells (Figure 2A–D). EPP85-181RNOV cells, despite their resistance to mitoxantrone, turned out to be more sensitive to the action of resveratrol compared to mitoxantrone-sensitive cells (EPP85-181P line). AsPC-1 cells were the least sensitive to the effects of resveratrol. A concentration- and time-dependent decrease in cell viability was also observed in normal H6c7 pancreatic cells. Based on the analysis of the results obtained, concentrations of 25 µM, 50 µM and 100 µM, as well as an incubation time of 48 h, were selected for further experiments on all the tested cell lines.

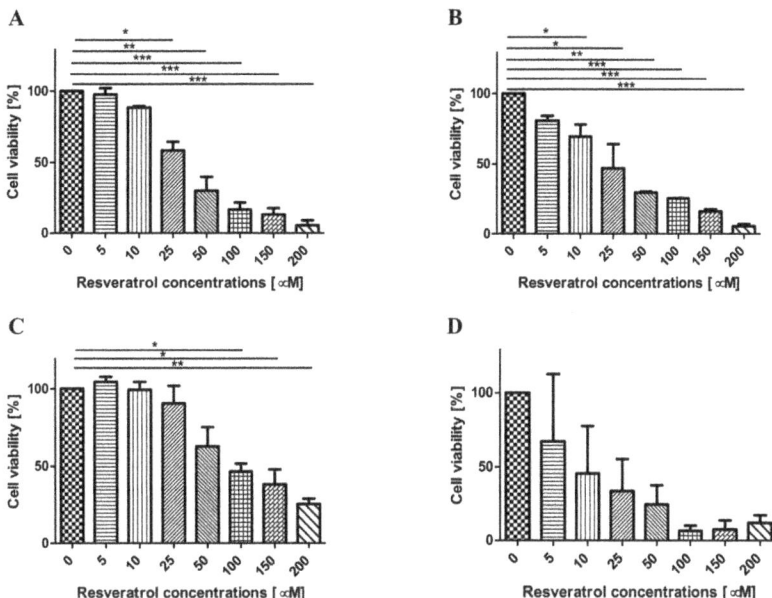

Figure 2. Effect of resveratrol on the proliferation of human cancer and normal pancreatic cells. Cells were treated with various concentrations of resveratrol for 48 h. Cell viability was assessed by MTT assays. (**A**) EPP85-181P cell line, (**B**) EPP85-181RNOV cell line, (**C**) AsPC-1 cell line, (**D**) H6c7 cell line. Values are expressed as mean ± SD, (n = 3), * $p < 0.01$; ** $p < 0.001$; *** $p < 0.0001$.

2.2. Analysis of the Effect of Resveratrol on the Cell Cycle of Pancreatic Cells Using Flow Cytometry (FACS)

The distribution of the cell cycle phases was observed using flow cytometry. Treatment with resveratrol resulted in cell accumulation in the G0/G1 or S phase, depending on the type of cells and the concentration of the compound. In the EPP85-181P cell line, after 48 h of exposure to resveratrol at a concentration of 50 µM, the cell cycle was inhibited in the S phase. However, at a higher concentration (100 µM), the cycle was inhibited in the G1 phase (Figure 3A). Similar relationships were observed in the EPP85-181RNOV line, in which the cycle was already inhibited in the S phase at concentrations of 25 and 50 µM, although more pronounced changes could be seen at a concentration of 50 µM. Cycle inhibition in the G1 phase was recorded at 100 µM (Figure 3B). In the case of the AsPC-1 cell line, there were no statistically significant differences in the inhibition of the cycle between concentrations in the range of 0–100 µM, but there was a significant change in the distribution of cells in the various phases of the cell cycle (Figure 3C). The effect of various concentrations of resveratrol in the range of 0–100 µM on normal pancreatic cells H6c7 did not change cell distribution throughout the phases of the cell cycle (Figure 3D) (Table 1).

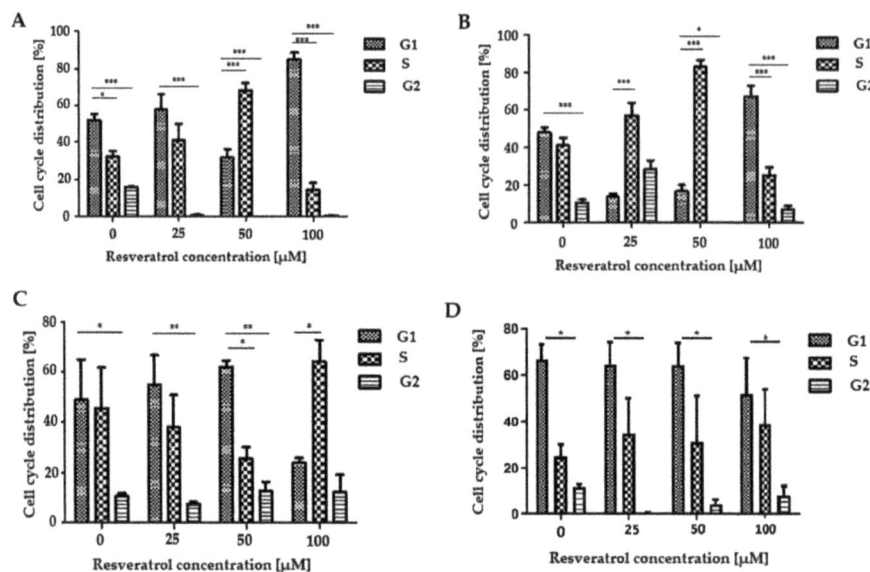

Figure 3. Cell distribution in particular phases of the cell cycle. (**A**) EPP85-181P cell line, (**B**) EPP85-181RNOV cell line, (**C**) AsPC-1 cell line, (**D**) H6c7 cell line, * $p < 0.05$; ** $p < 0.01$; *** $p < 0.001$.

Table 1. Change in cell cycle phase distribution after 48-h treatment with resveratrol (0–100 μM) on EPP85-181P, EPP85-181RNOV, AsPC-1 and H6c7 cells. Results are presented as mean of triplicate measurements.

Cell Line	Resveratrol Concentration [μM]	Percentage of Cell Breakdown in Different Phases of the Cell Cycle [%]		
		G1	S	G2
EPP85-181P	0	51.99 ± SD 5.47	32.28 ± SD 5.66	15.73 ± SD 0.44
	25	57.66 ± SD 14.31	4.40 ± SD 15.06	0.61 ± SD 1.05
	50	31.91 ± SD 7.54	68.09 ± SD 7.54	0.00 ± SD 0.0
	100	84.90 ± SD 6.42	14.78 ± SD 6.75	0.32 ± SD 0.56
EPP85-181RNOV	0	47.80 ± SD 5.37	41.70 ± SD7.10	10.50 ± SD 2.85
	25	13.61 ± SD 3.75	57.99 ± SD 11.56	28.40 ± SD 8.07
	50	16.52 ± SD 6.75	83.48 ± SD 6.75	0.00 ± SD 0.00
	100	67.32 ± SD 10.70	25.57 ± SD 7.74	7.11 ± SD 3.00
AsPC-1	0	48.85 ± SD 28.16	45.60 ± SD 28.29	10.52 ± SD 2.16
	25	54.77 ± SD 20.86	38.05 ± SD 22.19	7.18 ± SD 1.83
	50	62.02 ± SD 4.52	25.45 ± SD 8.65	12.53 ± SD 6.55
	100	23.78 ± SD 3.35	64.20 ± SD 15.36	12.02 ± SD 12.36
H6c7	0	66.68 ± SD 6.96	25.41 ± SD 5.86	11.87 ± SD 1.21
	25	64.40 ± SD 10.11	35.37 ± SD 10.41	0.23 ± SD 0.40
	50	64.33 ± SD 9.98	31.22 ± SD 10.86	4.45 ± SD 0.98
	100	51.84 ± SD 15.81	39.89 ± SD 15.80	8.27 ± SD 4.09

2.3. Analysis of the Percentage of Apoptotic Cells after 48 h of Incubation with Resveratrol Solution Measured by Flow Cytometry (FACS)

Flow cytometry analysis was performed to assess the ability of resveratrol to induce apoptosis in pancreatic cells. The tested cells were treated with various concentrations of resveratrol (0, 25, 50 and 100 μM) for 48 h. The obtained results indicated that resveratrol could induce apoptosis in a concentration-dependent manner (Table 2). The most prominent changes in early apoptosis markers were noted in the EPP85-181P cell line. In contrast, the smallest increase in the percentage of apoptotic cells was observed in the AsPC-1 cell line. The EPP85-181RNOV and H6c7 cell lines showed a moderate increase in the percentage of cells in the early phase of apoptosis (Figure 4).

Table 2. Apoptosis percentage in neoplastic and normal pancreatic cells induced by resveratrol. Results are presented as mean of triplicate measurements.

Resveratrol Concentration [µM]	Early Apoptosis Percentage [%]			
	EPP85-181P	EPP85-181RNOV	AsPC-1	H6c7
0	7.18 ± SD 1.62	4.04 ± SD 1.59	6.08 ± SD 1.38	2.06 ± SD 0.57
25	10.13 ± SD 2.24	4.92 ± SD 0.79	4.55 ± SD 1.85	6.94 ± SD 1.87
50	18.90 ± SD 1.35	10.40 ± SD 1.27	4.21 ± SD 1.82	10.73 ± SD 3.00
100	21.00 ± SD 2.40	11.64 ± SD 2.13	5.82 ± SD 1.24	36.73 ± SD 8.91

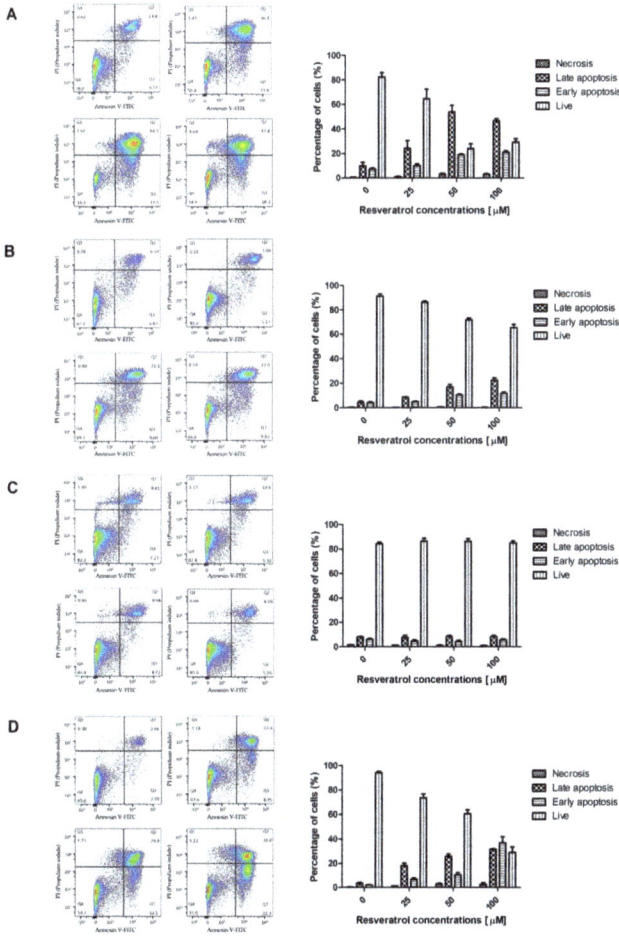

Figure 4. Analysis of apoptotic cells after incubation with resveratrol using flow cytometry. (**A**) EPP85-181P cell line, (**B**) EPP85-181RNOV cell line, (**C**) AsPC-1 cell line and (**D**) H6c7 cell line.

2.4. Analysis of the Percentage of Apoptotic Cells after 48 h of Incubation with Resveratrol Solution Measured Using the TUNEL Assay

The TUNEL reaction showed an increase in apoptosis in all of the cell groups after an incubation of 48 h with various concentrations of resveratrol (Figure 5). The increase in apoptosis in the tested cell lines was consistent with the increase in the concentration of the compound. The smallest increase in the number of apoptotic cells was noted in the AsPC-1 cell line. The EPP85-181P and EPP85-181RNOV cell lines were characterized by a moderate increase in the number of apoptotic cells. The highest number of apoptotic cells was observed in the H6c7 line, but only at the highest resveratrol concentration (100 µM). In vitro experiments have shown that resveratrol can induce apoptosis in pancreatic cells.

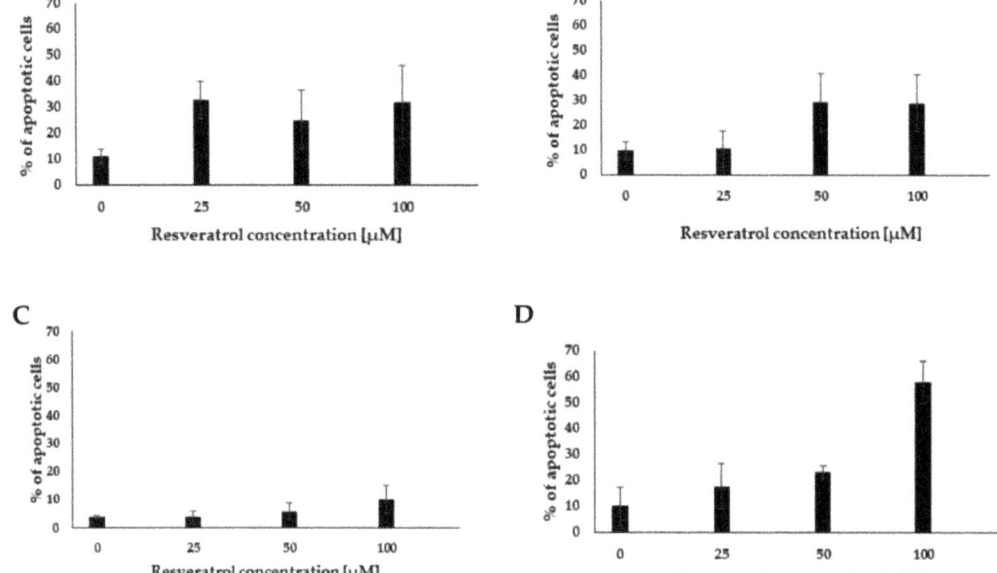

Figure 5. Detection of apoptotic cells using the TUNEL method. The number of apoptotic cells increases with the concentration of resveratrol in all cell lines: (**A**) EPP85-181P cell line, (**B**) EPP85-181RNOV cell line, (**C**) AsPC-1 cell line and (**D**) H6c7 cell line.

2.5. Detection of DNA Damage by Comet Assay

The Comet assay performed under neutral, nondenaturing conditions detects breaks in the double-stranded DNA chain, thus allowing the detection of apoptosis. Using this method, the percentage of apoptotic cells was estimated after 48 h of incubating individual cells with various concentrations of resveratrol. In all the cell lines tested, an increase in the number of damaged cells was observed after exposure to resveratrol. Moreover, this effect was most pronounced in cytostatic-resistant cells (EPP85-181RNOV). The EPP85-181P and H6c7 cell lines showed moderate sensitivity to the action of the compound. The lowest sensitivity was noted in the AsPC-1 cell line (Figure 6).

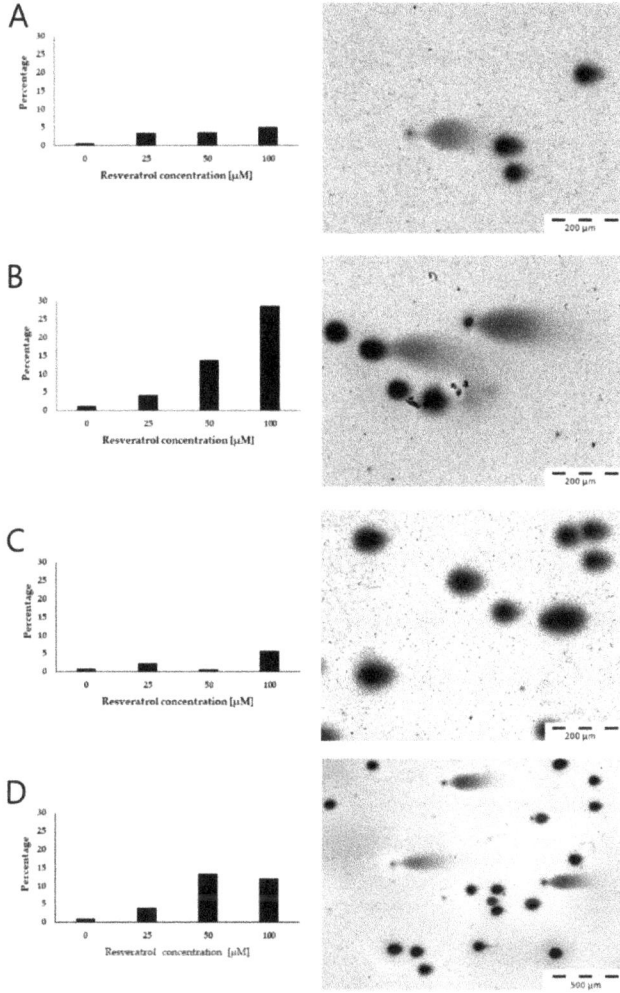

Figure 6. Percentage of nuclei with DNA damage in pancreatic cell lines after 48 h of incubation with different concentrations of resveratrol: (**A**) EPP85-181P cell line, (**B**) EPP85-181RNOV cell line, (**C**) AsPC-1 cell line and (**D**) H6c7 cell line.

2.6. Immunocytochemical Analysis of Resveratrol's Ability to Induce Apoptosis in Human Pancreatic Cells

To assess the ability of resveratrol to induce apoptotic in the tested cell lines, immunocytochemical reactions were performed; on this basis, the impact of the compound on the level of the Bcl-2, Bax and Caspase-3 proteins (which are related to the apoptosis process) was assessed (Figure 7). In the case of the anti-apoptotic protein Bcl-2, a significant decrease in the level of protein was observed after treatment with resveratrol in all of the tested cancer lines (Figure 7A–C). These changes were dependent on the concentration of the compound. The smallest changes were observed in the AsPC-1 cell line (Figure 7C). In turn, treatment with resveratrol caused a significant increase in the level of the Bax and Caspase-3 proteins, with changes depending on the concentration of the compound (Figure 7A–C). In the normal pancreatic cell line H6c7, resveratrol did not cause significant changes in the level of individual proteins.

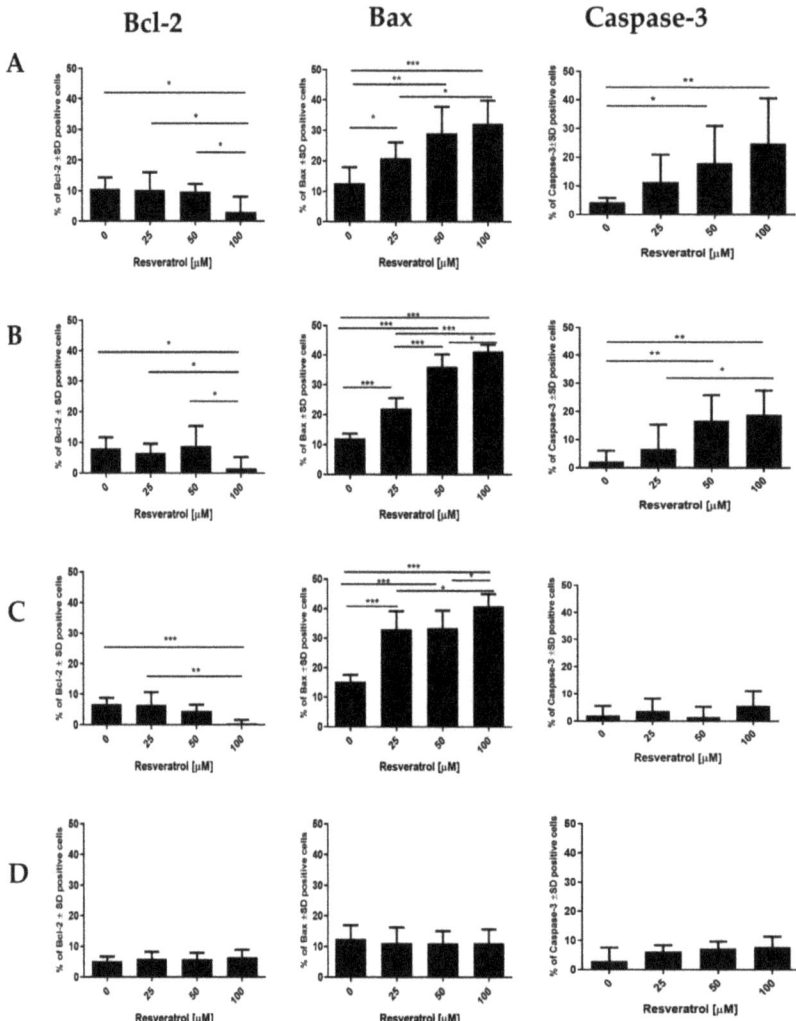

Figure 7. Analysis of resveratrol's ability to induce apoptosis in human pancreatic cells by immunocytochemistry. In the tested cell lines, the effect of resveratrol on the expression level of the Bcl-2, Bax and Caspase-3 proteins (related to the apoptotic process) was assessed. The cells of each cell line were exposed to 48 h of treatment with various concentrations of resveratrol. (**A**) EPP85-181P cell line, (**B**) EPP85-181RNOV cell line, (**C**) AsPC-1 cell line, (**D**) H6c7 cell line; * $p < 0.01$; ** $p < 0.001$; *** $p < 0.0001$.

2.7. Changes in the Expression Level of Genes Encoding Proteins of Bcl-2 Family in Pancreatic Cells by Real-Time PCR

The effect of resveratrol on the changes in the expression of the genes encoding proteins related to the apoptotic process was determined by real-time PCR. The analysis of mRNA expression showed that after 48 h of incubation of the cells with various concentrations of resveratrol, concentration-dependent changes in the expression of the *BAX* and *BCL2* genes appeared. In the case of the EPP85-181P cell line, a reduction in *BAX* expression was observed after treatment with resveratrol compared to untreated cells. In contrast, the level of *BCL2* expression after treatment with resveratrol increased at a concentration of

25 µM compared to untreated cells. Between concentrations of 50 and 100 µM, a decrease in the level of *BCL2* expression was observed. In the EPP85-181RNOV cell line, resveratrol reduced *BAX* expression in a concentration-dependent manner. On the other hand, a concentration of 25 µM caused a decrease in the level of *BCL2* expression, while an increase was observed between 50 and 100 µM. Similar results were obtained with the AsPC-1 cell line. The effect of resveratrol resulted in a concentration-dependent decrease in *BAX* expression and an increase in *BCL2* expression. In the H6c7 cell line, resveratrol increased the level of *BAX* expression at a concentration of 25 µM, while decreasing it between 50 and 100 µM. In the case of *BCL2*, a concentration of 25 µM caused a decrease in its expression, while concentrations of 50 and 100 µM led to an increase (left panel of Figure 8).

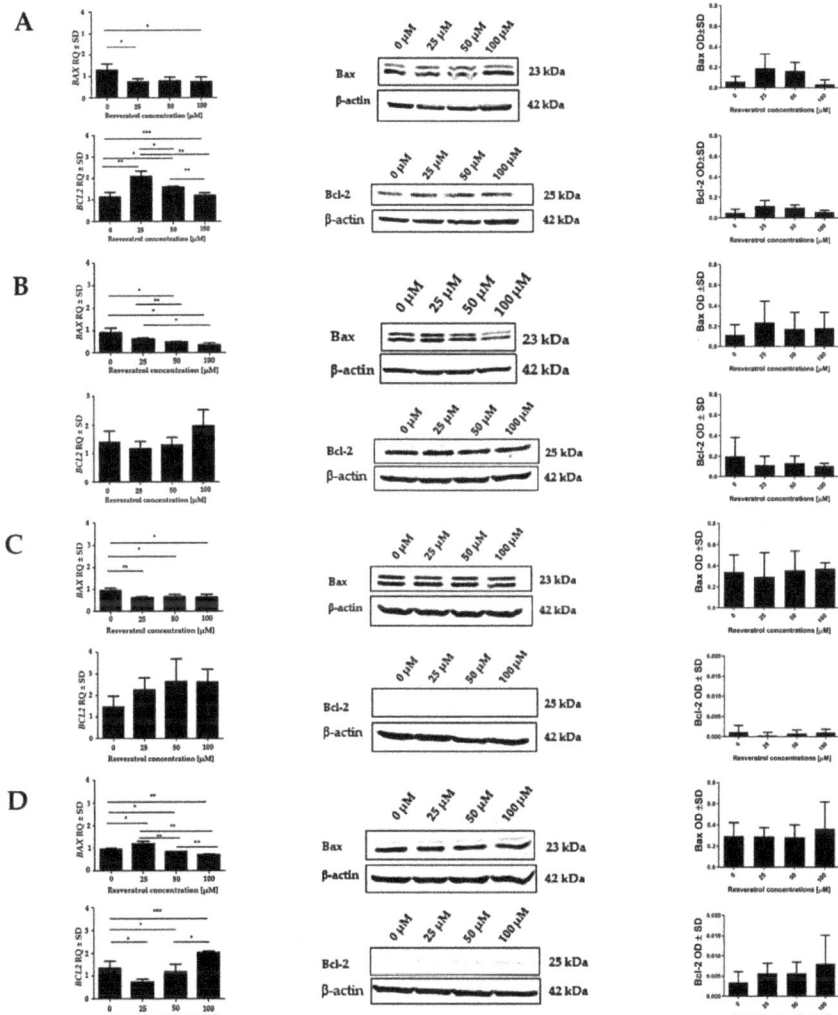

Figure 8. Effect of resveratrol on changes in the expression level of genes and proteins related to the apoptotic process assessed by real-time PCR (left panel) and Western Blot (middle and left panels). The analysis was performed on human pancreatic cell lines after 48 h of exposure to various concentrations of resveratrol. (**A**) EPP85-181P cell line, (**B**) EPP85-181RNOV cell line, (**C**) AsPC-1 cell line and (**D**) H6c7 cell line; * $p < 0.01$; ** $p < 0.001$; *** $p < 0.0001$.

2.8. Changes in the Level of Bcl-2 Proteins in Pancreatic Cells (WB)

Western Blot analysis was performed to assess the possible modulation of apoptotic proteins by resveratrol. The changes in the level of Bax and Bcl-2 proteins were examined after 48 h of incubation of human pancreatic cells with various concentrations of resveratrol. After treatment with resveratrol at a concentration of 25 µM, EPP85-181P cells showed a higher level of the pro-apoptotic protein Bax compared to untreated cells. Between 50 and 100 µM, a concentration-dependent decrease in the level of this protein was observed. In the case of the anti-apoptotic protein Bcl-2, an increase in the level was initially observed (25 µM), while higher concentrations of the compound caused a decrease in the level of the protein.

In the cell line showing resistance to mitoxantrone (EPP85-181RNOV), exposure to resveratrol at a concentration of 25 µM resulted in an increase in the level of the Bax protein compared to untreated cells. The effect of higher concentrations led to a decrease in the level of Bax in comparison to its level at 25 µM. However, in this case, the changes in the 50 and 100 µM concentrations were at a similar level. The level of the Bcl-2 protein at a concentration of 25 µM was lower compared to that in cells not treated with resveratrol, and no significant differences in the level of protein were observed with subsequent concentrations.

In the AsPC-1 cell line, slight changes in the level of the Bax protein were observed. There was a slight decrease in the level at a concentration of 25 µM in relation to cells not treated with resveratrol, and between 50 and 100 µM, an increase in the level of expression took place. A similar relationship was observed for the Bcl-2 protein. The action of resveratrol at a concentration of 25 µM reduced the level of protein, while at higher concentrations, an increase in Bcl-2 level was noted.

In the normal H6c7 pancreatic cell line, no significant changes in the level of the Bax protein were observed after treatment with resveratrol. Only at the highest concentration (100 µM), an increase in the level of this protein was noted. In the case of the anti-apoptotic protein Bcl-2, there was an increase in its level in the treated cells, with the changes being proportional to the concentration of the compound (middle and right panels of Figure 8).

2.9. Cell Morphological Changes Induced by Resveratrol

A 48-h treatment with resveratrol induced morphological changes in all the tested cell lines. A decrease in cell density and a change in cellular shape and size were observed (Figure 9).

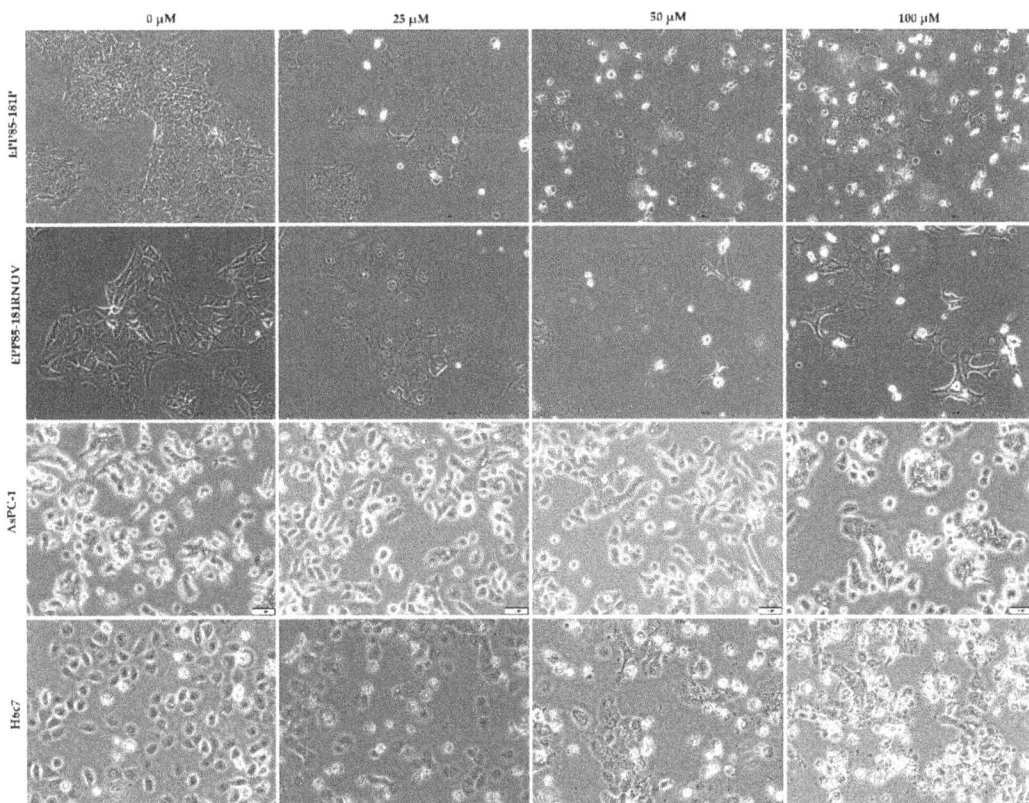

Figure 9. Resveratrol induces morphological changes in EPP85-181P, EPP85-181RNOV, AsPC-1 and H6c7 cells after 48 h incubation with different concentrations of the compound. As the concentration increases, a smaller number of cells can be observed compared to the control, as well as many cells detached (iridescent) from the substrate.

2.10. Bax and Bcl-2 Expression Levels by Confocal Microscopy

To visualize the effect of resveratrol on the level of the Bax and Bcl-2 proteins, an immunofluorescence reaction was performed on the AsPC-1 tumor cell line. The analysis of the results using a confocal microscope showed that 48-h treatment with resveratrol (100 μM) resulted in an increase in the level of the pro-apoptotic protein Bax in relation to untreated cells. In the case of the anti-apoptotic protein Bcl-2, the level was reduced compared to untreated cells (Figure 10).

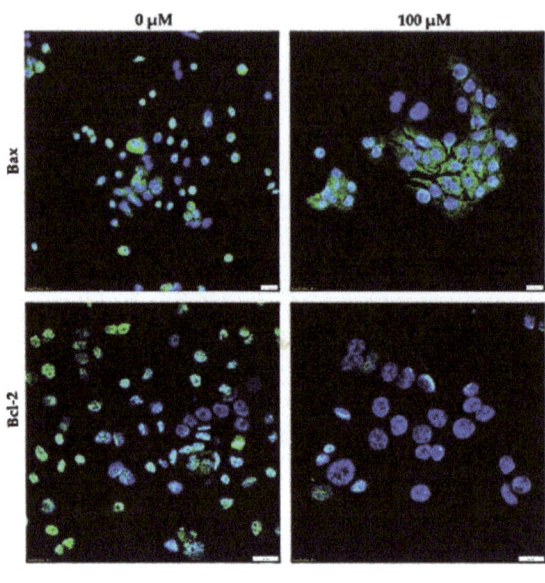

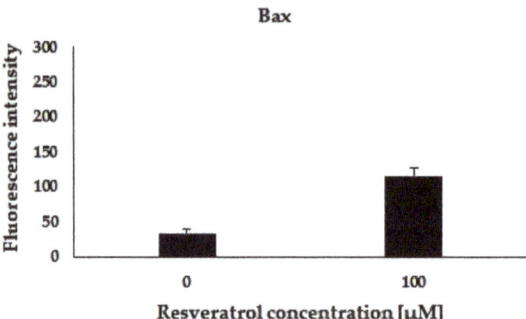

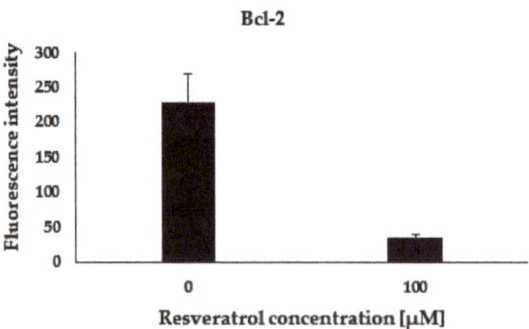

Figure 10. Confocal images showing changes in the level of the Bax and Bcl-2 proteins in the pancreatic cancer cell line AsPC-1 after treatment with 100 µM of resveratrol. Magnification 60×, scale = 20 µm.

3. Discussion

Cancer remains one of the leading causes of death worldwide. Pancreatic neoplasms pose a particular problem due to their late diagnosis because of the lack of early and characteristic symptoms [26]. Hence, there is an increasingly urgent need for compounds (especially of natural origin) that show anticancer activity while protecting normal cells [27]. An example of such a bioactive compound is resveratrol [28]. Even though it has been the subject of many studies, its mechanism of action is not fully understood and requires further research. However, it is known that resveratrol has a pleiotropic effect, and its action depends on many factors (concentration, duration of action, type of cell line).

The present study shows that resveratrol can significantly inhibit the proliferation of pancreatic cells, in a manner dependent both on the duration of the effect and the concentration of the compound. At the same time, changes in the distribution of neoplastic cells between different phases of the cell cycle were also noticed under the influence of different concentrations of resveratrol.

In one of the studies that analyzed the effect of resveratrol on the proliferation of the pancreatic cancer cells PANC-1 and AsPC-1, significant changes in cell survival were observed after incubations longer than 24 h and at a higher concentration of the compound (100 µM) [3]. Moreover, significant changes in AsPC-1 cell survival appeared only at higher resveratrol concentrations ($\geq$100 µM). The studies conducted by Cui et al. showed that the action of resveratrol inhibits the proliferation of the pancreatic neoplastic cell lines PANC-1, BxPC-3 and AsPC-1, and the changes depend on the concentration and duration of the compound's effect. There were differences in the sensitivity of cells to resveratrol between individual cell lines, with AsPC-1 being the least sensitive (concentration > 100 µM), which was consistent with our observations [29]. Another research team demonstrated the antiproliferative effect of resveratrol on the pancreatic cancer cells MIA PaCa-2, AsPC-1, PANC-1 and Hs766T. In this case, a 48-h incubation with various concentrations of resveratrol resulted in a concentration-dependent inhibition of cell growth. The cell lines differed in their sensitivity to the effects of resveratrol. As in previous studies, the AsPC-1 cell line was one of the least susceptible to the effects of resveratrol [30]. In their studies, Liu et al. assessed the effect of resveratrol on the proliferation of neoplastic (PANC-1, CFPAC-1 and MIA PaCa-2) and normal pancreatic cells (Pancreatic Duct Cells). Cells were exposed to various concentrations of resveratrol (10, 50 and 100 µM) for 72 h. Resveratrol was shown to have a concentration-dependent inhibitory effect on cell viability, which is consistent with our observations. Compared to neoplastic cells (PANC-1, CFPAC-1 and MIA PaCa-2), normal pancreatic duct cells showed greater resistance to the cytotoxic effect of resveratrol [31]. In our study, on the other hand, the normal pancreatic cell line H6c7 showed less tolerance to the compound.

The cell cycle is a basic process common to all living organisms, essential for reproduction and growth. It comprises two main phases: the interphase (G1, S and G2 phases) and mitosis (M) [32]. It was found that resveratrol influences the cell cycle by reducing the number of cells in the G1/S and S/G2 phases, which leads to the inhibition of cell proliferation [33,34]. The analysis of the cell cycle in the tumor lines EPP85-181P and EPP85-181RNOV showed that lower concentrations of resveratrol (25 and 50 µM) increase the number of cells in the S/G2 phase. In the mitoxantrone-resistant line, this effect was stronger. On the other hand, at a higher concentration (100 µM), a greater accumulation of cells in the G1/S phase was observed. These results are consistent with previous studies performed on the EPP85-181P and EPP85-181RNOV cell lines, treated for 72 h with two concentrations of resveratrol (30 and 50 µM) [25]. In the EPP85-181P and EPP85-181RNOV lines, at a concentration of 50 µM, an increase in the number of cells in the S/G2 phase was observed, while in the EPP85-181RNOV line, these changes were visible at a lower concentration (30 µM) [25]. In our study, no significant changes in the distribution of the different phases of the cell cycle were observed in the AsPC-1 line after 48 h of incubation with resveratrol (0–100 µM). In contrast, the team of Cui et al. showed an increase in cell accumulation in the S phase of the cell cycle. However, these changes were observed after 72 h of incubation with resveratrol at a concentration of 100 µM [3].

Apoptosis is a process involving the activation, expression, and regulation of a wide range of genes with a consequent programmed cell death. This process is aimed at ensuring and maintaining a stable internal environment by removing unwanted and abnormal cells from the body [35]. In neoplastic diseases, the balance between cell division and death is usually disturbed [36]. Therefore, understanding the process of apoptosis may prove helpful not only in assessing the pathogenesis of cancer, but also in developing a treatment strategy.

Along with the effect on the growth and changes in the distribution of cells among the various phases of the cell cycle under the action of resveratrol, the participation of the compound in the process of apoptotic induction has also been observed. In our studies, we have shown that resveratrol induces apoptosis in pancreatic cells, and that the observed changes are concentration dependent. These observations are consistent with research conducted by Roy et al., who showed a similar dependence on the neoplastic pancreatic cell lines PANC-1, MIA PaCa-2, Hs766T and AsPC-1. Additionally, the intensity of the changes depends on the pancreatic cell line. Both in our study and in the work of Roy et al., the AsPC-1 cell line was characterized by its low sensitivity to the action of resveratrol [30]. Furthermore, Cui et al. showed that, out of the three pancreatic cancer lines (PANC-1, AsPC-1 and BxPC-3) incubated for 48 h with various concentrations of resveratrol (0–200 µM), the AsPC-1 line showed the lowest susceptibility to the effect of the compound at lower concentrations. Significant changes appeared only at concentrations over 150 µM [29]. The team of Zhou et al. investigated the ability of resveratrol to induce apoptosis on the pancreatic cancer cell models Capan-1, Capan-2, BxPC-3, MIA PaCa-2 and Colo357. After 24 h of exposure of the cells to resveratrol at a concentration of 200 µM, Capan-1, MIA PaCa-2 and BxPC-3 turned out to be less sensitive to the compound compared to the other two, i.e., Capan-2 and Colo357. The same study also showed a slight effect of resveratrol on the induction of apoptosis in normal pancreatic cells (HPDE—Human Pancreatic Duct Epithelial Cell Line) [37]. In our study, we observed apoptotic changes in the normal pancreatic cell line, but these were most pronounced only at the highest concentration of resveratrol (100 µM). It is also worth noting that we analyzed the effect of the compound after a longer duration of the effect (48 h). The Comet assay results showed DNA damage typical of apoptosis, the trend was similar to that of the TUNEL method.

To better understand the effect of resveratrol on the inhibition of cell growth and the induction of the apoptotic process, Western Blot analyses were performed. Proteins from the Bcl-2 family play a key role in the control of the apoptotic execution process. Among the members of this family, there are pro-apoptotic proteins (e.g., Bid, Bax) and proteins that inhibit this process (e.g., Bcl-2). Thanks to these two opposite types of regulatory proteins, it is possible to maintain the homeostasis of the processes of this type of programmed cell death [38,39].

In studies performed on the PANC-1 and MIA PaCa-2 cell lines, 24-h incubation with different concentrations of resveratrol (0, 50, 10, 150 and 200 µM) resulted in an increase in the level of the Bax protein and a decrease in the level of the Bcl-2 protein [40]. The studies by Yang et al. on the Capan-2 cell line showed that a 24-h incubation of the cells with resveratrol at a concentration of 100 µM led to a significant increase in the level of the Bax protein [41]. An increase in the level of the Bax protein and a decrease in the level of the Bcl-2 protein (in direct proportion to the increase in resveratrol concentration 50, 200 and 400 µM) were also demonstrated in the gastric tumor cell line SGC-7901 after 24 h of incubation [42]. The team of Cui et al., in their studies performed on three pancreatic cell lines (PANC-1, BxPC-3, AsPC-1) exposed for 48 h to different concentrations of resveratrol (0–200 µM), observed changes in the level of pro- and anti-apoptotic proteins. In two of the analyzed cell lines (PANC-1 and BxPC-3), a concentration-dependent increase in the expression level of the pro-apoptotic protein (Bax) and a decrease in the level of the anti-apoptotic protein (Bcl-2) were observed. In the case of the AsPC-1 cell line, no significant changes in the level of the Bax protein were observed. However, there were changes in the level of the Bcl-2 protein, which were most visible at the highest concentration of resveratrol used [29]. Similarly, in our study, we did not observe significant changes in the level of the Bax protein in the AsPC-1 line after a 48-h incubation with different concentrations of the compound (0, 25, 50 and 100 µM). On the other hand, the most visible changes in the level of the Bcl-2 protein level were noticed at higher concentrations (50 and 100 µM). Immunofluorescence also allowed us to obtain confirmation of changes in the level of these proteins in cells that had been incubated with resveratrol. Confocal microscopy analysis showed an increase in the level of the Bax protein and a decrease in the Bcl-2 protein level in AsPC-1 cells after a 48-h incubation with resveratrol (100 µM).

Furthermore, the analysis of the real-time PCR reaction showed that a 48-h incubation of cells with resveratrol (0, 25, 50 and 100 µM) led to a decrease in the expression of the gene encoding the pro-apoptotic protein Bax (*BAX*) and an increase in the expression of the gene encoding the anti-apoptotic protein Bcl-2 (*BCL2*). This was confirmed by the results obtained by a research team that carried out similar studies on the pancreatic cancer cell line Panc 2.03. In that study, a real-time PCR reaction was performed after 12 and 24 h of exposure to resveratrol at a concentration of 40 µg/mL. The reaction showed an increase in the mRNA expression level of *BAX* and a decrease in the mRNA expression level of *BCL2*. Moreover, Western Blot studies performed on the same cell line after 48-h exposure to resveratrol (10, 20, 40 and 80 µg/mL) confirmed the same relationship we observed in the experiments carried out after the same incubation time [43]. It follows that 48 h is the optimal time to study Bcl-2 and Bax level changes.

4. Materials and Methods

4.1. Cell Lines and Culture Conditions

In vitro studies were carried out on three human pancreatic cancer cell lines: EPP85-181P, EPP85-181RNOV (cell lines were obtained from Institute of Pathology, Charité Campus Mitte, Humboldt University Berlin, Berlin, Germany) and AsPC-1 (ATCC, Manassas, VA, USA), as well as the normal pancreatic line H6c7 (Kerafast, Inc., Boston, MA, USA). The EPP85-181P cell line is sensitive to the action of cytostatics, while the EPP85-181RNOV line is resistant to the action of mitoxantrone. The appropriate culture media were selected for the cultivation of individual cell lines. Lines EPP85-181P and EPP85-181RNOV were grown in Leibovitz's L-15 medium (Sigma, St. Louis, MO, USA) enriched with the following supplements: 10% Fetal Bovine Serum (FBS), 1 mM L-glutamine, 6.25 mg/L fetuin, 80 IE/L insulin, 2.5 mg/L transferrin, 1 g/L glucose, 1.1 g/L NaHCO$_3$ and 1% minimal essential vitamins (Sigma, St. Louis, MO, USA). Mitoxantrone was present in the culture of EPP85-181RNOV cells at a dose of 0.02 µg/mL. RPMI-1640 medium (Gibco Life Technologies, Paisley, Scotland, UK) containing 10% FBS (Sigma, St. Louis, MO, USA) was used to culture AsPC-1 cells. The H6c7 cell line was grown in Keratinocyte serum-free medium SFM (Gibco Life Technologies, Paisley, Scotland, UK) supplemented with bovine pituitary extract (25 µg/mL) and recombinant human epidermal growth factor (0.25 ng/mL). Additionally, the media were supplemented with a 1% penicillin solution and streptomycin (Sigma, St. Louis, MO, USA). Cells were grown in monolayers in 75 cm^2 culture flasks (Thermo Scientific, Roskilde, Denmark) which were placed in an incubator (37 °C, 5% CO$_2$). A solution of 0.25% trypsin-ethylene diamine tetraacetic acid (Sigma, St. Louis, MO, USA) was used to pass the cells of the pancreatic cancer lines. The passage of normal pancreatic cells was performed with the TrypLETM Express Enzyme solution (Gibco Life Technologies, Paisley, Scotland, UK).

4.2. MTT Assay

The effect of resveratrol on cell proliferation was investigated using the MTT colorimetric assay [44]. The cells of the tested lines were plated in 96-well plates 24 h before the start of the experiment in the following amounts: EPP85-181P and AsPC-1 cells—5×10^3 cells/well, EPP85-181RNOV cells—2.5×10^3 cells/well and H6c7 cells—

1.2×10^4 cells/well. Dimethyl sulfoxide (DMSO) was used as an initial solvent. Resveratrol was subsequently dissolved in culture media for cell treatment. The cells were then treated with a solution of resveratrol at various concentrations (0, 5, 10, 25, 50, 100, 150 and 200 µM) at three-time regimens: 24, 48 and 72 h (37 °C, 5% CO_2). After incubation under the set conditions, cells were treated with a solution of MTT (3-(4,5-dimethylthiazol-2-yl)-2,5-diphenyltetrazolium bromide) (0.5 mg/mL) for 4 h (37 °C, 5% CO_2). The MTT cytotoxicity test is based on the color reaction of a tetrazole salt and the assessment of the mitochondrial activity of the cells. As a result of the reduction of the substrate in the mitochondria of living cells, a water-insoluble purple formazan compound is formed depending on the viability of the cells. After the formazan crystals were thoroughly dissolved in dimethylsulfoxide (DMSO), the absorbance was measured for each sample at 570 nm using a microplate reader (Infinite 200 Pro, TECAN, Männedorf, Switzerland). The experiment was repeated independently three times.

4.3. Cell Cycle Analysis, Flow Cytometry (FACS)

The distribution of the cell cycle phases following resveratrol treatment was assessed using the flow cytometric method. Twenty-four hours before the start of the experiment, the cell lines were plated in the following amounts: EPP85-181P—1.2×10^5 cells/well, EPP85-181RNOV—1.8×10^5 cells/well, AsPC-1—4.6×10^5 cells/well and H6c7—4.6×10^5 cells/well. They were then placed in an incubator (37 °C, 5% CO_2). After this time, cells were treated with resveratrol at concentrations of 0, 25, 50 and 100 µM for 48 h (37 °C, 5% CO_2). Afterwards, they were trypsinized and centrifuged in fresh culture medium (1050 rpm, 5 min), and then rinsed twice in ice-cold Phosphate Buffered Saline (PBS) and fixed in cold 70% ethanol overnight at 4 °C. After that, cells were centrifuged (1050 rpm, 5 min, 4 °C) and rinsed twice in PBS. The samples were stained with an FxCycle™ PI/RNase Staining Solution kit (Life Technologies, Carlsbad, CA, USA) and incubated for 30 min at 37 °C in the dark. Propidium iodide fluorescence was measured using a BD FACSCanto II flow cytometer on channel 630/22 (Beckton Dickinson, Franklin Lakes, NJ, USA). Data from at least 20,000 events per sample were collected and calculated using the ModFit LTTM software, version 4.0.5 (Verity Software House, Inc., Topsham, ME, USA). The experiment was carried out in three independent laboratory replications.

4.4. Apoptosis, Flow Cytometry Method (FACS)

The flow cytometry method was used to study the intensity of the apoptotic induction under the effect of resveratrol. The cells of the tested lines (EPP85-181P, EPP85-181RNOV, AsPC-1 and H6c7) were cultured in 25 cm^2 flasks for 24 h (37 °C, 5% CO_2). After this time, cells were treated with resveratrol at concentrations of 0, 25, 50 and 100 µM for 48 h (37 °C, 5% CO_2). Subsequently, they were trypsinized and then centrifuged (1050 rpm, 5 min) in fresh culture medium. Cells were then rinsed twice in PBS solution and centrifuged afterwards (1050 rpm, 5 min). Cells were diluted to 1×10^6 cells/mL and stained with the FITC Annexin V Apoptosis Detection Kit II (Beckton Dickinson, Franklin Lakes, NJ, USA) according to the manufacturer's instructions. Data from at least 10,000 events were collected for each sample. The results obtained were further analyzed with the FlowJo 10.5 software (FlowJo, Asham, OR, USA). The experiment was carried out in three independent laboratory replications.

4.5. Apoptosis, TUNEL Assay

The ability of resveratrol to induce the apoptotic process was also detected by using the TUNEL assay. The cells of the tested lines were plated on Millicell® EZ SLIDES eight-well glass slides (Merck Millipore, Gernsheim, Germany) in the following amounts: EPP85-181P—1×10^4 cells/well, EPP85-181RNOV—1×10^4 cells/well, AsPC-1—1.5×10^4 cells/well and H6c7—1.5×10^4 cells/well. After 24 h, cells were treated with resveratrol at concentrations of 0, 25, 50 and 100 µM for 48 h (37 °C, 5% CO_2). After this time, cells were fixed in cold methanol-acetone (1:1) for 10 min at 4 °C and then dried. Apoptosis was detected with the ApopTag® Peroxidase In Situ Apoptosis Detection Kit (Merck Millipore, Gernsheim, Germany) according to the manufacturer's instructions. Cells were rinsed with PBS solution (pH 7.4), then incubated with Proteinase K (5 min, room temperature) and rinsed again with PBS solution. Endogenous peroxidase blocking was done by incubation in 3% H_2O_2 in PBS (5 min, room temperature). Next, cells were rinsed again with PBS solution. Cells were then incubated, first with pre-incubation buffer (10 min, room temperature), then with incubation buffer (1 h, 37 °C). The reaction was stopped by adding a stop buffer (10 min, room temperature). Cells were then incubated with antidigoxigenin antibodies (30 min, room temperature). To visualize the nuclei of the apoptotic cells, cells were incubated with diaminobenzidine (DAB, 5 min, room temperature). Contrast staining with hematoxylin was performed. The expression of the nuclei of the apoptotic cells was assessed using a BX-41 light microscope (Olympus, Tokyo, Japan).

4.6. DNA-Damages Visualisation, Comet Assay

The detection of apoptosis-related DNA damage was assessed by using a neutral Comet assay. Cell lines EPP85-181P, EPP85-181RNOV, AsPC-1 and H6c7 were cultured in 25 cm^2 flasks for 24 h (37 °C, 5% CO_2). Afterwards, they were treated with resveratrol at concentrations of 0, 25, 50 and 100 μM for 48 h (37 °C, 5% CO_2). Cells were trypsinized, then centrifuged (1050 rpm, 5 min) in fresh culture medium and later rinsed twice in PBS and centrifuged (1050 rpm, 5 min). The method described by Collins [45] was used to detect DNA damage. Portions of the cells (min. 1×10^4) treated with the specified concentrations of the analyses compound for 48 h were combined with low melting point agarose (type VII) and transferred onto a glass slide precoated with high melting point agarose (type I). Then, the slides were placed in a lysis solution (2.5 M NaCl, 100 mM EDTA, 10 mM Tris base, 1% Triton X-100, pH 10) at 40 °C for 60 min. Afterwards, the slides were rinsed in electrophoresis buffer (TBE) for 30 min at 40 °C. Then, electrophoresis was carried out at a voltage of 1.0 V/cm, 490 mA intensity for 20 min at 40 °C. Staining was carried out with the silver method. 80–100 nuclei were counted on each slide. DNA damage was assessed, assigning each nucleus to the appropriate category: apoptosis, indirect damage, or no damage.

4.7. Immunocytochemistry (ICC)

To assess the ability of resveratrol to induce the apoptotic process, an ICC reaction was performed. The cells of the tested lines were plated on Millicell EZ SLIDES eight-well glass slides (Merck Millipore, Gernsheim, Germany) in the following amounts: EPP85-181P—1×10^4 cells/well, EPP85-181RNOV—1×10^4 cells/well, AsPC-1—1.5×10^4 cells/well and H6c7—1.5×10^4 cells/well. 24 h later, cells were treated with resveratrol at concentrations of 0, 25, 50 and 100 μM for 48 h. After this time, cells were fixed with methanol-acetone (1:1) for 10 min at 4 °C. The ICC reaction was performed on an Autostainer Link48 (Dako, Glostrup, Denmark). The following primary antibodies were used: Bcl-2 (Dako, Glostrup, Denmark), Bax (Santa Cruz Biotechnology, Dallas, TX, USA) and activated Caspase-3 (Cell Signaling Technology, Boston, MA, USA). Slides were first incubated with primary antibodies against Bcl-2 (ready-to-use), Bax (1:25) and activated Caspase-3 (1:400) for 20 min at room temperature, followed by 20 min with EnVision FLEX/HRP (Dako, Glostrup, Denmark). In the next step, the slides were incubated for 10 min with 3,3′-diaminobenzidine (DAB, Dako. Glostrup, Denmark). The slides were counterstained with EnVision FLEX Hematoxylin (Dako, Glostrup, Denmark) and sealed with coverslips in a mounting medium. The ICC reaction was assessed using a BX-41 light microscope (Olympus, Tokyo, Japan).

4.8. Real-Time PCR

An assessment of the changes in the *BAX* and *BCL2* gene expressions was performed after treatment with resveratrol at concentrations of 0, 25, 50 and 100 μM on the cell lines EPP85-181P, EPP85-181RNOV, AsPC-1 and H6c7. After 48 h of incubation with the compound, cells were trypsinized, as described in the Cell Lines and Culture Conditions section above. RNA was isolated with the RNeasy Mini Kit (Qiagen, Hilden, Germany) according to the manufacturer's instructions. The samples were digested with RNase DNset (Qiagen, Hilden, Germany) to remove genomic DNA. The concentration and quality of the isolated RNA was measured on a NanoDrop 1000 spectrophotometer (Thermo-Fischer Waltham, MA, USA). A reverse transcription reaction was then performed using the High-Capacity cDNA Reverse Transcription Kits (Applied Biosystems, Foster City, CA, USA). The assessment of the changes in the gene expression was performed by real-time PCR using a 7900HT Fast Real Time PCR System thermocycler with SDS 2.3 and RQ Manager 1.2 software (Applied Biosystems, Foster City, CA, USA). Primers *BAX* (Hs00180269_m1 BAX) and *BCL2* (Hs00608023_m1 BCL2) were obtained from Applied Biosystems (Foster City, CA, USA). *GUSB* (beta glucuronidase—Hs99999908_m1 GUSB, Applied Biosystems, Foster City, CA, USA) was used as a reference gene. The reaction was performed in triplicate under the following conditions: polymerase activation at 50 °C for 2 min, initial denaturation at 94 °C for 10 min, 40 cycles including denaturation at 94 °C for 15 s, annealing of primers and probes as well as synthesis at 60 °C for 1 min. The results were analyzed based on the expression of the GUSB reference gene. The relative expression (RQ) of *BCL2* and *BAX* mRNA was calculated using the ΔΔCt method (RQ = $2^{-\Delta\Delta Ct}$).

4.9. Western Blot

The Western Blot (WB) method was used to study the effect of resveratrol on the changes in the level of the proteins related to the process of apoptosis. The cells of the tested lines (EPP85-181P, EPP85-181RNOV, AsPC-1 and H6c7) were treated with various concentrations of resveratrol (0, 25, 50 and 100 µM) for 48 h. Total cellular protein was isolated from the cell lines tested. The procedure was performed at 4 °C using RIPA lysis buffer (50 mM Tris-HCl pH 8.0, 150 mM NaCl, 0.1% SDS, 1% IGEPAL CA-630, 0.5% sodium deoxycholate) with the addition of PMSF (2.5 µL/mL RIPA) and an inhibitor cocktail (2 µL/200 µL RIPA). The samples were incubated for 20 min on ice with vortexing every 5 min. After this time, the samples were centrifuged (4 °C, 12 min, 12,000× *g*). The supernatant was transferred to clean tubes and frozen at −80°C. Protein concentration was determined by the BCA method using the Pierce BCA Protein Assay kit (Thermo Fischer Scientific, Waltham MA, USA). Protein samples were loaded in GLB (4×) and denatured (95 °C, 10 min). Total protein (50 µg) was separated by SDS-PAGE in a 12% polyacrylamide gel (Bio-Rad, Hercules, CA, USA) at a voltage of 140 V. Subsequently, wet transfer was performed onto nitrocellulose membranes (Millipore, Billerica, MA, USA) in buffer (48 mM Tris, 39 mM glycine, 20% methanol, 0.1% SDS, pH 9.2) at 100 V for one hour. After transfer, the membranes were rinsed with distilled water then 0.1% TBST solution. After blocking for 1 h at room temperature (Bax: 5% milk in 0.1% TBST; Bcl-2: 4% BSA in 0.1% TBST), the membranes were incubated overnight at 4°C with specific primary antibodies: mouse anti-Bax (sc-7480; 1:200; Santa Cruz Biotechnology, Dallas, TX, USA) and mouse anti-Bcl-2 (124, 1:200, Novus Biologicals, Littleton, CO, USA). Additionally, the membranes were incubated with horseradish peroxidase-conjugated secondary antibodies (715-035-152; Jackson ImmunoResearch, Cambridgeshire, UK) at a dilution of 1:3000 (1 h, room temperature). After incubation with the secondary antibodies, the membranes were rinsed and then treated with a Luminata Classico chemiluminescent substrate (Merck KGaA, Darmstad, Germany). As an internal control, β-actin was used to normalize the amount of individual proteins levels. β-actin was detected with primary rabbit antihuman β-actin antibody (4970; Cell Signaling Technology, Danvers, MA, USA) at a dilution of 1:2000 (overnight incubation at 4 °C) and horseradish peroxidase conjugated secondary antibody (711-035-152; Jackson ImmunoResearch, Cambridgeshire, UK) at a dilution of 1:3000 (1 h, room temperature). The visualization was made with the ChemiDoc Imaging System with the ImageLab software (Bio-Rad Laboratories, Marnes-la-Coquette, France). A densitometry analysis of the results obtained was performed with the ImageLab software (Bio-Rad Laboratories, Marnes-la-Coquette, France).

4.10. Confocal Microscopy

For immunofluorescence, AsPC-1 cells were plated (1.5×10^4 cells/well) on Millicell® EZ SLIDES eight-well glass slides (Merck Millipore, Gernsheim, Germany). After 24 h, cells were treated with resveratrol (0 and 100 µM) for 48 h. Cells were then fixed in 4% paraformaldehyde (12 min, room temperature). The membranes were permeabilized with 0.2% Triton X-100 (10 min, room temperature). Nonspecific binding sites were blocked with 3% BSA in PBS (1 h, room temperature). Cells were incubated overnight at 4 °C with primary antibodies: Bax (1:25 dilution, Santa Cruz Biotechnology, Dallas, TX, USA) in 3% BSA/PBS and Bcl-2 (ready-to-use, Dako, Glostrup, Denmark). Protein detection was performed with Alexa Fluor 488 conjugated antibody secondary antimouse (dilution 1:2000, Abcam, Cambridge, UK, Cat# ab150113, RRID: AB_2756499), incubation 1 h, temp. 4 °C. The slides were sealed in a medium containing DAPI (Invitrogen, Carlsbad, CA, USA). The analysis of the proteins levels was performed using a Fluoview FV3000 confocal microscope (Olympus, Tokyo, Japan, RRID: SCR_017015) with the cellSens software (Olympus, Tokyo, Japan, RRID: SCR_016238).

4.11. Statistical Analysis

The experiments were performed in three independent laboratory replications. The unpaired t-test was used to compare two groups of data. The one-way ANOVA with post hoc analysis using the Dunn's or Bonferroni multiple comparison tests were used to compare 3 or more groups. Statistical analysis was performed using the Prism 5.0 software (Graphpad Software, Inc., La Jolla, CA, USA). The differences were regarded as significant when $p < 0.05$.

5. Conclusions

The results of our research show the antitumor potential of resveratrol in terms of antiproliferative and pro-apoptotic effects on human pancreatic cells by changing the expression of proteins related to the apoptotic process. At the same time, resveratrol has been shown to have a stronger effect on cancer cells than on normal cells, which is extremely important in the context of possibly using this compound not only in the prevention, but also in the treatment, of pancreatic tumors while protecting normal tissues. Additionally, each cell line is characterized by a different sensitivity to the effect of the compound, which confirms the validity of separate studies for different types of cancer. The action of resveratrol may also be important in the process of overcoming multidrug resistance (MDR) due to the induction of larger changes in cytostatic-resistant cancer cells compared to cytostatic-sensitive cells.

The results of our in vitro study are the basis for planning the direction of further in vivo and clinical research. Due to the low bioavailability of orally administered resveratrol, it is necessary to determine the appropriate dosage and method of administration of the compound, e.g., intravenous (IV) injection or encapsulation.

Author Contributions: Conceptualization, K.R. and S.B.; methodology, K.R. and S.B.; software, K.R.; validation, K.N.; investigation, K.R., N.G.-P. and K.R.-W.; resources, K.R.; data curation, K.R. and S.B.; writing—original draft preparation, K.R.; writing—review and editing, K.R. and S.B.; visualization, K.R.; supervision, S.B.; project administration, K.R. and S.B.; funding acquisition, K.R. All authors have read and agreed to the published version of the manuscript.

Funding: This research was funded by Wroclaw Medical University, ID No. STM.A110.17.029.

Institutional Review Board Statement: Not applicable.

Informed Consent Statement: Not applicable.

Data Availability Statement: Data sharing not applicable to this article. No new data were created or analyzed in this study.

Acknowledgments: Many thanks to Piotr Dzięgiel (Wroclaw Medical University; University School of Physical Education in Wroclaw, Wroclaw, Poland) for valuable substantive tips on this research. Many thanks to Małgorzata Drąg-Zalesińska, Agnieszka Gomułkiewicz and Aleksandra Piotrowska (Wroclaw Medical University, Wroclaw, Poland) for their assistance in experiments. We would like to thank H. Lage and M. Dietel (Humboldt University Berlin, Wroclaw, Poland) for the possibility of using cancer cells lines EPP85-181P and EPP85-181RNOV.

Conflicts of Interest: The authors declare no conflict of interest.

Sample Availability: Not applicable.

References

1. Bray, F.; Ferlay, J.; Soerjomataram, I.; Siegel, R.L.; Torre, L.A.; Jemal, A. Global cancer statistics 2018: GLOBOCAN estimates of incidence and mortality worldwide for 36 cancers in 185 countries. *CA Cancer J. Clin.* **2018**, *68*, 394–424. [CrossRef]
2. Ilic, M.; Ilic, I. Epidemiology of pancreatic cancer. *World J. Gastroenterol.* **2016**, *22*, 9694–9705. [CrossRef] [PubMed]
3. Mo, W.; Xu, X.; Xu, L.; Wang, F.; Ke, A.; Wang, X.; Guo, C. Resveratrol Inhibits Proliferation and Induces Apoptosis through the Hedgehog Signaling Pathway in Pancreatic Cancer Cell. *Pancreatology* **2011**, *11*, 601–609. [CrossRef] [PubMed]
4. El-Zahaby, S.A.; Elnaggar, Y.S.R.; Abdallah, O.Y. Reviewing two decades of nanomedicine implementations in targeted treatment and diagnosis of pancreatic cancer: An emphasis on state of art. *J. Control. Release* **2019**, *293*, 21–35. [CrossRef]
5. McGuigan, A.; Kelly, P.; Turkington, R.C.; Jones, C.; Coleman, H.G.; McCain, R.S. Pancreatic cancer: A review of clinical diagnosis, epidemiology, treatment and outcomes. *World J. Gastroenterol.* **2018**, *24*, 4846–4861. [CrossRef]
6. Zhang, L.; Sanagapalli, S.; Stoita, A. Challenges in diagnosis of pancreatic cancer. *World J. Gastroenterol.* **2018**, *24*, 2047–2060. [CrossRef]
7. Housman, G.; Byler, S.; Heerboth, S.; Lapinska, K.; Longacre, M.; Snyder, N.; Sarkar, S. Drug resistance in cancer: An overview. *Cancers* **2014**, *6*, 1769–1792. [CrossRef]
8. Ghorbani, A.; Hosseini, A. Cancer therapy with phytochemicals: Evidence from clinical studies. *Avicenna J. Phytomed.* **2015**, *5*, 84–97. [CrossRef]
9. Elshaer, M.; Chen, Y.; Wang, X.J.; Tang, X. Resveratrol: An overview of its anti-cancer mechanisms. *Life Sci.* **2018**, *207*, 340–349. [CrossRef]
10. Campbell, K.J.; Tait, S.W.G. Targeting BCL-2 regulated apoptosis in cancer. *Biol. Open* **2018**, *8*, 180002. [CrossRef] [PubMed]
11. Pannu, N.; Bhatnagar, A. Resveratrol: From enhanced biosynthesis and bioavailability to multitargeting chronic diseases. *Biomed. Pharmacother.* **2019**, *109*, 2237–2251. [CrossRef]
12. Xu, Q.; Zong, L.; Chen, X.; Jiang, Z.; Nan, L.; Li, J.; Duan, W.; Lei, J.; Zhang, L.; Ma, J.; et al. Resveratrol in the treatment of pancreatic cancer. *Ann. N. Y. Acad. Sci.* **2015**, *1348*, 10–19. [CrossRef] [PubMed]
13. Li, X.; Wu, B.; Wang, L.; Li, S. Extractable Amounts of *trans*-Resveratrol in Seed and Berry Skin in Vitis Evaluated at the Germplasm Level. *J. Agric. Food Chem.* **2006**, *54*, 8804–8811. [CrossRef] [PubMed]
14. Anisimova, N.Y.U.; Kiselevsky, M.V.; Sosnov, A.V.; Sadovnikov, S.V.; Stankov, I.N.; Gakh, A.A. *Trans*-, *cis*-, and *dihydro*-resveratrol: A comparative study. *Chem. Cent. J.* **2011**, *5*, 88. [CrossRef]
15. Trela, B.C.; Waterhouse, A.L. Resveratrol: Isomeric molar absorptivities and stability. *J. Agric. Food Chem.* **1996**, *44*, 1253–1257. [CrossRef]
16. Roupe, K.A.; Remsberg, C.M.; Yanez, J.A.; Davies, N.M. Pharmacometrics of Stilbenes: Seguing Towards the Clinic. *Curr. Clin. Pharmacol.* **2008**, *1*, 81–101. [CrossRef]
17. Watson, R.; Preedy, V.; Zibadi, S. *Polyphenols in Human Health and Disease*; Academic Press: Cambridge, MA, USA, 2013; Volume 1–2.
18. Kundu, J.K.; Surh, Y.-J. Molecular basis of chemoprevention by resveratrol: NF-κB and AP-1 as potential targets. *Mutat. Res.-Fund. Mol. Mech. Mutagenesis* **2004**, *555*, 65–80. [CrossRef]
19. Aggarwal, B.B.; Bhardwaj, A.; Aggarwal, R.S.; Seeram, N.P.; Shishodia, S.; Takada, Y. Role of Resveratrol in Prevention and Therapy of Cancer: Preclinical and Clinical Studies. *Anticancer Res.* **2004**, *24*, 2783–2840.
20. Wu, X.; Li, Q.; Feng, Y.; Ji, Q. Antitumor Research of the Active Ingredients from Traditional Chinese Medical Plant Polygonum Cuspidatum. *Evid. Based Complementary Altern. Med.* **2018**, *2018*, 2313021. [CrossRef]
21. Jang, M.; Cai, L.; Udeani, G.O.; Slowing, K.V.; Thomas, K.F.; Beecher, C.W.W.; Fong, H.H.S.; Farnsworth, N.R.; Kinghorn, A.D.; Mehta, R.G.; et al. Cancer Chemopreventive Activity of Resveratrol, a Natural Product Derived from Grapes. *Science* **1997**, *275*, 218–220. [CrossRef]
22. Thyagarajan, A.; Forino, A.S.; Konger, R.L.; Sahu, R.P. Dietary Polyphenols in Cancer Chemoprevention: Implications in Pancreatic Cancer. *Antioxidants* **2020**, *9*, 651. [CrossRef]
23. Ratajczak, K.; Borska, S. Cytotoxic and Proapoptotic Effects of Resveratrol in In Vitro Studies on Selected Types of Gastrointestinal Cancers. *Molecules* **2021**, *26*, 4350. [CrossRef]
24. Mieszala, K.; Rudewicz, M.; Gomulkiewicz, A.; Ratajczak-Wielgomas, K.; Grzegrzolka, J.; Dziegiel, P.; Borska, S. Expression of genes and proteins of multidrug resistance in gastric cancer cells treated with resveratrol. *Oncol. Lett.* **2018**, *15*, 5825–5832. [CrossRef]

25. Borska, S.; Pedziwiatr, M.; Danielewicz, M.; Nowinska, K.; Pula, B.; Drag-Zalesinska, M.; Olbromski, M.; Gomulkiewicz, A.; Dziegiel, P. Classical and atypical resistance of cancer cells as a target for resveratrol. *Oncol. Rep.* **2016**, *36*, 1562–1568. [CrossRef]
26. Loveday, B.P.T.; Lipton, L.; Thomson, B.N.J. Pancreatic cancer: An update on diagnosis and management. *Aust. J. Gen. Pract.* **2019**, *48*, 826–831. [CrossRef] [PubMed]
27. Luo, H.; Vong, C.T.; Chen, H.; Gao, Y.; Lyu, P.; Qiu, L.; Zhao, M.; Liu, Q.; Cheng, Z.; Zou, J.; et al. Naturally occurring anti-cancer compounds: Shining from Chinese herbal medicine. *Chin. Med.* **2019**, *14*, 48. [CrossRef]
28. Xiao, Q.; Zhu, W.; Feng, W.; Lee, S.S.; Leung, A.W.; Shen, J.; Gao, L.; Xu, C. A Review of Resveratrol as a Potent Chemoprotective and Synergistic Agent in Cancer Chemotherapy. *Front. Pharmacol.* **2019**, *9*, 1534. [CrossRef] [PubMed]
29. Cui, J.; Sun, R.; Yu, Y.; Gou, S.; Zhao, G.; Wang, C. Antiproliferative effect of resveratrol in pancreatic cancer cells. *Phyther. Res.* **2010**, *24*, 1637–1644. [CrossRef] [PubMed]
30. Roy, S.K.; Chen, Q.; Fu, J.; Shankar, S.; Srivastava, R.K. Resveratrol Inhibits Growth of Orthotopic Pancreatic Tumors through Activation of FOXO Transcription Factors. *PLoS ONE* **2011**, *6*, e25166. [CrossRef]
31. Liu, P.; Liang, H.; Xia, Q.; Li, P.; Kong, H.; Lei, P.; Wang, S.; Tu, Z. Resveratrol induces apoptosis of pancreatic cancers cells by inhibiting miR-21 regulation of BCL-2 expression. *Clin. Transl. Oncol.* **2013**, *15*, 741–746. [CrossRef] [PubMed]
32. Wenzel, E.S.; Singh, A.T.K. Cell-cycle Checkpoints and Aneuploidy on the Path to Cancer. *In Vivo* **2018**, *32*, 1–5. [CrossRef] [PubMed]
33. Wu, H.; Chen, L.; Zhu, F.; Han, X.; Sun, L.; Chen, K. The Cytotoxicity Effect of Resveratrol: Cell Cycle Arrest and Induced Apoptosis of Breast Cancer 4T1 Cells. *Toxins* **2019**, *11*, 731. [CrossRef]
34. Singh, S.K.; Banerjee, S.; Acosta, E.P.; Lillard, J.W.; Singh, R. Resveratrol induces cell cycle arrest and apoptosis with docetaxel in prostate cancer cells via a p21$^{WAF1/CIP1}$ and p27^{KIP1} pathway. *Oncotarget* **2017**, *8*, 17216–17228. [CrossRef] [PubMed]
35. Pistritto, G.; Trisciuoglio, D.; Ceci, C.; Garufi, A.; D'Orazi, G. Apoptosis as anticancer mechanism: Function and dysfunction of its modulators and targeted therapeutic strategies. *Aging* **2016**, *8*, 603–619. [CrossRef]
36. Wong, R.S.Y. Apoptosis in cancer: From pathogenesis to treatment. *J. Exp. Clin. Cancer Res.* **2011**, *30*, 87. [CrossRef] [PubMed]
37. Zhou, J.-H.; Cheng, H.-Y.; Yu, Z.-Q.; He, D.-W.; Pan, Z.; Yang, D.-T. Resveratrol induces apoptosis in pancreatic cancer cells. *Chin. Med. J. (Engl.)* **2011**, *124*, 1695–1699. [CrossRef]
38. Singh, R.; Letai, A.; Sarosiek, K. Regulation of apoptosis in health and disease: The balancing act of BCL-2 family proteins. *Nat. Rev. Mol. Cell Biol.* **2019**, *20*, 175–193. [CrossRef] [PubMed]
39. Aniogo, E.C.; George, B.P.A.; Abrahamse, H. Role of Bcl-2 Family Proteins in Photodynamic Therapy Mediated Cell Survival and Regulation. *Molecules* **2020**, *25*, 5308. [CrossRef] [PubMed]
40. Cheng, L.; Yan, B.; Chen, K.; Jiang, Z.; Zhou, C.; Cao, J.; Qian, W.; Li, J.; Sun, L.; Ma, J.; et al. Resveratrol-induced downregulation of NAF-1 enhances the sensitivity of pancreatic cancer cells to gemcitabine via the ROS/Nrf2 signaling pathways. *Oxid. Med. Cell. Longev.* **2018**, *2018*, 9482018. [CrossRef]
41. Yang, L.; Yang, L.; Tian, W.; Li, J.; Liu, J.; Zhu, M.; Zhang, Y.; Yang, Y.; Liu, F.; Zhang, Q.; et al. Resveratrol plays dual roles in pancreatic cancer cells. *J. Cancer Res. Clin. Oncol.* **2014**, *140*, 749–755. [CrossRef]
42. Wu, X.; Xu, Y.; Zhu, B.; Liu, Q.; Yao, Q.; Zhao, G. Resveratrol induces apoptosis in SGC-7901 gastric cancer cells. *Oncol. Lett.* **2018**, *16*, 2949–2956. [CrossRef]
43. Kaewdoungdee, N.; Hahnvajanawong, C.; Chitsomboon, B.; Boonyanugomol, W.; Sripa, B.; Pattanapanyasat, K.; Maitra, A. Molecular mechanisms of resveratrol-induced apoptosis in human pancreatic cancer cells. *Maejo Int. J. Sci. Technol.* **2014**, *8*, 251–263. [CrossRef]
44. Mosmann, T. Rapid colorimetric assay for cellular growth and survival: Application to proliferation and cytotoxicity assays. *J. Immunol. Methods* **1983**, *65*, 55–63. [CrossRef]
45. Collins, A.R. The Comet assay for DNA damage and repair: Principles, applications, and limitations. *Mol. Biotechnol.* **2004**, *26*, 249–261. [CrossRef]

Article

Effects of a Semisynthetic Catechin on Phosphatidylglycerol Membranes: A Mixed Experimental and Simulation Study

Elisa Aranda [1,†], José A. Teruel [1], Antonio Ortiz [1], María Dolores Pérez-Cárceles [2], José N. Rodríguez-López [1] and Francisco J. Aranda [1,*]

[1] Departamento de Bioquímica y Biología Molecular-A, Facultad de Veterinaria, Universidad de Murcia, 30100 Murcia, Spain
[2] Departamento de Medicina Legal y Forense, Facultad de Medicina, Instituto de Investigación Biomédica (IMIB-Arrixaca), Universidad de Murcia, 30120 Murcia, Spain
* Correspondence: fjam@um.es; Tel.: +34-868-884-760
† Present Address: Hospital Universitario Virgen de la Arrixaca, Área de Salud 1, 30120 Murcia, Spain.

Abstract: Catechins have been shown to display a great variety of biological activities, prominent among them are their chemo preventive and chemotherapeutic properties against several types of cancer. The amphiphilic nature of catechins points to the membrane as a potential target for their actions. 3,4,5-Trimethoxybenzoate of catechin (TMBC) is a modified structural analog of catechin that shows significant antiproliferative activity against melanoma and breast cancer cells. Phosphatidylglycerol is an anionic membrane phospholipid with important physical and biochemical characteristics that make it biologically relevant. In addition, phosphatidylglycerol is a preeminent component of bacterial membranes. Using biomimetic membranes, we examined the effects of TMBC on the structural and dynamic properties of phosphatidylglycerol bilayers by means of biophysical techniques such as differential scanning calorimetry, X-ray diffraction and infrared spectroscopy, together with an analysis through molecular dynamics simulation. We found that TMBC perturbs the thermotropic gel to liquid-crystalline phase transition and promotes immiscibility in both phospholipid phases. The modified catechin decreases the thickness of the bilayer and is able to form hydrogen bonds with the carbonyl groups of the phospholipid. Experimental data support the simulated data that locate TMBC as mostly forming clusters in the middle region of each monolayer approaching the carbonyl moiety of the phospholipid. The presence of TMBC modifies the structural and dynamic properties of the phosphatidylglycerol bilayer. The decrease in membrane thickness and the change of the hydrogen bonding pattern in the interfacial region of the bilayer elicited by the catechin might contribute to the alteration of the events taking place in the membrane and might help to understand the mechanism of action of the diverse effects displayed by catechins.

Keywords: catechin; dimyristoylphosphatidylglycerol; DSC; FTIR; X-ray diffraction; molecular dynamics

1. Introduction

The number of healthful effects attributed to green tea catechins is remarkable. The health promoting properties of catechins include protection from inflammatory and neurodegenerative diseases, obesity, metabolic syndrome, diabetes, and hypertension [1,2]. In addition, different studies have provided evidence that catechins display antimicrobial effects on both Gram-positive and Gram-negative bacteria [3], and that they impair the infectivity of a series of both animal and human viruses [4].

A most outstanding characteristic of catechins is that they show both chemo-preventive and chemotherapeutic activities against a great variety of different cancers [5]. The exceptional anticancer activity of catechins is exerted by modulating different hallmarks and suppressing characteristics of cancer, including sustaining proliferative signals, evading growth suppressors, avoiding immune destruction, inducing angiogenesis, resisting cell death, and tumor promoting inflammation [6,7]. Almost all of these anticancer achievements are fulfilled essentially as a result of the interaction between catechins and a variety of intracellular targets, membrane proteins, and the plasma membrane [8].

However, the exact molecular mechanism through which catechins produce all of these beneficial effects still remain to be addressed. There is increasing evidence that the membrane is a potential target for the action of catechins. They alter the properties of phospholipid membranes [9], modify the rigidity of the membrane [10], and change the organization of lipid rafts [11,12]. The concept of the membrane as a simple barrier has evolved to include the membrane as a complex structure with biological functions and an identity intrinsic to the type of cell or disease. In this way, it is possible to look at the mechanism of action of catechins from a lipid and membrane centered perspective [13]. By incorporating into membranes, catechins can alter the conformational dynamics of the membrane, and these changes may have a variety of effects on cellular functions through the indirect modulation of membrane proteins such as receptors, channels, enzymes, and regulatory signals [14]. In this context, the study of the interaction between catechins and membranes is of the utmost importance.

Phosphatidylglycerol is a minor anionic phospholipid component of nearly all natural membranes and has remarkable physical and biochemical characteristics that make it biologically important [15,16]. In eukaryotic cells, phosphatidylglycerol is largely restricted to the mitochondrial membrane, and it is interesting as catechins have been shown to regulate mitochondrial membrane permeability [17] and to protect mitochondria against various insults [18]. Phosphatidylglycerol acts as a lipid signal that promotes early keratinocyte differentiation suppressing skin inflammation [19] and it inhibits Toll-like receptor activation, thereby reducing inflammatory signals [20]. It has been shown that phosphatidylglycerol is able to inhibit inflammatory responses when located in the lung surfactant [21] and in the mitochondria [22], and also to stimulate α-synuclein amyloid formation [23] and to suppress influenza A virus infection [24]. It is important to note that phosphatidylglycerol is a main constituent of virtually all bacterial membranes [25] and thus it has become a good biomimetic model for these membranes [26,27]. This last feature is important in connection with the known antibacterial activity of catechins [28]. It should be highlighted that there are numerous studies that have demonstrated selective toxicity of catechins against different bacterial pathogens, and which have suggested promising use in the treatment of bacterial infections [29,30]. Catechins have been shown to inhibit bacterial toxins, they inhibit the hemolytic activity of *S. aureus* α-toxin preventing the secretion of the toxin by binding to the cytoplasmic membrane and decreasing its permeability, or by blocking signal transduction processes [31]. A mechanism via interaction with the outer cell membrane has been suggested for the inhibitory effect of catechins on enterohemorrhagic Vero toxin from *E. coli* [32]. Catechins also hold promise as biofilm inhibitors [33]. A main mechanism of the antibacterial activity of catechins is the modification of cell membrane [34]. Catechins bind to bacterial cell membrane causing the membrane to burst and release the cytoplasmic content, with subsequent cell death [35], they decrease membrane fluidity that eventually results in membrane breakage [36]. These polyphenols can also inhibit multidrug bacterial efflux pumps restoring the antibacterial activity of antibiotics and acting in synergy with them [37].

Regardless of their diverse advantageous characteristics, the therapeutic effect of catechins is restricted as a result of their low stability, poor absorption, limited membrane permeability, and low bioavailability [3,38]. An important strategy to improve the properties of catechins is the structural modification of the catechin molecule through the synthesis of a catechin-based analog in order to obtain more effective, stable, and specific active molecules [5,39]. TMBC (Figure 1) is a structural analog of catechin that has been shown to exert high antiproliferative activity against melanoma and breast cancer cells [40,41]. It has been shown that TMBC perturbs the structural properties of the bilayers composed of phospholipids bearing different polar head groups, including phosphatidylcholine [42], phosphatidylethanolamine [43], and phosphatidylserine [44]. In this work, in order to advance the knowledge of the molecular interaction between catechins and individual membrane phospholipid species, we present a study on the effect of TMBC on the structural and dynamic properties of biomimetic model systems composed of 1,2-dimyristoyl-sn-glycero-3-phospho-(1′-rac-glycerol) (DMPG), by using differential scanning calorimetry (DSC), X-ray diffraction, Fourier transform infrared (FTIR) spectroscopy, and molecular dynamics simulation.

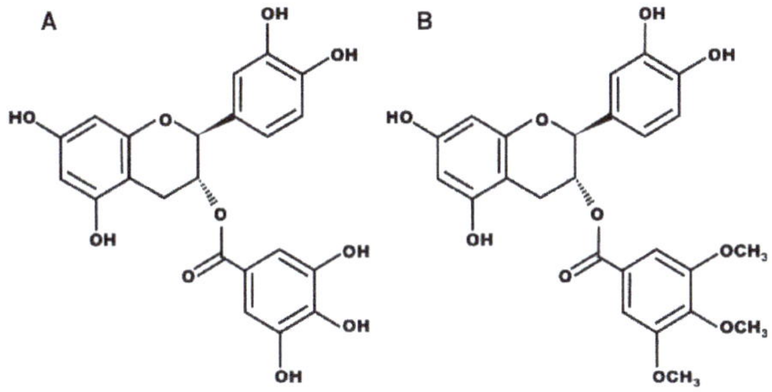

Figure 1. Chemical structure of (**A**) catechin gallate and (**B**) 3,4,5-trimethoxybenzoate of catechin (TMBC).

2. Results and Discussion

2.1. Differential Scanning Calorimetry

DSC is a straightforward and potent nonperturbing physical technique, which is well appropriate to observe and depict the thermotropic phase transition of membranes [45]. In order to investigate the molecular interaction between TMBC and membranes we used model bilayer systems formed by DMPG. DSC was used to describe the effect of this semisynthetic catechin on the thermotropic properties of this phospholipid. The perturbation exerted by TMBC on the thermotropic phase transition of DMPG is shown in Figure 2.

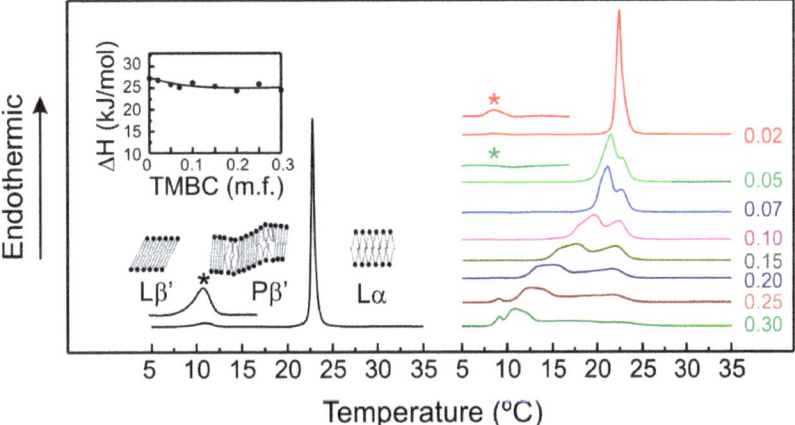

Figure 2. DSC heating thermograms for pure DMPG (left) and DMPG containing TMBC at different concentrations (right). Inset shows the enthalpy change for the main gel to liquid-crystalline phase transition. TMBC mole fraction is expressed on the right side of the thermograms. Asterisks indicate the enlarged region (×7) of the pretransition.

The heating thermogram corresponding to pure DMPG showed two transitions, a peak to lower temperature starting at 9 °C corresponding to the weakly energetic pretransition from the gel tilted phase (Lβ′) to the gel ripple phase (Pβ′), and a peak to higher temperature starting at 22.3 °C corresponding to the highly energetic main transition from the ripple phase to the liquid-crystalline phase (Lα). These values are in accordance with previous data [46,47]. The presence of TMBC at very low concentrations such as 0.02 mole fraction makes the pretransition broaden and shift to lower temperatures, and the increase of TMBC to 0.05 mole fraction made the pretransition undetectable. There is a possibility that the pretransition had already disappeared and then the phospholipid directly underwent the transition from the gel tilted to the fluid phase. However, it is most probable that the pretransition had already started at such a low temperature that was out of the range under study and that it was so broad that it could not be observed. The presence of increasing concentrations of TMBC produced the broadening of the main transition and the appearance of a second peak with a temperature that was lower when the presence of TMBC in the bilayer was greater. The presence of different peaks in the thermograms, may indicate the presence of different lipid domains in the bilayer. The enthalpy change associated with the main gel to liquid-crystalline phase transition of pure DMPG was determined to be 27.2 kJ/mol. As the inset in Figure 2 shows, the presence of low proportions of TMBC produced a decrease of nearly 10% of the enthalpy change; this value did not decrease further when the concentration of the compound increased above 0.07 mole fraction.

The broadening of the transition and the appearance of additional components, indicate that TMBC incorporates into the phosphatidylglycerol bilayer, where it modifies the organization of the acyl chains of the phospholipid and shifts the phase transition temperature to lower values. It is interesting to note that the ending temperature of the transition did not change with the presence of TMBC; even in the case of the most concentrated sample there was still a portion of the phospholipids that finished its phase transition at the same temperature as the pure phospholipid. Additionally, a new peak emerged at a fixed temperature, near 8 °C, when TMBC reached 0.20 mole fraction. The appearance of a transition peak at a lower and fixed temperature has also been detected in zwitterionic bilayers containing elevated concentrations of TMBC [42,43].

2.2. X-ray Diffraction

X-ray diffraction is an acknowledged non-interfering exploratory technique which allows the examination of the overall structural organization of model membranes [48]. We used small- and wide-angle X-ray diffraction (SAXD and WAXD) to address the effect of TMBC on the overall structural properties of DMPG bilayers. Measurements in the wide angle (WAXD) region provide information about the packing of the phospholipid acyl chains. Figure 3 displays the WAXD patterns corresponding to pure DMPG and DMPG containing TMBC. At 6 °C, pure DMPG gave a sharp reflection at 4.18 Å and a broad one at 4.10 Å. This asymmetrical pattern is representative of lipids organized in the Lβ′ phase with orthorhombic packing and the hydrocarbon chains tilted to the membrane surface [49,50]. At 14 °C, pure DMPG showed a symmetrical reflection near 4.16 Å ascribed to the Pβ′ phase in which the hydrocarbon chains were oriented normal to the bilayer plane in a two-dimensional hexagonal lattice [51,52]. Finally, at 35 °C, a diffuse scattering reflection was observed, which is representative of the fluid Lα phase [53].

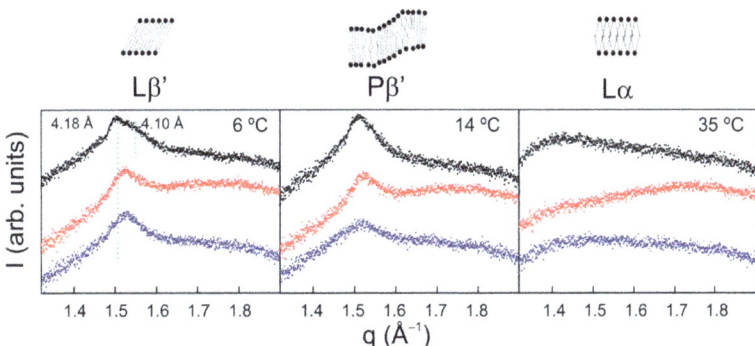

Figure 3. Intensity (arbitrary units lineal scale) vs. scattering vector (q) for WAXD profiles of pure DMPG (top black) and DMPG containing TMBC at 0.07 (middle red) and 0.20 mole fraction (bottom blue) at different temperatures.

At 6 °C, in the presence of TMBC, the asymmetric reflection characteristic of the Lβ′ phase was replaced by a symmetric reflection at 4.13 Å corresponding to the Pβ′ phase, which is consistent with the shifting of the pretransition to lower temperatures as observed by DSC (Figure 2). At 14 °C, all the systems displayed the symmetric reflection characteristic of the Pβ′ phase, though the reflection in the presence of TMBC appeared at 4.13 Å instead of 4.16 Å, as is the case for pure DMPG. At 35 °C, all the systems presented the diffuse reflection characteristic of the Lα fluid phase.

The SAXD patterns for pure DMPG and DMPG containing TMBC, at different temperatures are shown in Figure 4. All the systems exhibited broad scattering at all temperatures that originated from positionally uncorrelated bilayers. This has been interpreted by the general negative surface charge that drive the formation of positionally uncorrelated bilayers, most likely vesicles with fewer lamellae, because of electrostatic repulsion [47,54]. All systems show a broad bilayer peak around $q = 0.12$ Å^{-1} which arose from the electron density contrast between the bilayer and the solvent, similar to that which has been described for pure DMPG [55].

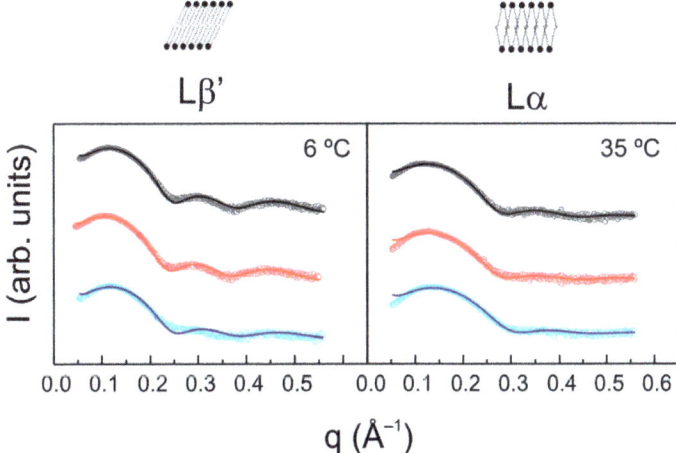

Figure 4. Intensity (arbitrary units log scale) vs. scattering vector (q) for SAXD profiles of pure DMPG (top, black) and DMPG containing TMBC at 0.07 (middle, red) and 0.20 mole fraction (bottom, blue) at different temperatures. Solid lines represent the best fit to the experimental patterns using the GAP program.

The analysis of the SAXD patterns using the Global Analysis Program (GAP) enabled us to determine the bilayer thickness (d_B) of the different systems. We found d_B values of 50.16 ± 0.15 Å in the gel phase (6 °C) and 45.20 ± 0.35 Å in the liquid-crystalline phase (35 °C) for pure DMPG, in accordance with previous data [50,55]. The presence of TMBC at 0.07 mole fraction induced a small decrease in the bilayer thickness to 49.23 ± 0.15 Å and 44.80 ± 0.20 Å for the gel and the liquid-crystalline phases. However, the presence of TMBC at 0.2 mole fraction produced a marked decrease in the bilayer thickness, with dB values of 48.16 ± 0.15 Å in the gel phase and 42.60 ± 0.25 Å in the liquid-crystalline phase.

The phospholipid acyl chains were in contact with the hydrophobic parts of integral membrane proteins, and these interactions have been proposed to be crucial for the balanced integration of the protein into the bilayer [56]. Hydrophobic mismatch occurs when the hydrophobic thickness of the membrane does not match with the hydrophobic length of the integral protein. This modification of the membrane properties could be capable of altering the function of lipid-dependent proteins because it could produce changes in the structure of the protein [57]. Considering that integral membrane proteins are involved in crucial cellular processes, the decrease in the bilayer thickness exerted by TMBC might be decisive when considering the hydrophobic mismatch and may have an influence on the mechanism of some of the effects of the catechin. The thinning effect of TMBC was observed at relatively high concentration of the compound. We believe that low concentrations of catechins in the blood stream would correspond to a much greater availability in the membrane fraction and that they may accumulate over time to produce cellular concentrations that are much higher than that observed in serum samples. Moreover, the molar ratios studied in our biomimetic membranes are not necessarily required to be homogeneous in the whole cellular membrane, it would be enough that this TMBC/phospholipid be fulfilled locally in certain part of the membrane. In this respect, the described propensity of TMBC to form enriched domains in the bilayer may help to locally attain higher concentrations of the molecule where it is needed.

We used the phase transitions temperatures obtained from the DSC measurements and the structural information from the X-ray diffraction experiments to construct the partial phase diagram for the DMPG component in mixtures with TMBC, which are presented in Figure 5. When an incorporated compound in the phospholipid bilayer shows good mixing behavior, i.e., it is miscible with the lipid, the interaction between them will cause the phospholipid transition temperature to change. In this case, the higher the concentration of the compound in the mixture the larger the change in the transition temperature. If the presence of an increasing concentration of a compound in the bilayer does not result in a transition temperature change, i.e., a constant transition temperature is observed, it means that there is always pure phospholipid undergoing transition and suggests that the compound is immiscible with the phospholipid. In this case, an immiscibility was produced with phase separation between the compound and the phospholipid, and with the formation of different domains containing different amounts of compound.

The behavior of the solidus line was different from that of the fluidus line. The solidus line displayed good mixing behavior with its temperature decreasing as more TMBC was present in the bilayer. When a 0.2 mole fraction was reached, the temperature remained constant suggesting the presence of a gel phase immiscibility. This gel phase immiscibility was not observed in mixtures of TMBC and another anionic phospholipid such as phosphatidylserine [44]. The temperature of the fluidus line remained constant in the whole range of TMBC concentrations which suggests that an immiscibility in the liquid-crystalline phase was present. The TMBC-induced fluid-phase immiscibility has not been observed in mixtures of TMBC with any other glycerophospholipids with different polar head groups [42–44]. The DMPG system evolves from a gel phase, which shows immiscibility from a certain catechin concentration, to an immiscible fluid phase through a coexistence region which is wider as more TMBC is present in the bilayer. The phase diagram for the TMBC/DMPG mixture seemed to be singular as it showed immiscibility both in the gel and the liquid-crystalline phases.

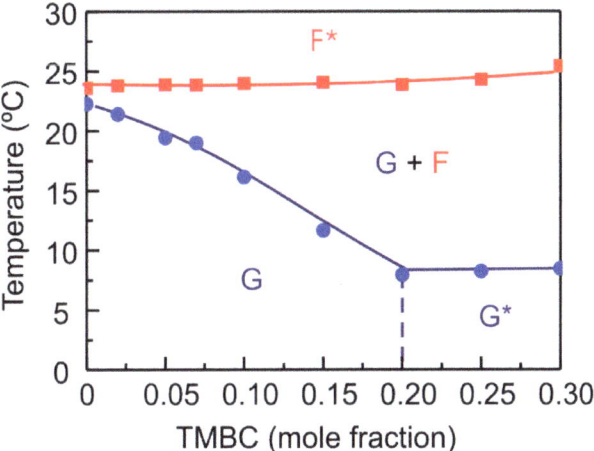

Figure 5. Partial phase diagram for DMPG in DMPG/TMBC mixtures. Circles and squares were obtained from the onset and completion temperatures of the main gel to liquid-crystalline phase transition, respectively. Blue circles, solidus line; red squares, fluidus line. The phase designations are as follows: G, gel phase; F, liquid-crystalline phase (fluid phase); asterisk indicates that immiscible phases are present.

2.3. FTIR Spectroscopy

Infrared spectroscopy determines the energy transitions between the electronic vibrational levels arising from the absorption of radiation in the infrared spectrum. These vibrational levels are produced by distinctive motions taking place within the different chemical bonds present in the various functional groups of a molecule. The infrared spectrum of phospholipids contains abundant data about both the chemical structure of the molecule and the membrane physical state (chain ordering, phase transition). The gel to liquid-crystalline phase transition of phospholipids goes by apparent changes in the absorption bands originating from moieties in the hydrophobic and interfacial regions of these phospholipid membranes [58]. We used infrared spectroscopy to study the interfacial interaction between the catechin derivative and the bilayer. Figure 6 shows the temperature dependence of the wavenumber of the maximum of the carbonyl stretching band of the infrared spectra corresponding to pure DMPG and DMPG/TMBC systems.

The thermotropic phase changes undergone by phospholipids can be followed by very apparent changes in the contours of the ester carbonyl stretching band, ν (C=O). The features of this absorption band are sensitive to the conformation, hydration state, and the degree and nature of hydrogen-bonding interactions in the polar/apolar interfaces of phospholipids bilayers [59]. A pure DMPG ester carbonyl stretching band was considered to be a summation of two component bands centered near 1742 cm^{-1} and 1728 cm^{-1}, and their relative intensities reflect the contribution of a subpopulation of non-hydrogen bonded and hydrogen bonded carbonyl groups [46].

For pure DMPG, the gel to liquid-crystalline phase transition produced a shift in the wavenumber of the maximum of the band to lower wavenumbers. This was due to the increase in intensity of the underlying component band at 1728 cm^{-1}. This increase is attributed to a higher amount of hydrogen bonded carbonyl groups that resulted from the increase in the hydration of the polar/apolar interface in the liquid-crystalline phase [60]. The shift in the phase transition to lower temperatures produced by the presence of TMBC can be seen following the wavenumber of the maximum of the carbonyl band illustrated in Figure 6. It is interesting to note that in the liquid-crystalline phase, the presence of increasing concentrations of TMBC produced a shift in the maximum of the carbonyl band to lower wavenumbers, as compared with the pure phospholipid. The latter indicated an increase in the proportion of the hydrogen bonded carbonyl groups, and this could have been due to a direct interaction of TMBC with the interfacial region of the DMPG bilayer or to an indirect mechanism through the TMBC disordering the membrane and increasing the hydration of the carbonyl groups of the phospholipid.

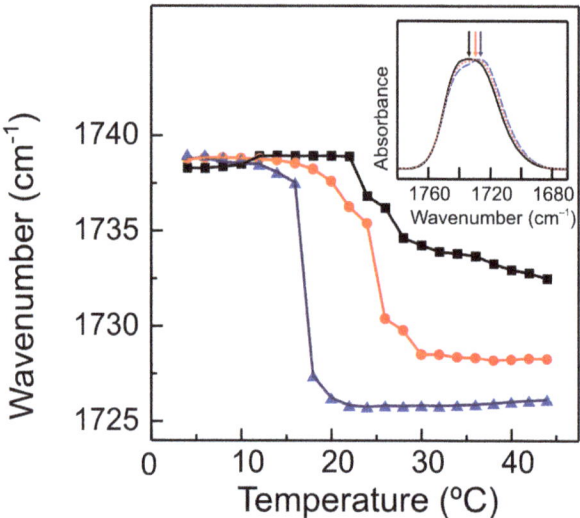

Figure 6. Temperature dependence of the wavenumber of the maximum of the ester carbonyl stretching band, ν (C=O), exhibited by pure DMPG (black squares) and DMPG containing TMBC 0.07 (red circles) and 0.20 (blue triangles) mole fraction. Inset shows the 1780–1670 cm^{-1} spectral region containing the absorption band originating from the ester carbonyl stretching band of pure DMPG (black solid line) and DMPG containing TMBC at 0.07 (red dotted line) and 0.20 (blue dashed line) mole fraction, at 35 °C. Arrows point to the wavenumber of the maximum of each band at this temperature.

2.4. Molecular Dynamics

Computer simulation, such as molecular dynamics, has proven to be an important contribution to biophysical research on the physicochemical properties of lipid membranes, as it provides atomic detail of the simulated system [61]. The area per lipid at the membrane aqueous interface is frequently used as a property of the lipid bilayer for validating molecular dynamics simulations and as a proof of convergence [62]. Figure 7 shows the progression of the area per lipid of the simulation runs, where it can be observed that the area per lipid reached convergence and kept constant in the time range used for all the analyses (last 60 ns). The area per lipid was calculated as the area of the x y plane of the simulation box divided by the number of lipids in each leaflet. For the pure DMPG bilayer in the liquid-crystalline phase the area per lipid was 0.63 ± 0.01 nm^2, in accordance with reported data [63], and in the presence of TMBC this value increased to 0.66 ± 0.01 nm^2.

The bilayer thickness was computed calculating the phosphorous atoms distance between both leaflets. For pure DMPG, we obtained a bilayer thickness of 3.37 ± 0.07 nm, while in the presence of TMBC we observed a decrease in the bilayer thickness to 3.29 ± 0.07 nm, the latter data being in agreement with the X-ray diffraction experiments discussed above.

The number of hydrogen bonds between the DMPG carbonyl groups and water and the TMBC molecules were measured in the simulation box. The data show that the total number of hydrogen bonds per lipid increased from 202.2 ± 4.6 for pure DMPG to 212.5 ± 5.7 in the presence of TMBC. This increase was mostly due to the new hydrogen bonds established between the carbonyl groups of the phospholipid and the hydroxyl groups of TMBC (7.10 ± 2.15), this being in agreement with the increase in the number of hydrogen bonds determined by the shift of the wavenumber of the maximum of the carbonyl absorption band to lower values as obtained by FTIR (Figure 6).

The mass density profiles of the simulated DMPG bilayer in the presence of TMBC are shown in Figure 8A. The non-symmetrized mass density profiles correspond to the profiles along the z-axis of the simulation box over the entire analyzed time trajectory. The lipid phosphorous atoms are included to label the polar head region, the lipid terminal methyl groups to label the center of the membrane and the lipid carbonyl groups to label the position of the hydrogen bonding. The TMBC molecules were mainly distributed across the middle region of each monolayer approaching the carbonyl moiety of DMPG. In the different simulations, TMBC molecules were located at different random starting locations in the lipid phase, but this did not produce differences in the final output of the location of TMBC molecules across the phospholipid bilayer.

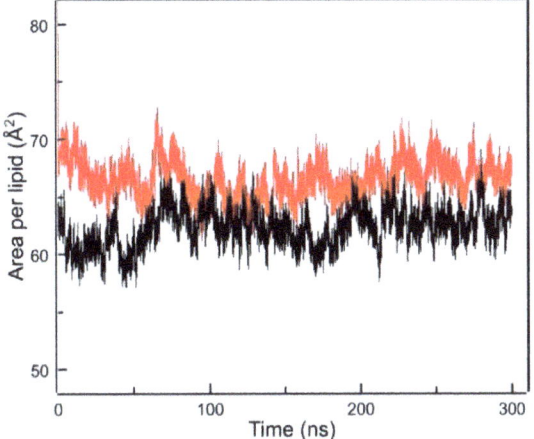

Figure 7. Area per lipid vs. simulated time for pure DMPG (black line) and DMPG containing TMBC (red line). Last 60 ns were used for all MD analysis.

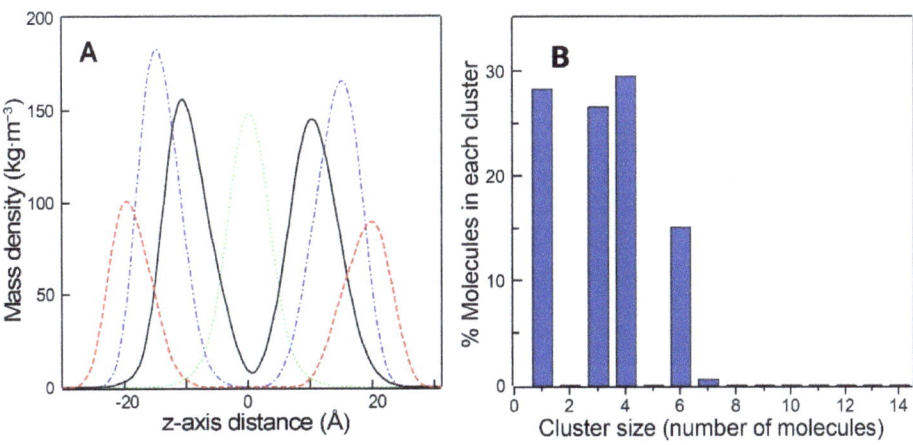

Figure 8. (**A**) Non-symmetrized mass density profiles along the z-axis of the simulation box of DMPG/TMBC system at 308 K. TMBC molecule in solid black line, phosphorus atoms in dashed red line, lipid carbonyl groups in blue dash one dot line and lipid terminals methyl carbon atoms in green dotted lines. (**B**) Cluster size distribution of TMBC molecules in the DMPG bilayer.

The propensity of TMBC to form aggregates was examined by determining the cluster size distribution of TMBC in the bilayer, and it was calculated as the number of TMBC molecules that were found in the analyzed trajectory within a distance of 0.25 nm. Figure 8B shows that the proportion of TMBC molecules present as monomers was 28.30 ± 0.05%, and the rest of TMBC forms aggregates of 3–6 molecules. The proportion of TMBC monomers in the DMPG bilayer was lower than the in case of phosphatidylserine bilayer [44], where more than 50% of TMBC was present as monomers.

In order to gain insight into the differences observed between phosphatidylglycerol and phosphatidylserine systems, we determined the hydrogen bonds of the phospholipid headgroups and TMBC, and the data are presented in Table 1. There were more hydrogen bonds between the headgroups of dimyristoylphosphatidylserine (DMPS) than between those of DMPG, both in the absence and presence of TMBC. In the presence of TMBC, there were more hydrogen bonds between TMBC and the headgroup of DMPG than between TMBC and those of DMPS, probably reflecting the higher availability of DMPG headgroups to form hydrogen bonds with other molecules than the phospholipid itself. Table 1 also shows the hydrogen bonds formed between different TMBC molecules. It was observed that TMBC formed more intermolecular hydrogen bonds in the DMPG bilayer than in the DMPS one. These data contribute to explaining the different effects exerted by TMBC on the different phospholipids, and the higher cluster formation in the case of DMPG. The presence of these different clusters in the liquid-crystalline bilayer may explain the presence of different domains in the DSC thermograms (Figure 2) and the strong tendency of TMBC to form clusters in DMPG systems may explain the presence of immiscibility in the liquid-crystalline phase (Figure 5).

Figure 9 shows a snapshot of the simulation box at 308 K of the DMPG/TMBC mixture where the location of TMBC in the bilayer can be observed. This is the expected location for TMBC considering the experimental results reported above. The location near the center of each monolayer allows TMBC to perturb the gel to the liquid-crystalline phase transition and the proximity to the carbonyl region of DMPG enables the catechin to interfere with the hydrogen bonding pattern of the interfacial region of the bilayer.

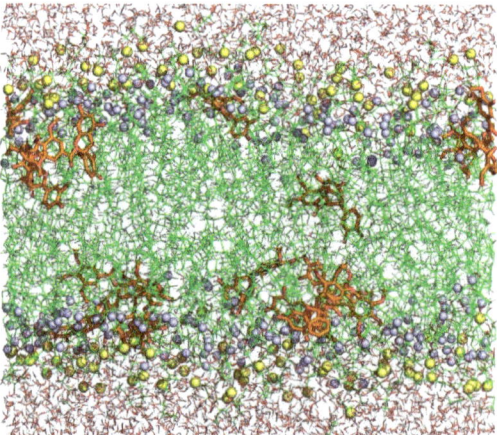

Figure 9. Final snapshot of the simulation box at 308 K of DMPG + TMBC. Water molecules are shown with purple lines, TMBC with orange and red sticks, DMPG with green lines, lipid carbonyl groups with blue spheres, and phosphorous atoms with yellow spheres.

Table 1. Hydrogen bonds of the phospholipid polar headgroups and TMBC. The dimyristoylphosphatidylserine (DMPS) data presented were obtained from previously reported simulations [44].

		Hydrogen Bonds	S.E. ($n = 3$)
DMPS	DMPS-DMPS	193.59	5.21
DMPS + TMBC	DMPS-DMPS	185.13	6.26
	TMBC-DMPS	13.51	0.88
	TMBC-TMBC	1.26	0.48
DMPG	DMPG-DMPG	147.89	4.36
DMPG + TMBC	DMPG-DMPG	145.49	4.39
	TMBC-DMPG	16.55	1.13
	TMBC-TMBC	4.95	0.83

3. Materials and Methods

3.1. Materials

1,2-Dimyristoyl-sn-glycero-3-phospho-(1′-rac-glycerol) (sodium salt, dimyristoylphosphatidylglycerol, DMPG) (>99% TLC) was purchased from Avanti Polar Lipids Inc. (Birmingham, AL, USA). Phosphorous analysis was used to determine the phospholipid concentration [64]. (-)-Catechin and 3,4,5-trimethoxybenzoyl chloride were purchased from Sigma Chemical Co. (Madrid, Spain), and TMBC was synthesized from catechin as detailed previously [40]. All other reagents were of the highest purity available.

The ratios between TMBC and phospholipid used in this study were similar to those commonly used in previous studies on the interaction between catechins and membranes [9,65] and ranged from low TMBC concentration in the membrane (0.02 mole fraction) to high concentration of TMBC in the membrane (0.30 mole fraction). TMBC is a synthetically modified catechin and no data is yet available concerning physiological concentrations. However, a correlation between these ratios and the concentrations of TMBC exhibiting anticancer activity can be established. It has been recently reported for an epithelial cell line that the phospholipid content was around 2 μg Pi/10^6 cells [66]. If we assume that the phospholipid content in melanoma cells is similar to this value and we consider the IC$_{50}$ of 1.5 μM for TMBC in melanoma cells [40], it renders that under the cell culture conditions (number of cells and volume of the medium) the TMBC/phospholipid ratio in the antiproliferative studies was around 0.3 mole fraction. Hence, the molar fraction used in our study was in the range of those expressing biological activity.

3.2. Differential Scanning Calorimetry

Samples for DSC were prepared by drying organic solvent solutions containing convenient quantities of DMPG and TMBC, and forming model bilayer vesicles in 150 mM NaCl, 0.1 mM EDTA, 10 mM Hepes, and pH 7.4 buffer, essentially as described previously [42]. In the case of DMPG, due to the electrostatic repulsion that is generated by the negative surface charge of the phospholipid, this thin-film hydration and manual agitation method produced vesicles with fewer lamellae. The experiments were carried out in a MicroCal PEAQ-DSC calorimeter (Malvern Panalytical, Malvern, UK) at 1.5 mM final phospholipid concentration, and heating scan rate of 60 °C h^{-1}. Data were analyzed using ORIGIN v7 (Northampton, MA, USA). Areas under the thermograms were used to determine the enthalpy change of the transitions. The onset and completion temperatures for each transition peak were obtained from the heating thermograms taken at the points of intersection of the tangents to the leading edges of the endotherms and the baselines, and were plotted as a function of the mole fraction of TMBC to construct a partial phase diagram.

3.3. X-ray Diffraction

Samples containing 10 μmol of DMPG and a convenient amount of TMBC were prepared similarly to those described for DSC. The suspensions were centrifuged for 30 min at 12,000 rpm in order to obtain concentrated samples to ensure that the diffraction intensities were high enough to be usable. Pellets were placed in a steel holder and were measured in a modified Kratky compact camera (MBraum-Graz-Optical Systems, Graz, Austria). Nickel-filtered Cu Kα X-rays were generated by a Philips PW3830 X-ray Generator operating at 50 kV and 30 mA. SAXD and WAXD were accomplished at the same time essentially as previously described [31]. The q (scattering vector) range covered ($q = 4\pi \sin \theta / \lambda$; where 2θ is the scattering angle and $\lambda = 1.54$ Å the selected X-ray wavelength) was between 0.05 and 0.6 Å^{-1} for SAXD and from 1.32 to 1.95 Å^{-1} for WAXD. Background corrected SAXD data were analyzed using the program GAP (Global Analysis Program) written by Prof. Georg Pabst (University of Graz, Austria) and obtained from the author [67,68]. In this program, the membrane is modeled as a sheet of infinite lateral extent with an electron density profile that is taken to be given by the summation of two headgroup Gaussians of width σ_H and position $\pm Z_H$, as well as a hydrocarbon chain Gaussian of width σ_C and negative amplitude located at the center of the bilayer at $Z = 0$. For randomly oriented bilayers that exhibit no positional correlations, such as DMPG vesicles, the scattered intensity is given by

$$I(q) = \frac{|F(q)|^2}{q^2}$$

where the form factor $F(q)$ is the Fourier transform of the electron density profile [40]. This program allows the membrane thickness to be retrieved, $d_B = 2 (Z_H + 2\sigma_H)$ from a full q-range analysis of the SAXD patterns [69]. The width σ_H of the Gaussian peak applied to model electron density profile of the head group region was fixed to 3 Å. Data were presented as mean values $\pm$ S.E. ($n = 3$).

3.4. Infrared Spectroscopy

Samples for the infrared measurements containing 10 µmol of DMPG and convenient amount of TMBC were formed in 75 µL amounts of the same buffer prepared in D$_2$O as described above. Infrared spectra were collected in a Nicolet 6700 FTIR spectrometer (Thermo Fisher Scientific, Madison, WI, USA) essentially as described previously [42]. Spectra were analyzed using the software Grams (Galactic Industries, Salem, NH, USA).

3.5. Molecular Dynamics

The molecular structure of TMBC was constructed from the chemical structure of (-)-catechin gallate obtained from the PubChem Substance and Compound data base [70] through the identifier number 6419835. All molecular dynamics simulations were carried out using GROMACS 5.0.7 and 2018.1 [71] with the aid of the Computational Service of the Universidad de Murcia (Spain).

CHARMM36 force field parameters for DMPG, TMBC, water, chloride and sodium ions were obtained from CHARMM-GUI [72–74]. Packmol software [75] was used to build the initial membrane structures formed by two leaflets oriented normal to the z-axis. The bilayer membrane was built with 128 molecules of DMPG with and without 14 molecules of TMBC, with a water layer containing a total of 6400 water molecules (TIP3 model), 144 sodium ions, and 144 chloride ions. DMPG and TMBC were randomly distributed in each phospholipid layer keeping the DMPG molecules oriented normal to z-x plane, All systems were simulated using the NpT-ensemble at 308 K constant average temperature. Pressure was controlled semi-isotropically at 1 bar of pressure and 4.5×10^{-5} bar^{-1} of compressibility. The cutoffs for van der Waals and short-range electrostatic interactions were set to 1.2 nm, and a force switch function was applied between 1.0 and 1.2 nm. Equilibration was undertaken for 3 ns using the V-rescale temperature coupling method, and Berendsen pressure coupling method [76]. Equilibration was followed by production runs of 300 ns using the Nose-Hoover thermostat [77] and the Parrinello-Rahman barostat [78]. Graphical representation and inspection of all molecular structures were carried out with PyMOL 2.3.0 [79]. The last 60 ns of the production run were used for the analysis by using Gromacs tools. The used timestep was 2 fs. The reported hydrogen bonds were calculated with the corresponding GROMACS tool with distances between donor and acceptor of ≤0.35 nm and an angle between hydrogen-donor and donor-acceptor of 30°. The mass density profile was calculated with the corresponding GROMACS tool, assuming no symmetry between both monolayers and centered to the origin Z = 0. Three replica simulations for the DMPG/TMBC system were performed. In the different simulations the TMBC molecules were at different random starting locations in the lipid phase. Data were presented as mean values ± S.E. (n = 3).

4. Conclusions

We investigated the molecular interactions between TMBC and biomimetic bilayer membranes of DMPG employing a mixed experimental and computational approach. The DSC experiments showed that TMBC incorporated into the DMPG bilayer where it was able to perturb the gel to liquid-crystalline phase transition, giving rise to the formation of immiscible lateral domains both in the gel and the liquid-crystalline phase. X-ray diffraction measurements indicated that TMBC promoted the formation of the ripple gel phase in DMPG, and it was able to produce a decrease in the bilayer thickness. The FTIR experiments illustrated how TMBC established an alteration of the hydrogen bonding pattern in the interfacial region of the bilayer. The experimental results support the simulation data, where a decrease in the bilayer thickness and an increase in the number of hydrogen bonds were determined. Simulation experiments locate the semisynthetic catechin molecules as monomers and small clusters in the middle region of the DMPG acyl chain palisade reaching the interfacial carbonyl region in agreement with the effect observed by experimental techniques. We believe that the observed interactions between TMBC and DMPG generate physical disturbances that might alter membrane function, and may help to discern the mechanism of action of the increasing list of biological action of catechins.

Author Contributions: Investigation, E.A.; conceptualization, M.D.P.-C. and F.J.A.; data curation, E.A. and J.A.T.; formal analysis, A.O. and J.A.T.; funding acquisition, J.N.R.-L.; resources, J.N.R.-L. and M.D.P.-C.; software, J.A.T.; validation, A.O. and J.A.T.; visualization, E.A. and F.J.A.; writing—original draft, F.J.A.; writing—review and editing, J.A.T. and F.J.A.; supervision, F.J.A. All authors have read and agreed to the published version of the manuscript.

Funding: This research was funded by a grant from the Fundación Séneca, Región de Murcia, Spain (FS-RM) (20809/PI/18).

Institutional Review Board Statement: Not applicable.

Informed Consent Statement: Not applicable.

Data Availability Statement: Not applicable.

Acknowledgments: Computational Service of the Universidad de Murcia (Spain) is acknowledged for the allocated computational time on its supercomputing facilities.

Conflicts of Interest: The authors declare no conflict of interest.

References

1. Singh, B.N.; Shankar, S.; Srivastava, R.K. Green tea catechin, epigallocatechin-3-gallate (EGCG): Mechanisms, perspectives and clinical applications. *Biochem. Pharmacol.* **2011**, *82*, 1807–1821. [CrossRef] [PubMed]
2. Musial, C.; Kuban-Jankowska, A.; Gorska-Ponikowska, M. Beneficial properties of green tea catechins. *Int. J. Mol. Sci.* **2020**, *21*, 1744. [CrossRef] [PubMed]
3. Wu, M.; Brown, A.C. Applications of catechins in the treatment of bacterial infections. *Pathogens* **2021**, *10*, 546. [CrossRef]
4. Wang, L.; Song, J.; Liu, A.; Xiao, B.; Li, S.; Wen, Z.; Lu, Y.; Du, G. Research progress of the antiviral bioactivities of natural flavonoids. *Nat. Products Bioprospect.* **2020**, *10*, 271–283. [CrossRef]
5. Cheng, Z.; Zhang, Z.; Han, Y.; Wang, J.; Wang, Y.; Chen, X.; Shao, Y.; Cheng, Y.; Zhou, W.; Lu, X.; et al. A review on anti-cancer effect of green tea catechins. *J. Funct. Foods* **2020**, *74*, 104172. [CrossRef]
6. Cadoná, F.C.; Dantas, R.F.; de Mello, G.H.; Silva, F.P., Jr. Natural products targeting into cancer hallmarks: An update on caffeine, theobromine, and (+)-catechin. *Crit. Rev. Food Sci. Nutr.* **2022**, *62*, 7222–7241. [CrossRef]

7. Shirakami, Y.; Shimizu, M. Possible mechanisms of green tea and its constituents against cancer. *Molecules* **2018**, *23*, 2284. [CrossRef] [PubMed]
8. Negri, A.; Naponelli, V.; Rizzi, F.; Bettuzzi, S. Molecular targets of epigallocatechin—Gallate (EGCG): A special focus on signal transduction and cancer. *Nutrients* **2018**, *10*, 1936. [CrossRef]
9. Caturla, N.; Vera-Samper, E.; Villalaín, J.; Mateo, C.R.; Micol, V. The relationship between the antioxidant and the antibacterial properties of galloylated catechins and the structure of phospholipid model membranes. *Free Radic. Biol. Med.* **2003**, *34*, 648–662. [CrossRef]
10. Watanabe, T.; Kuramochi, H.; Takahashi, A.; Imai, K.; Katsuta, N.; Nakayama, T.; Fujiki, H.; Suganuma, M. Higher cell stiffness indicating lower metastatic potential in B16 melanoma cell variants and in (2)-epigallocatechin gallate-treated cells. *J. Cancer Res. Clin. Oncol.* **2012**, *138*, 859–866. [CrossRef]
11. Takahashi, A.; Watanabe, T.; Mondal, A.; Suzuki, K.; Kurusu-Kanno, M.; Li, Z.; Yamazaki, T.; Fujiki, H.; Suganuma, M. Mechanism-based inhibition of cancer metastasis with (-)-epigallocatechin gallate. *Biochem. Biophys. Res. Commun.* **2014**, *443*, 1–6. [CrossRef] [PubMed]
12. Duhon, D.; Bigelow, R.L.H.; Coleman, D.T.; Steffan, J.J.; Yu, C.; Langston, W.; Kevil, C.G.; Cardelli, J.A. The polyphenol epigallocatechin-3-gallate affects lipid rafts to block activation of the c-met receptor in prostate cancer cells. *Mol. Carcinog.* **2010**, *49*, 739–749. [CrossRef] [PubMed]
13. Zalba, S.; ten Hagen, T.L.M. Cell membrane modulation as adjuvant in cancer therapy. *Cancer Treat. Rev.* **2017**, *52*, 48–57. [CrossRef] [PubMed]
14. Ingólfsson, H.I.; Koeppe, R.E.; Andersen, O.S. Effects of green tea catechins on gramicidin channel function and inferred changes in bilayer properties. *FEBS Lett.* **2011**, *585*, 3101–3105. [CrossRef]
15. Stillwell, W. *An Introduction to Biological Membranes: Composition, Structure and Function*, 2nd ed.; Academic Press: London, UK, 2016. [CrossRef]
16. Furse, S. Is phosphatidylglycerol essential for terrestrial life? *J. Chem. Biol.* **2017**, *10*, 1–9. [CrossRef]
17. Veiko, A.G.; Sekowski, S.; Lapshina, E.A.; Wilczewska, A.Z.; Markiewicz, K.H.; Zamaraeva, M.; Zhao, H.C.; Zavodnik, I.B. Flavonoids modulate liposomal membrane structure, regulate mitochondrial membrane permeability and prevent erythrocyte oxidative damage. *Biochim. Biophys. Acta-Biomembr.* **2020**, *1862*, 183442. [CrossRef]
18. Kicinska, A.; Jarmuszkiewicz, W. Flavonoids and mitochondria: Activation of cytoprotective pathways? *Molecules* **2020**, *25*, 3060. [CrossRef]
19. Bollag, W.B.; Xie, D.; Zheng, X.; Zhong, X. A potential role for the phospholipase D2-aquaporin-3 signaling module in early keratinocyte differentiation: Production of a phosphatidylglycerol signaling lipid. *J. Investig. Dermatol.* **2007**, *127*, 2823–2831. [CrossRef]
20. Choudhary, V.; Uaratanawong, R.; Patel, R.R.; Patel, H.; Bao, W.; Hartney, B.; Cohen, E.; Chen, X.; Zhong, Q.; Isales, C.M.; et al. Phosphatidylglycerol inhibits toll-like receptor–mediated inflammation by danger-associated molecular patterns. *J. Investig. Dermatol.* **2019**, *139*, 868–877. [CrossRef]
21. Kuronuma, K.; Mitsuzawa, H.; Takeda, K.; Nishitani, C.; Chan, E.D.; Kuroki, Y.; Nakamura, M.; Voelker, D.R. Anionic pulmonary surfactant phospholipids inhibit inflammatory responses from alveolar macrophages and U937 cells by binding the lipopolysaccharide-interacting proteins CD14 and MD-2. *J. Biol. Chem.* **2009**, *284*, 25488–25500. [CrossRef]
22. Chen, W.W.; Chao, Y.J.; Chang, W.H.; Chan, J.F.; Hsu, Y.H.H. Phosphatidylglycerol incorporates into cardiolipin to improve mitochondrial activity and inhibits inflammation. *Sci. Rep.* **2018**, *8*, 4949. [CrossRef] [PubMed]
23. Jiang, Z.; Flynn, J.D.; Teague, W.E.; Gawrisch, K.; Lee, J.C. Stimulation of α-synuclein amyloid formation by phosphatidylglycerol micellar tubules. *Biochim. Biophys. Acta-Biomembr.* **2018**, *1860*, 1840–1847. [CrossRef] [PubMed]
24. Numata, M.; Kandasamy, P.; Nagashima, Y.; Posey, J.; Hartshorn, K.; Woodland, D.; Voelker, D.R. Phosphatidylglycerol suppresses influenza a virus infection. *Am. J. Respir. Cell Mol. Biol.* **2012**, *46*, 479–487. [CrossRef] [PubMed]
25. Dowhan, W. Molecular basis for membrane phospholipid diversity: Why are there so many lipids? *Annu. Rev. Biochem.* **1997**, *66*, 199–232. [CrossRef]
26. Elmore, D.E. Molecular dynamics simulation of a phosphatidylglycerol membrane. *FEBS Lett.* **2006**, *580*, 144–148. [CrossRef]
27. Sosa Morales, M.C.; Álvarez, R.M.S. Structural characterization of phosphatidylglycerol model membranes containing the antibiotic target lipid II molecule: A raman microspectroscopy study. *J. Raman Spectrosc.* **2017**, *48*, 170–179. [CrossRef]
28. Renzetti, A.; Betts, J.W.; Fukumoto, K.; Rutherford, R.N. Antibacterial green tea catechins from a molecular perspective: Mechanisms of action and structure-activity relationships. *Food Funct.* **2020**, *11*, 9370–9396. [CrossRef]
29. Fathima, A.; Rao, J.R. Selective toxicity of Catechin—A natural flavonoid towards bacteria. *Appl. Microbiol. Biotechnol.* **2016**, *100*, 6395–6402. [CrossRef]
30. Taylor, P.W. Interactions of tea-derived catechin gallates with bacterial pathogens. *Molecules* **2020**, *25*, 1986. [CrossRef]
31. Shah, S.; Stapleton, P.D.; Taylor, P.W. The polyphenol (−)-epicatechin gallate disrupts the secretion of virulence-related proteins by *Staphylococcus aureus*. *Lett. App. Microbiol.* **2008**, *46*, 181–185. [CrossRef]
32. Sugita-Konishi, Y.; Hara-Kudo, Y.; Amano, F.; Okubo, T.; Aoi, N.; Iwaki, M.; Kumagai, S. Epigallocatechin gallate and gallocatechin gallate in green tea catechins inhibit extracellular release of Vero toxin from enterohemorrhagic *Escherichia coli* O157:H7. *Biochim. Biophys. Acta* **1999**, *1472*, 42–50. [CrossRef] [PubMed]
33. Hengge, R. Targeting bacterial biofilms by the green tea polyphenol EGCG. *Molecules* **2019**, *24*, 2403. [CrossRef] [PubMed]

34. Ikigai, H.; Nakae, T.; Hara, Y.; Shimamura, T. Bactericidal catechins damage the lipid bilayer. *Biochim. Biophys. Acta* **1993**, *1147*, 132–136. [CrossRef] [PubMed]
35. Shigemune, N.; Nakayama, M.; Tsugukuni, T.; Hitomi, J.; Yoshizawa, C.; Mekada, Y.; Kurahachi, M.; Miyamoto, T. The mechanisms and effect of epigallocatechin gallate (EGCg) on the germination and proliferation of bacterial spores. *Food Control* **2012**, *27*, 269–274. [CrossRef]
36. He, M.; Wu, T.; Pan, S.; Xu, X. Antimicrobial mechanism of flavonoids against *Escherichia coli* ATCC 25922 by model membrane study. *Appl. Surf. Sci.* **2014**, *305*, 515–521. [CrossRef]
37. Mahmood, H.Y.; Jamshidi, S.; Mark Sutton, J.M.; Rahman, K.M. Current advances in developing inhibitors of bacterial multidrug efflux pumps. *Curr. Med. Chem.* **2016**, *23*, 1062–1081. [CrossRef]
38. Mehmood, S.; Maqsood, M.; Mahtab, N.; Khan, M.I.; Sahar, A.; Zaib, S.; Gul, S. Epigallocatechin gallate: Phytochemistry, bioavailability, utilization challenges, and strategies. *J. Food Biochem.* **2022**, *46*, 14189. [CrossRef]
39. Cai, Z.Y.; Li, X.M.; Liang, J.P.; Xiang, L.P.; Wang, K.R.; Shi, Y.L.; Yang, R.; Shi, M.; Ye, J.H.; Lu, J.L.; et al. Bioavailability of tea catechins and its improvement. *Molecules* **2018**, *23*, 2346. [CrossRef]
40. Sáez-Ayala, M.; Sánchez-Del-Campo, L.; Montenegro, M.F.; Chazarra, S.; Tárraga, A.; Cabezas-Herrera, J.; Rodríguez-López, J.N. Comparison of a pair of synthetic tea-catechin-derived epimers: Synthesis, antifolate activity, and tyrosinase-mediated activation in melanoma. *Chem. Med. Chem.* **2011**, *6*, 440–449. [CrossRef]
41. Montenegro, M.F.; Sáez-Ayala, M.; Piñero-Madrona, A.; Cabezas-Herrera, J.; Rodríguez-López, J.N. Reactivation of the tumour suppressor RASSF1A in breast cancer by simultaneous targeting of DNA and E2F1 methylation. *PLoS ONE* **2012**, *7*, e52231. [CrossRef]
42. How, C.W.; Teruel, J.A.; Ortiz, A.; Montenegro, M.F.; Rodríguez-López, J.N.; Aranda, F.J. Effects of a synthetic antitumoral catechin and its tyrosinase-processed product on the structural properties of phosphatidylcholine membranes. *Biochim. Biophys. Acta-Biomembr.* **2014**, *1838*, 1215–1224. [CrossRef] [PubMed]
43. Casado, F.; Teruel, J.A.; Casado, S.; Ortiz, A.; Rodríguez-López, J.N.; Aranda, F.J. Location and effects of an antitumoral catechin on the structural properties of phosphatidylethanolamine membranes. *Molecules* **2016**, *21*, 829. [CrossRef] [PubMed]
44. Aranda, E.; Teruel, J.A.; Ortiz, A.; Pérez-Cárceles, M.-D.; Rodríguez-López, J.N.; Aranda, F.J. 3,4,5-trimethoxybenzoate of catechin, an anticarcinogenic semisynthetic catechin, modulates the physical properties of anionic phospholipid membranes. *Molecules* **2022**, *27*, 2910. [CrossRef] [PubMed]
45. Lewis, R.N.A.H.; Mannock, D.A.; McElhaney, R.N. Differential scanning calorimetry in the study of lipid phase transitions in model and biological membranes. *Methods Mol. Biol.* **2007**, *400*, 171–195. [CrossRef] [PubMed]
46. Zhang, Y.P.; Lewis, R.N.A.H.; McElhaney, R.N. Calorimetric and spectroscopic studies of the thermotropic phase behavior of the N-saturated 1,2-diacylphosphatidylglycerols. *Biophys. J.* **1997**, *72*, 779–793. [CrossRef]
47. Pabst, G.; Danner, S.; Karmakar, S.; Deutsch, G.; Raghunathany, V.A. On the propensity of phosphatidylglycerols to form interdigitated phases. *Biophys. J.* **2007**, *93*, 513–525. [CrossRef]
48. Semeraro, E.F.; Marx, L.; Frewein, M.P.K.; Pabst, G. Increasing complexity in small-angle X-ray and neutron scattering experiments: From biological membrane mimics to live cells. *Soft Matter.* **2021**, *17*, 222–232. [CrossRef]
49. Tardieu, A.; Luzzati, V.; Reman, F.C. Structure and polymorphism of the hydrocarbon chains of lipids: A study of lecithin-water phases. *J. Mol. Biol.* **1973**, *75*, 711–733. [CrossRef]
50. Pabst, G.; Grage, S.L.; Danner-Pongratz, S.; Jing, W.; Ulrich, A.S.; Watts, A.; Lohner, K.; Hickel, A. Membrane thickening by the antimicrobial peptide PGLa. *Biophys. J.* **2008**, *95*, 5779–5788. [CrossRef]
51. Lohner, K.; Latal, A.; Degovics, G.; Garidel, P. Packing characteristics of a model system mimicking cytoplasmic bacterial membranes. *Chem. Phys. Lipids* **2001**, *111*, 177–192. [CrossRef]
52. Ortiz, A.; Teruel, J.A.; Manresa, A.; Espuny, M.J.; Marqués, A.; Aranda, F.J. Effects of a bacterial trehalose lipid on phosphatidylglycerol membranes. *Biochim. Biophys. Acta-Biomembr.* **2011**, *1808*, 2067–2072. [CrossRef] [PubMed]
53. Kriechbaum, M.; Laggner, P. States of phase transitions in biological structures. *Prog. Surf. Sci.* **1996**, *51*, 233–261. [CrossRef]
54. Riske, K.A.; Amaral, L.Q.; Lamy-Freund, M.T. Thermal transitions of DMPG bilayers in aqueous solution: SAXS structural studies. *Biochim. Biophys. Acta-Biomembr.* **2001**, *1511*, 297–308. [CrossRef] [PubMed]
55. Fernandez, R.M.; Riske, K.A.; Amaral, L.Q.; Itri, R.; Lamy, M.T. Influence of salt on the structure of DMPG studied by SAXS and optical microscopy. *Biochim. Biophys. Acta-Biomembr.* **2008**, *1778*, 907–916. [CrossRef] [PubMed]
56. Killian, J.A. Hydrophobic mismatch between proteins and lipids in membranes. *Biochim. Biophys. Acta-Rev. Biomembr.* **1998**, *1376*, 401–416. [CrossRef] [PubMed]
57. Cybulski, L.E.; de Mendoza, D. Bilayer Hydrophobic thickness and integral membrane protein function. *Curr. Protein Pept. Sci.* **2011**, *12*, 760–766. [CrossRef] [PubMed]
58. Mantsch, H.H.; McElhaney, R. Phospholipid phase transitions in model and biological membranes as studied by infrared spectroscopy. *Chem. Phys. Lipids* **1991**, *57*, 213–226. [CrossRef] [PubMed]
59. Lewis, R.N.A.H.; McElhaney, R.N. Fourier transform infrared spectroscopy in the study of lipid phase transitions in model and biological membranes: Practical considerations. *Methods Mol. Biol.* **2007**, *400*, 207–226. [CrossRef]
60. Blume, A.; Hübner, W.; Messner, G. Fourier transform infrared spectroscopy of $^{13}C=0$-labeled phospholipids hydrogen bonding to carbonyl groups. *Biochemistry* **1988**, *27*, 8239–8249. [CrossRef]

61. Friedman, R.; Khalid, S.; Aponte-Santamaría, C.; Arutyunova, E.; Becker, M.; Boyd, K.J.; Christensen, M.; Coimbra, J.T.; Daday, C.; van Eerden, F.J.; et al. Understanding conformational dynamics of complex lipid mixtures relevant to biology. *J. Membr. Biol.* **2018**, *251*, 609–631. [CrossRef]
62. Venable, R.M.; Krämer, A.; Pastor, R.W. Molecular dynamics simulations of membrane permeability. *Chem. Rev.* **2019**, *119*, 5954–5997. [CrossRef] [PubMed]
63. Pan, J.; Heberle, F.A.; Tristram-Nagle, S.; Szymanski, M.; Koepfinger, M.; Katsaras, J.; Kučerka, N. Molecular structures of fluid phase phosphatidylglycerol bilayers as determined by small angle neutron and X-ray scattering. *Biochim. Biophys. Acta-Biomembr.* **2012**, *1818*, 2135–2148. [CrossRef] [PubMed]
64. Böttcher, C.; Gent, C.; Pries, C. A rapid and sensitive sub-micro phosphorus determination. *Anal. Chim. Acta* **1961**, *24*, 203–204. [CrossRef]
65. Sun, Y.; Hung, W.-C.; Chen, F.-Y.; Lee, C.-C.; Huang, H.W. Interaction of tea catechin (−)-epigallocatechin gallate with lipid bilayers. *Biophys. J.* **2009**, *96*, 1026–1035. [CrossRef]
66. Casali, C.I.; Weber, K.; Favale, N.O.; Fernández Tome, M.C. Environmental hyperosmolality regulates phospholipid biosynthesis in the renal epithelial cell line MDCK. *J. Lipid Res.* **2013**, *54*, 677–691. [CrossRef]
67. Pabst, G.; Rappolt, M.; Amenitsch, H.; Laggner, P. Structural Information from multilamellar liposomes at full hydration: Full q-range fitting with high quality X-ray data. *Phys. Rev. E-Stat. Phys. Plasmas Fluids Relat. Interdiscip. Top.* **2000**, *62*, 4000–4009. [CrossRef]
68. Pabst, G.; Koschuch, R.; Pozo-Navas, B.; Rappolt, M.; Lohner, K.; Laggner, P. Structural analysis of weakly ordered membrane stacks. *J. Appl. Crystallogr.* **2003**, *36*, 1378–1388. [CrossRef]
69. Pabst, G. Global properties of biomimetic membranes: Perspectives on molecular features. *Biophys. Rev. Lett.* **2006**, *01*, 57–84. [CrossRef]
70. Kim, S.; Thiessen, P.A.; Bolton, E.E.; Chen, J.; Fu, G.; Gindulyte, A.; Han, L.; He, J.; He, S.; Shoemaker, B.A.; et al. PubChem substance and compound databases. *Nucleic Acids Res.* **2016**, *44*, D1202–D1213. [CrossRef]
71. Abraham, M.J.; Murtola, T.; Schulz, R.; Páll, S.; Smith, J.C.; Hess, B.; Lindah, E. Gromacs: High performance molecular simulations through multi-level parallelism from laptops to supercomputers. *SoftwareX* **2015**, *1–2*, 19–25. [CrossRef]
72. Jo, S.; Kim, T.; Iyer, V.G.; Im, W. CHARMM-GUI: A web-based graphical user interface for CHARMM. *J. Comput. Chem.* **2008**, *29*, 1859–1865. [CrossRef] [PubMed]
73. Brooks, B.R.; Brooks, C.L.; Mackerell, A.D.; Nilsson, L.; Petrella, R.J.; Roux, B.; Won, Y.; Archontis, G.; Bartels, C.; Boresch, S.; et al. CHARMM: The biomolecular simulation program. *J. Comput. Chem.* **2009**, *30*, 1545–1614. [CrossRef] [PubMed]
74. Lee, J.; Cheng, X.; Swails, J.M.; Yeom, M.S.; Eastman, P.K.; Lemkul, J.A.; Wei, S.; Buckner, J.; Jeong, J.C.; Qi, Y.; et al. CHARMM-GUI input generator for NAMD, GROMACS, AMBER, OpenMM, and CHARMM/OpenMM simulations using the CHARMM36 additive force field. *J. Chem. Theory Comput.* **2016**, *12*, 405–413. [CrossRef]
75. Martínez, L.; Andrade, R.; Birgin, E.G.; Martínez, J.M. PACKMOL: A package for building initial configurations for molecular dynamics simulations. *J. Comput. Chem.* **2009**, *30*, 2157–2164. [CrossRef] [PubMed]
76. Berendsen, H.J.C.; Postma, J.P.M.; Van Gunsteren, W.F.; Dinola, A.; Haak, J.R. Molecular dynamics with coupling to an external bath. *J. Chem. Phys.* **1984**, *81*, 3684–3690. [CrossRef]
77. Hoover, W.G. Canonical dynamics: Equilibrium phase-space distributions. *Phys. Rev. A* **1985**, *31*, 1695–1697. [CrossRef] [PubMed]
78. Parrinello, M.; Rahman, A. Polymorphic transitions in single crystals: A new molecular dynamics method. *J. Appl. Phys.* **1981**, *52*, 7182–7190. [CrossRef]
79. Schrödinger, L. *The PyMOL Molecular Graphics System*, version 2.3; Schrödinger, Inc.: New York, NY, USA, 2010.

Disclaimer/Publisher's Note: The statements, opinions and data contained in all publications are solely those of the individual author(s) and contributor(s) and not of MDPI and/or the editor(s). MDPI and/or the editor(s) disclaim responsibility for any injury to people or property resulting from any ideas, methods, instructions or products referred to in the content.

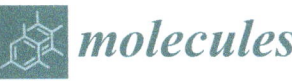

Review

Phytochemicals Derived from Agricultural Residues and Their Valuable Properties and Applications

Marta Oleszek [1,*], Iwona Kowalska [1], Terenzio Bertuzzi [2] and Wiesław Oleszek [1]

[1] Department of Biochemistry and Crop Quality, Institute of Soil Science and Plant Cultivation, State Research Institute, 24-100 Puławy, Poland
[2] DIANA, Department of Animal Science, Food and Nutrition, Faculty of Agricultural, Food and Environmental Sciences, Università Cattolica del Sacro Cuore, Via E. Parmense, 84, 29122 Piacenza, Italy
* Correspondence: moleszek@iung.pulawy.pl

Abstract: Billions of tons of agro-industrial residues are produced worldwide. This is associated with the risk of pollution as well as management and economic problems. Simultaneously, non-edible portions of many crops are rich in bioactive compounds with valuable properties. For this reason, developing various methods for utilizing agro-industrial residues as a source of high-value by-products is very important. The main objective of the paper is a review of the newest studies on biologically active compounds included in non-edible parts of crops with the highest amount of waste generated annually in the world. The review also provides the newest data on the chemical and biological properties, as well as the potential application of phytochemicals from such waste. The review shows that, in 2020, there were above 6 billion tonnes of residues only from the most popular crops. The greatest amount is generated during sugar, oil, and flour production. All described residues contain valuable phytochemicals that exhibit antioxidant, antimicrobial and very often anti-cancer activity. Many studies show interesting applications, mainly in pharmaceuticals and food production, but also in agriculture and wastewater remediation, as well as metal and steel industries.

Keywords: bioactive compounds; antioxidants; agricultural residues; fruits; vegetables; mass spectrometry; extraction

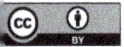

1. Introduction

The agricultural industry generates billions of tonnes of waste from the tillage and processing of various crops. The crops with the largest amounts of produced residues are rice, maize, soybean, sugarcane, potato, tomato, and cucumber, as well as some fruits, mainly bananas, oranges, grapes, and apples [1,2]. It has been estimated that European food processing companies generate annually approximately 100 Mt of waste and by-products, mostly during the production of drinks (26%), dairy and ice cream (21.3%), and fruits and vegetables (14.8%) [3].

In Table 1, the amounts of particular wastes generated worldwide are presented. Many of them are rich in biologically active compounds and have the potential to become important raw materials for obtaining valuable phytochemicals. Vegetable and fruit processing by-products are promising sources of valuable phytochemicals having antioxidant, antimicrobial, anti-inflammatory, anti-cancer, and cardiovascular protection activities [4]. The applications of these agro-industrial residues and their bioactive compounds in functional food and cosmetics production were presented in many studies [5–7]. Moreover, due to the potential health risk of some synthetic antioxidants such as BHA, the identification and isolation of natural antioxidants from waste has become increasingly attractive. Important criteria to decide if a product or by-product can be of interest to recover phytochemicals are the absolute concentration and preconcentration factor, as well as the total amount of product or by-product per batch [8].

Table 1. Amount of residues from some crops produced in the world in 2020.

Crop	Global Crop Production * [Million Ton]	Residue to Crop Ratio	Amount of Residue ** [Million Ton]	References
Sugarcane	1869.7	0.1	189.1	Jiang et al. [9]
Maize	1162.4	2.0	2324.8	Jiang et al. [9]
Wheat	760.9	1.18	897.9	Searle and Malins [10]
Rice	756.7	1.0	756.7	Jiang et al. [9]
Potato	359.1	0.4	143.6	Ben Taher et al. [11]
Soybean	353.5	1.5	530.3	Yanli et al. [12]
Sugar beet	253.0	0.27	68.3	Searle and Malins [10]
Tomato	186.8	3.5	653.8	Oleszek et al. [13]
Barley	157.0	1.18	185.3	Searle and Malins [10]
Banana	119.8	0.6	71.9	Gabhane et al. [14]
Cucumber	91.3	4.5	410.9	Oleszek et al. [13]
Apples	86.4	0.25	21.6	Cruz et al. [15]
Grapes	78.0	0.3	23.4	Muhlack et al. [16]
Oranges	75.5	0.5	37.8	Rezzadori et al. [17]
Olives	23.6	0.12	2.8	Searle and Malins [10]

* based on FAOSTAT, 2022, ** calculated based on the global crop production in 2020 and the residue-to-crop ratio according to cited references.

As interest in waste processing has been growing in recent years, many scientific papers have been published on new compounds in agro-industrial waste, new properties of valuable phytochemicals contained in crop residues and their applications. It seems necessary to summarize and collect the latest knowledge on this subject. In this work, an overview of the recent knowledge on the phytochemicals in some of the most popular food by-products, with the highest amount generated in the world, as well as on their properties and potential applications, have been presented in more detail (Figure 1).

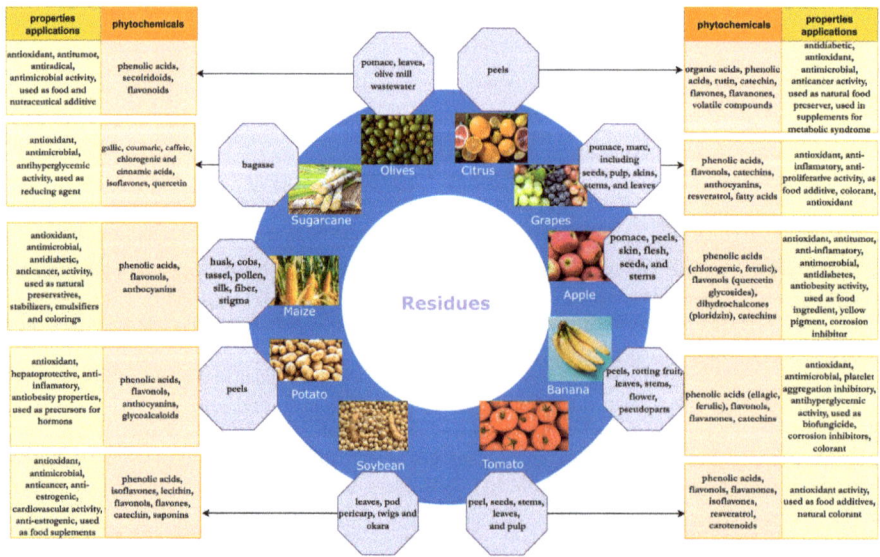

Figure 1. Agricultural residues and the properties and applications of their phytochemicals.

2. Phytochemicals from Crop Residues
2.1. Sugarcane Bagasse

Large amounts of waste are generated during the processing of sugarcane. In fact, one metric ton of sugarcane generates 280 kg of bagasse. Sugarcane bagasse is one of the most abundant agro-food by-products and is a very promising raw material available at low cost for recovering bioactive substances [18,19]. Sugarcane bagasse consists mainly of cellulose (35–50%), hemicellulose (26–41%), lignin (11–25%), but also some amount of plant secondary metabolites (PSM), mainly anthocyanins and mineral substances [20–25].

Phenolic compounds are a very important group of natural substances identified in sugarcane waste. Nonetheless, steam explosion and ultrasound-assisted extraction (UAE) pretreatment was applied for the production of valuable phenolic compounds from the lignin included in this residue. Chromatographic analysis revealed that sugarcane bagasse is a good feedstock for the generation of phenolic acids. The concentration of total phenolics with the Folin-Ciocalteau method was between 2.8 and 3.2 g/L. Zhao et al. [26] have identified many phenolics, mainly flavonoids and phenolic acids, in sugarcane bagasse extract (Table 2). The total polyphenol content was detected as higher than 4 mg/g of dry bagasse, with total flavonoid content of 470 mg quercetin/g of polyphenol. The most abundant phenolic acids identified in the sugarcane bagasse extract were gallic acid (4.36 mg/g extract), ferulic acid (1.87 mg/g extract) and coumaric acid (1.66 mg/g extract). Spectroscopic analysis showed that a predominant amount of p-coumaric acid is ester-linked to the cell wall components, mainly to lignin. On the other hand, about half of the ferulic acid is esterified to the cell wall hemicelluloses. The purified sugarcane bagasse hydrolysate consisted mainly of p-coumaric acid. Besides, the purified products showed the same antioxidant activity, reducing power and free radical scavenging capacity as the standard p-coumaric acid. Al Arni et al. [27] stated that the major natural products contained in the lignin fraction were p-coumaric acid, ferulic acid, syringic acid, and vanillin.

Table 2. Phytochemicals derived from sugarcane bagasse.

Name	MW * [g mol^{-1}]	C$_x$H$_y$O$_z$	References
Phenolic acids—hydroxybenzoic acids			
p-Hydroxybenzoic acid	138.12	C$_7$H$_6$O$_3$	Zheng et al. [19]
Vanillic acid	168.14	C$_8$H$_8$O$_4$	Zheng et al. [19]
Benzoic acid	122.12	C$_7$H$_6$O$_2$	Zheng et al. [19]
Protocatechuic acid	154.12	C$_7$H$_6$O$_4$	Zheng et al. [19]
Gallic acid	170.12	C$_7$H$_6$O$_5$	Zhao et al. [26]
Syringic acid	198.17	C$_9$H$_{10}$O$_5$	Zhao et al. [26]
Phenolic acids—hydroxycinnamic acids			
p-Coumaric acid	164.04	C$_9$H$_8$O$_3$	González–Bautista et al. [28]
Cinnamic acid	148.16	C$_9$H$_8$O$_2$	González–Bautista et al. [28]
Ferulic acid	194.18	C$_{10}$H$_{10}$O$_4$	González–Bautista et al. [28]
Caffeic acid	180.16	C$_9$H$_8$O$_4$	González–Bautista et al. [28]
Chlorogenic acids	354.31	C$_{16}$H$_{18}$O$_9$	Zhao et al. [26]
Sinapic acid	224.21	C$_{11}$H$_{12}$O$_5$	Zhao et al. [26]
Flavonoids—flavonols			
Quercetin	302.24	C$_{15}$H$_{10}$O$_7$	Zheng et al. [19]
Flavonoids—flavones			
Luteolin	286.24	C$_{15}$H$_{10}$O$_6$	Zheng et al. [29]
Tricin	330.29	C$_{17}$H$_{14}$O$_7$	Zheng et al. [29]
Flavonoid glycosides			
Diosmetin 6-C-glucoside	462.40	C$_{22}$H$_{22}$O$_{11}$	Zheng et al. [29]
Tricin 7-O-β-glucopyranoside	492.43	C$_{23}$H$_{24}$O$_{12}$	Zheng et al. [29]
Isoflavone			
Genistin	432.37	C$_{21}$H$_{20}$O$_{10}$	Zheng et al. [19]
Genistein	270.24	C$_{15}$H$_{10}$O$_5$	Zheng et al. [19]

Table 2. Cont.

Name	MW * [g mol^{-1}]	C$_x$H$_y$O$_z$	References
Others			
Catechol	110.11	C$_6$H$_6$O$_2$	Zheng et al. [19]
Phenol	94.11	C$_6$H$_6$O	Zheng et al. [19]
Guaiacol	124.14	C$_7$H$_8$O$_2$	Zheng et al. [19]
Vanillin	152.15	C$_8$H$_8$O$_3$	Zheng et al. [19]
Isovanillin	152.15	C$_8$H$_8$O$_3$	Van der Pol et al. [30]
Syringaldehyde	182.17	C$_9$H$_{10}$O$_4$	Zheng et al. [19]
Piceol	136.15	C$_8$H$_8$O$_2$	Van der Pol et al. [30]
Apocynin	166.17	C$_9$H$_{10}$O$_3$	Van der Pol et al. [30]
Acetosyringone	196.19	C$_{10}$H$_{12}$O$_4$	Van der Pol et al. [30]
Syringaldehyde	182.17	C$_9$H$_{10}$O$_4$	Van der Pol et al. [30]
Creosol	138.16	C$_8$H$_{10}$O$_2$	Lv et al. [31]
4-Ethylguaiacol	152.19	C$_9$H$_{12}$O$_2$	Lv et al. [31]
Chavicol	134.17	C$_9$H$_{10}$O	Lv et al. [31]
4-Vinylguaiacol	150.17	C$_9$H$_{10}$O$_2$	Lv et al. [31]
4-Allylsyringol	194.23	C$_{11}$H$_{14}$O$_3$	Lv et al. [31]

* MW—molecular weight.

Gallic, coumaric, caffeic, chlorogenic, and cinnamic acids were the main phenolic compounds extracted from raw and alkaline pretreated sugarcane bagasse and identified by high-performance liquid chromatography (HPLC) [28]. The aromatic phenolic compounds (p-coumaric acid, ferulic acid, p-hydroxybenzaldehyde, vanillin, and vanillic acid) were reported in sugarcane bagasse pith. Five phenolic compounds (tricin 4-O-guaiacylglyceryl ether-7-O-glucopyranoside, genistin, p-coumaric acid, quercetin, and genistein) in 30% hydroalcoholic fraction of sugarcane bagasse were identified using ultra-high performance liquid chromatography/high-resolution time of flight mass spectrometry (UHPLC-HR-TOF-MS); (Table 2). The total phenolic content was 170.68 mg gallic acid/g dry extract [19].

Phenolic compounds derived from sugarcane bagasse exhibited many biological activities, which were used in various applications. The most important biological activities and the newest and most interesting applications have been summarized in Table 3.

Table 3. Biological activities and potential applications of phytochemicals obtained from sugarcane bagasse.

Material	Extract/Compound	Biological Activity/Application	References
Sugarcane bagasse	phenolic compounds	- natural antioxidant - used in pharmacology	Al Arni et al. [27]
		- antibacterial agents against the foodborne pathogens Escherichia coli, Listeria monocytogenes, Staphylococcus aureus, Salmonella typhimurium	Zhao et al. [26]
	gallic and tannic acids	- deactivate cellulolytic and hemicellulolytic enzymes	Michelin et al. [32]
	extract	- antioxidant and radical scavenging activity - antimicrobial activity against Staphylococcus aureus TISTR029 and Escherichia coli O157:H7 - added value for the sugar industry	Juttuporn et al. [33]
		- antihyperglycemic ability - useful therapeutic agents to treat T2D patients	Zheng et al. [19]
		- used for the low-cost bio-oil production	Treedet and Suntivarakorn [34]
		- feedstock for ethanol (bioethanol) production	Krishnan et al. [35] Zhu et al. [36]
		- raw material for the production of industrial enzymes, xylose, glucose, methane	Guilherme et al. [37]
		- raw material for the production of xylitol and organic acids	Chandel et al. [38]
		- used to prepare highly valued succinic acid	Xi et al. [23]
		- used as a reducing agent in synthesizing biogenic platinum nanoparticles	Ishak et al. [20]
		- used as a fuel to power sugar mills	Mohan et al. [22]

2.2. Maize Residues

Maize (corn *Zea mays* L.) bran, husk, cobs, tassel, pollen, silk, and fiber are residues of corn production. They contain substantial amounts of phytochemicals, such as phenolic compounds, carotenoid pigments and phytosterols [39] (Table 4).

Table 4. Phytochemicals identified in corn waste.

Name	MW [g mol^{-1}]	Molecular Formula	References
Phenolic acids—hydroxycinnamic acids			
p-Coumaric acid	164.04	$C_9H_8O_3$	Guo et al. [39]
Ferulic acid	194.18	$C_{10}H_{10}O_4$	Guo et al. [39]
trans-ferulic acid	194.18	$C_{10}H_{10}O_4$	Guo et al. [39]
trans-ferulic acid methyl ester	208.21	$C_{11}H_{12}O_4$	Guo et al. [39]
cis-ferulic acid	194.18	$C_{10}H_{10}O_4$	Guo et al. [39]
cis-ferulic acid methyl ester	208.21	$C_{11}H_{12}O_4$	Guo et al. [39]
Flavonoids—flavonols			
Rutin	610.52	$C_{27}H_{30}O_{16}$	Bujang et al. [40]
Quercetin-3-*O*-glucoside	463.37	$C_{21}H_{19}O_{12}$	Dong et al. [41]
Isorhamnetin-3-*O*-glucoside	478.41	$C_{22}H_{22}O_{12}$	Dong et al. [41]
Kaempferol-3-*O*-glucoside	447.37	$C_{21}H_{19}O_{11}$	Li et al. [42]
Maysin	576.50	$C_{27}H_{28}O_{14}$	Haslina and Eva [43]
Isoorientin-2″-*O*-α-L-rhamnoside	594.50	$C_{27}H_{30}O_{15}$	Haslina and Eva [43]
Maysin-3′-methyl ether	590.50	$C_{28}H_{30}O_{15}$	Tian et al. [44]
ax-4″–OH–3′-Methoxymaysin	592.50	$C_{28}H_{32}O_{14}$	Tian et al. [44]
2″-*O*-α-L-Rhamnosyl-6-*C*-fucosylluteolin	578.50	$C_{27}H_{30}O_{14}$	Tian et al. [44]
Flavonoids—anthocyanins			
Pelargonidin-3-*O*-glucoside	433.40	$C_{21}H_{21}O_{10}$	Lao and Giusti [45]
Pelargonidin-3-(6″malonylglucoside)	519.23	$C_{24}H_{23}O_{13}$	Chen et al. [46]
Cyanidin-3-*O*-glucoside	449.39	$C_{21}H_{21}O_{11}$	Barba et al. [47]
Cyanidin 3-(6″-malonylglucoside)	535.11	$C_{24}H_{23}O_{14}$	Fernandez-Aulis et al. [48]
Peonidin-3-*O*-glucoside	463.41	$C_{22}H_{23}O_{11}$	Barba et al. [47]
Peonidin-3-(6″malonylglucoside)	549.50	$C_{25}H_{25}O_{14}$	Fernandez-Aulis et al. [48]
Other compounds			
p-Hydroxybenzaldehyde	122.12	$C_7H_6O_2$	Guo et al. [39]
β-Sitosterol glucoside	576.85	$C_{35}H_{60}O_6$	Guo et al. [39]
Indole-3-acetic acid	175.06	$C_{10}H_9NO_2$	Wille and Berhow [49]
Vanillin	154.05	$C_8H_8O_3$	Guo et al. [39]

Corn bran is produced as a plentiful by-product during the corn dry milling process. Similar to other cereal grains, phenolics in corn bran exist in free insoluble bound and soluble-conjugated forms. Corn bran is a rich source of ferulic acid compared to other cereals, fruits and vegetables. Guo et al. [39] isolated four forms of ferulic acid and its derivates from corn bran. On the other hand, it has been reported that the hexane-derived extract from corn bran contains high levels of ferulate-phytosterol esters, similar in composition and function to oryzanol.

Another corn waste is a husk. It is the outer leafy covering of an ear of *Zea mays* L. The main constituents of the maize husk extracts determined in various phytochemical studies are phenolic compounds, e.g., flavonoids [41,50]. Saponins, glycosides, and alkaloids are present mainly in the aqueous and methanolic extracts, while phenols and tannins are numerous in methanolic ones [51]. Moreover, corn husk has high contents of anthocyanins [48,52]. Simla et al. [53] reported that anthocyanins concentration in corn husks ranges from 0.003 to 4.9 mg/g. The major anthocyanins of corn husk were identified as malonylation products of cyanidin, pelargonidin, and peonidin derivatives [54].

Important by-products of the corn industry are cobs. For every 100 kg of corn grain, approximately 18 kg of corn cobs are produced. Corn cob is one of the food waste-material having a phytochemical component that has a healthy benefit [55]. They contain cyanidin-3-glucoside and cyanidin-3-(6″malonylglucoside) as main anthocyanins, as well as pelargonidin-3-glucoside, peonidin-3-glucoside and their malonyl counterparts [48].

Corn tassel is a by-product from hybrid corn seed production and an excellent source of phytochemicals (the flavonol glycosides of quercetin, isorhamnetin and kaempferol) with beneficial properties [56]. In Thailand, purple waxy corn is considered a special corn type because it is rich in phenolics, anthocyanins, and carotenoids in the tassel [57]. Besides, corn tassels could be considered a great source of valuable products such as volatile oils.

Corn pollen is another corn waste. Significant amounts of phytochemicals, including carotenoids, steroids, terpenes and flavonoids, are present in maize pollen [52]. Bujang et al. (2021) showed that maize pollen contains a high total phenolic content and total flavonoid content of 783.02 mg gallic acid equivalent (GAE)/100 g and 1706.83 mg quercetin equivalent (QE)/100 g, respectively. The flavonoid pattern of maize pollen is characterized by an accumulation of the predominant flavonols, quercetin and traces of isorhamnetin diglycosides and rutin. According to Žilić et al. [58], the quercetin values in maize pollen were 324.16 µg/g and 81.61 to 466.82 µg/g, respectively.

Corn silk, another by-product from corn processing, contains a wide range of bioactive compounds in the form of volatile oils, steroids, saponins, anthocyanins [59], and other natural antioxidants, such as flavonoids [52] and phenolic compounds [41,58,59]. In the corn silk powder, the high phenolic content (94.10 ± 0.26 mg GAE/g) and flavonoid content (163.93 ± 0.83 mg QE/100 g) are responsible for its high antioxidant activity [60]. About 29 flavonoids have been isolated from corn silk. Most of them are C-glycoside compounds and have the same parent nucleus as luteolin [44]. Ren et al. [61] successfully isolated and separated compounds such as 2″-O-α-L-rhamnosyl-6-C-3″-deoxyglucosyl-3′-methoxyluteolin, ax-5′-methane-3′-methoxymaysin, ax-4″-OH-3′-methoxymaysin, 6,4′-dihydroxy-3′-methoxyflavone-7-O-glucoside, and 7,4′-dihydroxy-3′-methoxyflavone-2″-O-α-L-rhamnosyl-6-C fucoside from corn silk. Moreover, among flavonoids, Haslina and Eva [43] determined in corn silk: apigmaysin, maysin, isoorientin-2″-O-α-L-rhamnoside, 3-methoxymaysine, and ax-4-OH maysin.

This richness of biologically active compounds results in advantageous properties and applications. The most important properties and the newest studies on the application are listed in Table 5.

Table 5. Biological activity and potential applications of phytochemicals obtained from corn wastes.

Material	Extract/Compound	Biological Activity/Application	References
Corn bran	tocopherols and polyphenolic compounds	- antioxidant properties - used as bioactive compounds in cosmetics or natural substitutes (antioxidants, preservatives, stabilizers, emulsifiers, and colorings) in foods to prevent potential adverse effects associated with the consumption of artificial ingredients	Galanakis [62]
Corn husk	extract	- used in the treatment of diabetes because it has shown high: - antidiabetic potential	Brobbey et al. [51]
		- anti-inflammatory effects	Roh et al. [63]
Corn stigma	extract	- antifungal and antibacterial activities against 23 of the studied microorganisms - use as a functional ingredient in the food and pharmaceutical industry	Boeira et al. [64]
Corn tassel	extract	- used as a traditional medicine in China - antioxidant capacity - the high ability to inhibit the proliferation of MGC80-3 gastric cancer cells	Wang et al. [65]
	tasselin A	- inhibition of melanin production - used as an ingredient in skin care whitener	Wille and Berhow [49]
Corn pollen	phenolic compounds	- antiradical activity	Bujang et al. [40]
	extract	- the source of functional and bioactive compounds for the nutraceutical and pharmaceutical industries	Bujang et al. [40]
		- the source of antioxidants and is high in nutrients	Žilić et al. [58]

2.3. Potato Waste

Approximately 40–50% of potatoes are not suitable for human consumption. Industrial processing of potatoes (mashed and canned potatoes, chips, fries and ready meals) creates huge amounts of peel as waste [66,67]. Potato peel is a non-edible residue generated in considerable amounts by food processing plants. Depending on the peeling process, e.g., abrasion, lye or steam peeling, the amount of waste can range between 15 and 40% of the number of processed potatoes [68]. Industrial processing produces between 70 to 140 thousand tons of peels worldwide annually, which are available to be used in other applications [69].

Potato peels differ greatly from other agricultural by-products because they are revalorized as a source of functional and bioactive compounds, including phenolic compounds, glycoalkaloids, vitamins and minerals [70] (Table 6).

Table 6. Phytochemicals identified in potato waste.

Name	MW [g mol^{-1}]	Molecular Formula	References
Phenolic acids—hydroxycinnamic acids			
p-Coumaric acid	164.04	$C_9H_8O_3$	Frontuto et al. [71]
Ferulic acid	194.18	$C_{10}H_{10}O_4$	Javed et al. [72]
Caffeic acid	180.16	$C_9H_8O_4$	Samarin et al. [73]
Chlorogenic acid	354.31	$C_{16}H_{18}O_9$	Javed et al. [72]
Sinapic acid	224.21	$C_{11}H_{12}O_5$	Mohdaly et al. [67]
Cinnamic acid	148.16	$C_9H_8O_2$	Mohdaly et al. [67]
Phenolic acids—hydroxybenzoic acids			
Gallic acid	170.12	$C_7H_6O_5$	Javed et al. [72]
Vanillic acid	168.15	$C_8H_8O_4$	Javed et al. [72]
Protocatechic acid	154.12	$C_7H_6O_4$	Frontuto et al. [71]
p-Hydroxybenzoic acid	138.12	$C_7H_6O_3$	Chamorro et al. [74]
3-Hydroxybenzoic acid	138.12	$C_7H_6O_3$	Paniagua–García et al. [75]
4-Hydroxybenzoic acid	138.12	$C_7H_6O_3$	Paniagua–García et al. [75]
2,5-Dihydroxybenzoic acid	154.12	$C_7H_6O_4$	Paniagua–García et al. [75]
Syringic acid	198.17	$C_9H_{10}O_5$	Sarwari et al. [76]
Cyclohexanecarboxylic acids			
Quinic acid	192.17	$C_7H_{12}O_6$	Wu et al. [77]
Flavonoids—flavonols			
Rutin	610.52	$C_{27}H_{30}O_{16}$	Silva–Beltran et al. [78]
Quercetin	302.24	$C_{15}H_{10}O_7$	Silva–Beltran et al. [78]
Flavonoids—anthocyanin			
Pelargonidin-3-(p-coumaryoly rutinoside)-5-glucoside	919.81	$C_{42}H_{47}O_{23}$	Chen et al. [79]
Petunidin-3-(p-coumaroyl rutinoside)-5-glucoside	933.86	$C_{43}H_{49}O_{23}$	Chen et al. [79]
Alkaloids			
α-Chaconine	852.06	$C_{45}H_{73}NO_{14}$	Ji et al. [80]
α-Solanine	868.06	$C_{45}H_{73}NO_{15}$	Ji et al. [80]
Solanidine	397.64	$C_{27}H_{43}NO$	Hossain et al. [81]
Demissidine	399.65	$C_{27}H_{45}NO$	Hossain et al. [81]
Commersonine	1048.20	$C_{51}H_{85}NO_{21}$	Rodríguez–Martínez et al. [82]
α-Tomatine	1034.19	$C_{50}H_{83}NO_{21}$	Rodríguez–Martínez et al. [82]

Potato peel is a good source of phenolic compounds because almost 50% of potato phenolics are located in the peel and adjoining tissues [74,83]. The results obtained by Wu et al. [77] showed that the potato peels contained a higher amount of phenolics than the flesh. Moreover, the polyphenols in potato peel are ten times higher than those in the pulp. Potato peel extract contains 70.82 mg of catechin equivalent (CE)/100 g of phenolic and had a high level of phenolic compounds (2.91 mg GAE/g dry weight) that was found to be greater than carrot (1.52 mg GAE/g dry weight), wheat bran (1.0 mg GAE/g dry weight), and onion (2.5 mg GAE/g dry weight) [67]. The results of Javed et al. [72] showed that the total phenolic content in potato peel ranged from 1.02 to 2.92 g/100 g and total flavonoids ranged from 0.51 to 0.96 g/100 g. Phenolic acids are the most abundant phenolic compounds in potato peel. They include derivatives of hydroxycinnamic and hydroxybenzoic acids (Table 6). Kumari et al. [84], using UHPLC-MS/MS, showed that chlorogenic and caffeic acids are important components of the free-form phenolics in potato peel. The results show that phenolic acids in potato peals are not only present in their free form but also occur in bound form. Javed et al. [72] showed that the extract of potato peel contains chlorogenic acid (753.0–821.3 mg/100 g), caffeic acid (278.0–296.0 mg/100 g), protocatechuic acid (216.0–256.0 mg/100 g), p-hydroxybenzoic acid (82.0–87.0 mg/100 g), gallic acid (58.6–63.0 mg/100 g), vanillic acid (43.0–48.0 mg/100 g), and p-coumaric acid (41.8–45.6 mg/100 g). Silva–Beltran et al. [78] showed that flavonoids such as rutin and quercetin were present in potato peel at low concentrations of 5.01 and 11.22 mg/100 g dry weight, respectively.

Many studies have noted that potato peels are excellent untapped source of steroidal alkaloids, e.g., glycoalkaloids (α-solanine and α-chaconine) and aglycone alkaloids (solanidine and demissidine; Table 6) [80,81,85]. α-solanine, α-chaconine, and the glycosides of solanidine constitute about 95% of the total potato peel glycoalkaloid content [86]. Higher amounts of these compounds were found in potato peel, unlike potato flesh [87]. There are various cultural, genetic and storage factors that influence the concentration of glycoalkaloids in potato peel [88]. Concerning cultivars, it was shown that the variety with blue flesh showed the highest concentration (5.68 mg/100 g fresh weight), followed by the red-leaved (5.26 mg/100 g fresh weight), while yellow or cream flesh. In the study of Singh et al. [89] of potato peel, glycoalkaloids were detected as 1.05 mg/100 g. The results of Rytel et al. [88] showed that the glycoalkaloid content of potato peel depends on the potato cultivar and ranges from 181 mg/kg to 3526 mg/kg of fresh potato tubers.

Besides, the peel of pigmented potatoes is an excellent source of anthocyanins, e.g., pelargonidin-3-(p-coumaryoly rutinoside)-5-glucoside and petunidin-3-(p-coumaroyl rutino side)-5-glucosid e. It has been proven that their content depends on the cultivar [90]. Ji et al. [80] showed that anthocyanidin levels were higher in the peel than in the tuber. The most important beneficial properties and potential applications of phytochemicals identified in potato waste are listed in Table 7.

Table 7. Biological activity and potential applications of phytochemicals obtained from potato wastes.

Material	Extract/Compound	Biological Activity/Application	References
Potato peel	phenolic compounds	- antioxidant activity	Singh et al. [91] Albishi et al. [83]
	extract	- used as a food preservative - pharmaceutical ingredient	Maldonado et al. [92]
		- natural food additives as an antioxidant for fresh-cut fruits	Akyol et al. [93] Venturi et al. [94]
		- food preservative - pharmaceutical ingredient	Gebrechristos and Chen [95]
		- limit oil oxidation	Amado et al. [96]
		- hepatoprotective effects, - protects erythrocytes against oxidative damage - lowers the toxicity of cholesterol oxidation products - attenuate diabetic alterations	Hsieh et al. [97]
		- protects atopic dermatitis	Yang et al. [98]
		- amylase and feed-stock for bioethanol production	Khawla et al. [99]
		- antioxidant, antibacterial, apoptotic, chemopreventive and anti-inflammatory	Wu [100]
		- bio-oil production	Liang et al. [101]
		- production of bacterial cellulose - biopolymer production	Abdelraof et al. [102]

Table 7. *Cont.*

Material	Extract/Compound	Biological Activity/Application	References
Potato waste		- antiobesity properties - used in the production of antiobesity functional food	Elkahoui et al. [103] Chimonyo [104]
		- a source of natural antioxidants against human enteric viruses (antiviral effect on the inhibition of Av-05 and MS2 bacteriophages, which were used as human enteric viral surrogates)	Silva-Beltran et al. [78]
	freeze-dried aqueous extracts	- use as food additives	Singh et al. [91]
	glycoalkaloids	- the potential of being used by the pharmaceutical industry	Apel et al. [105]
	extract	- as additives to biscuit	Khan et al. [106]
	glycoalkaloids	- precursors for the production of hormones, antibiotics and anticancer drugs - precursors for neurological and gastrointestinal disorders - anti-cancer and anti-proliferative activities in vitro	Hossain et al. [81] Hossain et al. [87] Ding et al. [107] Alves–Filho et al. [86]
	steroidal alkaloids	- biological properties such as antimicrobial, anti-inflammatory and anticarcinogenic activities	Kenny et al. [108]

2.4. Soybean Residues

Soybean waste has the potential as a sustainable source of phytochemicals and functional foods. It includes both leaves, pod pericarp, and twigs, as well as the residues after seeds processing, so-called okara. Okara is the residue of soybean milling after extraction of the aqueous fraction used for producing tofu and soy drink and presents high nutritional value [109]. The results of the last studies showed that an okara contains enough bioactive compounds that make it useful to obtain value-added products for use in food production, oil extraction, nutraceutical, pharmaceutical, and cosmetic formulations. Moreover, it was stated that okara isoflavones have good antioxidant activity. Although some nutrients like protein decrease in okara during soymilk processing, it still has many other phytochemicals and nutrients, making it their least expensive and most excellent source. Since it has good antimicrobial activity, it can be used in pharmaceutical industries, thus opening up new frontiers for drug exploration [109]. Various food enriched with okara, such as biscuits and cookies, have been mentioned in the literature [110,111]. Guimarães et al. [112] reported that food products enriched with okara contained 0.411 mg/100 mL of β-carotene and 0.15 μm/g isoflavones.

One of the main phytochemicals in soybean waste are isoflavones: daidzein, genistein, glycitein, and their glycosides (e.g., acetyl-, malonyl-, and β-glycosides) [113]. Isoflavones are compounds belonging to the flavonoid group. In addition to the well-established antioxidant effect, isoflavones exhibit estrogenic activity because of their similar structure to estrogen [113,114]. The beneficial effects of isoflavones are the prevention of hormone-dependent cancer, coronary heart disease, osteoporosis, and menopausal symptoms [114]. Kumar et al. [115] proved that daidzein expressed anticancer activity against human breast cancer cells MCF-7. The extract from soybean waste material showed total phenolic content (TPC) in the range of 27.4–167 mg GAE/g, total flavonoids from 10.4 to 63.8 mg QE/g and antioxidant activity (AOA) from 26.5% to 84.7% [114]. Moreover, their values were highest in the leaves, followed by pod pericarp and twigs. As was stated by Šibul et al. [113], soybean roots are also a good source of daidzein and genistein, as well as other phenolic compounds. The concentrations of isoflavones in roots were higher than in herbs, 1584.5 and 93.48 μg/g of dry extract, respectively. The newest study on soybean pods stated that its ethanolic extract and fractions exhibited anticancer potential against human colorectal carcinoma (HTC-116) and prostate cancer (PC-3) [116]. Moreover, it was the first analysis of this material using ultra-*high-performance liquid chromatography* coupled with electrospray ionization quadrupole time-of-flight mass spectrometry (UPLC-ESI-QTOF-MS), resulting in the identification of 50 polyphenols belonging to phenolic acids, flavonoids and other groups. The authors stated that soybean pods might be useful material as an active food additive or a component in dietary supplements and preparations with anti-radical and anti-cancer properties.

Soybean by-products are a good source of lecithin. Lecithin is a natural emulsifier that stabilizes fat and improves the texture of many food products, such as salad dressings, desserts, margarine, chocolate, and baking and cooking goods [117]. Moreover, it also has health benefits such as lowering cholesterol and low-density lipoprotein level in the human blood, improving digestion, cognitive and immune function, as well as aiding in the prevention of gall bladder and liver diseases.

Saponins are another important group of phytochemicals derived from soybean waste [113]. Soyasaponins have been linked to anti-obesity, antioxidative stress, and anti-inflammatory properties, as well as preventive effects on hepatic triacylglycerol accumulation [118]. One of the latest applications of saponins derived from soybean by-products was as eco-friendly agents for washing pesticide residues in the vegetable and fruit industries [119].

Compounds identified and quantified in soybean waste are specified in Table 8. The newest studies on the applications and properties of soybean waste are presented in Table 9.

Table 8. Phytochemicals identified and quantified in soybean waste.

Name	Soybean Residue	MW [g mol^{-1}]	$C_xH_yO_z$	Concentration	References
	Phenolic acids—hydroxybenzoic acids				
	herb			22.2–38.3 [a,b]	Šibul et al. [113]
p-Hydroxybenzoic acid	root	138.12	$C_7H_6O_3$	4.1–32.5 [a,b]	Šibul et al. [113]
	meal			51 [a]	Freitas et al. [120]
Salicylic acid	meal	138.12	$C_7H_6O_3$	38 [a]	Freitas et al. [120]
Protocatechuic acid	herb	154.12	$C_7H_6O_4$	4.4–14.4 [a,b]	Šibul et al. [113]
	root			2.35–4.71 [a,b]	
Gentisic acid	herb	154.12	$C_7H_6O_4$	<0.08–4.78 [a,b]	Šibul et al. [113]
	root			<0.08–7.17 [a,b]	
Vanillic acid	herb	168.14	$C_8H_8O_4$	<0.4–44.9 [a,b]	Šibul et al. [113]
	root			43.0–75.2 [a,b]	
	meal			91 [a]	Freitas et al. [120]
Syringic acid	herb	198.17	$C_9H_{10}O_5$	12.0–14.2 [a,b]	Šibul et al. [113]
	root			20.6–42.0 [a,b]	
	meal			81 [a]	Freitas et al. [120]
Gallic acid	meal	170.12	$C_7H_6O_5$	77 [a]	Freitas et al. [120]
	Phenolic acids—hydroxycinnamic acids				
p-Coumaric acid	herb	164.04	$C_9H_8O_3$	7.45–14.5 [a,b]	Šibul et al. [113]
	root			1.61–2.89 [a,b]	
	meal			20 [a]	Freitas et al. [120]
Ferulic acid	herb	194.18	$C_{10}H_{10}O_4$	5.89–14.0 [a,b]	Šibul et al. [113]
	root			4.55–7.66 [a,b]	
	meal			3 [a]	Freitas et al. [120]
Caffeic acid	herb	180.16	$C_9H_8O_4$	14.2–24.9 [a,b]	Šibul et al. [113]
	root			<0.08 [a]	
	meal			61 [a]	Freitas et al. [120]
Sinapic acid	meal	224.21	$C_{11}H_{12}O_5$	27 [a]	Freitas et al. [120]
	Cyclohexanecarboxylic acids				
Quinic acid	herb	192.17	$C_7H_{12}O_6$	399–532 [a,b]	Šibul et al. [113]
	root			111–249 [a,b]	

Table 8. Cont.

Name	Soybean Residue	MW [g mol^{-1}]	C$_x$H$_y$O$_z$	Concentration	References
5-O-Caffeoylquinic acid	herb	354.31	C$_{16}$H$_{18}$O$_9$	<8–235 [a,b]	Šibul et al. [113]
	root			<8 [a]	
	meal			35 [a]	Freitas et al. [120]
Flavonoids—flavonols					
Kaempferol	herb	286.23	C$_{15}$H$_{10}$O$_6$	<16–21.1 [a,b]	Šibul et al. [113]
	root			<16 [a]	
	meal			4 [a]	Freitas et al. [120]
Quercetin	herb	302.24	C$_{15}$H$_{10}$O$_7$	<16–278 [a,b]	Šibul et al. [113]
	root			<16 [a]	
Isorhamnetin	herb	316.26	C$_{16}$H$_{12}$O$_7$	<40–159 [a,b]	Šibul et al. [113]
	root			<40 [a]	
Quercitrin	herb	448.38	C$_{21}$H$_{20}$O$_{11}$	<0.06 [a]	Šibul et al. [113]
	root			<0.06 [a]	
Kaempferol 3-O-glucoside	herb	448.38	C$_{21}$H$_{20}$O$_{11}$	59.3–140 [a,b]	Šibul et al. [113]
	root			1.50–2.64 [a,b]	
Hyperoside	herb	464.38	C$_{21}$H$_{20}$O$_{12}$	<0.1–825 [a,b]	Šibul et al. [113]
	root			<0.06 [a]	
Quercetin 3-O-glucoside	herb	464.10	C$_{21}$H$_{20}$O$_{12}$	<0.06–967 [a,b]	Šibul et al. [113]
	root			<0.06 [a,b]	
Rutin	herb	610.52	C$_{27}$H$_{30}$O$_{16}$	7.05–4636 [a,b]	Šibul et al. [113]
	root			<2 [a]	
	meal			49 [a]	Freitas et al. [120]
Flavonoids—flavones					
Apigenin	herb	270.24	C$_{15}$H$_{10}$O$_5$	17.4–759 [a,b]	Šibul et al. [113]
	root			<8–22.3 [a,b]	
Baicalein	herb	270.24	C$_{15}$H$_{10}$O$_5$	27.8–745 [a,b]	Šibul et al. [113]
	root			<16–24.7 [a,b]	
Luteolin	herb	286.24	C$_{15}$H$_{10}$O$_6$	<40–194 [a,b]	Šibul et al. [113]
	root			<40 [a]	
Chrysoeriol	herb	300.26	C$_{16}$H$_{12}$O$_6$	<4–9.57 [a,b]	Šibul et al. [113]
	root			<4 [a]	
Vitexin	herb	432.38	C$_{21}$H$_{20}$O$_{10}$	1.37–2.36 [a,b]	Šibul et al. [113]
	root			1.81–3.57 [a,b]	
Apigenin 7-O-glucoside	herb	432.38	C$_{21}$H$_{20}$O$_{10}$	14.3–261 [a,b]	Šibul et al. [113]
	root			<0.2–1.99 [a,b]	
Luteolin 7-O-glucoside	herb	448.37	C$_{21}$H$_{20}$O$_{11}$	<4–145 [a,b]	Šibul et al. [113]
	root			<4 [a]	
Apiin	herb	564.49	C$_{26}$H$_{28}$O$_{14}$	<0.06–20.8 [a,b]	Šibul et al. [113]
	root			<0.06 [a]	
Flavonoids—flavanones					
Naringenin	herb	272.26	C$_{15}$H$_{12}$O$_5$	3.46–8.46 [a,b]	Šibul et al. [113]
	root			6.52–15.9 [a,b]	
	meal			25 [a]	Freitas et al. [120]
Hesperidin	meal	610.19	C$_{28}$H$_{34}$O$_{15}$	91 [a]	Freitas et al. [120]
Flavonoids—flavanols					
Catechin	herb	290.27	C$_{15}$H$_{14}$O$_6$	<0.4 [a]	Šibul et al. [113]
	root			<0.4 [a]	
Epicatechin	herb	290.27	C$_{15}$H$_{14}$O$_6$	<0.4 [a]	Šibul et al. [113]
	root			<0.4–36.3 [a,b]	
Isoflavones					
Daidzin	okara	416.38	C$_{21}$H$_{20}$O$_9$	920–1530 [b,c]	Anjum et al. [109]
	meal			350 [a]	Freitas et al. [120]

Table 8. Cont.

Name	Soybean Residue	MW [g mol^{-1}]	C$_x$H$_y$O$_z$	Concentration	References
Daidzein	okara herb root meal	254.23	C$_{15}$H$_{10}$O$_4$	310–639 [b,c] 40.7–122 [a,b] 40.5–1702 [a,b] 30 [a]	Anjum et al. [109] Šibul et al. [113] Freitas et al. [120]
Genistin	okara meal	432.37	C$_{21}$H$_{20}$O$_{10}$	3280–8360 [b,c] 490 [a]	Anjum et al. [109] Freitas et al. [120]
Genistein	okara herb root meal	270.24	C$_{15}$H$_{10}$O$_5$	380–650 [b,c] 15.1–39.2 [a,b] 159–270 [a,b] 50 [a]	Anjum et al. [109] Šibul et al. [113] Freitas et al. [120]
Glycitin	okara meal	446.40	C$_{22}$H$_{22}$O$_{10}$	450 [c] 160 [a]	Anjum et al. [109] Freitas et al. [120]
Glycitein	okara meal	284.26	C$_{16}$H$_{12}$O$_5$	58 [c] 3 [a]	Anjum et al. [109] Freitas et al. [120]
Soyasaponin B I Soyasaponin B II + III	meal meal	Saponins 943.12	C$_{48}$H$_{78}$O$_{18}$	2510 [c] 780 [c]	Silva et al. [121] Silva et al. [121]

[a] expressed in mg per kg of dry extract, [b] depending on cultivar, [c] expressed in mg per kg of residues.

Table 9. Biological activity and potential applications of phytochemicals obtained from soybean residues.

Material	Extract/Compound	Biological Activity/Application	References
okara	methanolic and ethanolic extracts	- antioxidant activity - antibacterial activity against *Bacillus subtilis, Bacillus megaterium, Escherichia coli*, and *Serratia marcescens*	Anjum et al. [109]
pod	Ethanolic extract and its 3 fractions	- antioxidant activity - anticancer activity against human colorectal carcinoma (HCT116) and prostate adenocarcinoma (PC-3)	Pabich et al. [116]
soybean by-product	saponins	- used to remove pesticides residues in fruits and vegetables	Hsu et al. [119]
defatted soy meal	isoflavones	- anti-cancerous, anti-estrogenic, anti-oxidant, anti-inflammatory, and phytoestrogen activities - preventions of cardiovascular and neurological disorders	Wang et al. [122]
soybean by-products	saponins	- insecticidal properties	
soybean meal	aqueous extract	- antioxidant activity - inhibition of lipid peroxidation - antimicrobial activity against several foodborne pathogens - antitumoral activity towards a human glioblastoma cell line	Freitas et al. [120]
soybean cake	soyasapogenol A and its microbial transformation products	- application as anti-inflammatory food supplements	Zhou et al. [123]

2.5. Tomato Residues

During the industrial processing of tomatoes, a considerable amount of waste is generated. Tomato waste consists mainly of peel, seeds, stems, leaves, fibrous parts and pulp residues [124]. The wet tomato pomace constitutes the major part of this waste, which consists of 33% seed, 27% peel and 40% pulp, while the dried pomace contains 44% seed and 56% pulp and peel [125]. When tomatoes are processed into products like ketchup, juice or sauces, 3–7% of their weight becomes waste. The management of tomato by-products is considered an important problem faced by tomato processing companies due to their disposal into the environment [126,127].

Although tomato waste has no commercial value, it is a rich source of nutrients, colorants and highly biologically active compounds such as polyphenols, carotenes, sterols, tocopherols, terpenes, and others (Table 10) [128–132]. The number of these compounds depends on tomato variety, part of the tomato residues (seed, peels, and pulp), time and extraction method, used solvent, as well as fractions gained after the isolation procedure, e.g., alkaline-hydrolyzable, acid-hydrolyzable, and bound phenolics [133]. They reported a total phenolics average of 1229.5 mg GAE/kg, of which flavonoids accounted for 415.3 mg QE/kg. The most abundant phenolic acids quantified in dried tomato waste were ellagic (143.4 mg/kg) and chlorogenic (76.3 mg/kg) acids. Other phenolic acids determined in lower concentrations were gallic, salicylic, coumaric, vanillic and syringic [133]. The levels of vanillic (26.9 mg/kg) and gallic (17.1 mg/kg) was lower than those found by Elbadrawy and Sello [134] in tomato peel (33.1 and 38.5 mg/kg, respectively). Ćetković et al. [135] identified phenolic acids (chlorogenic, p-coumaric, ferulic, caffeic and rosmarinic acid), flavonols (quercetin and rutin and its derivatives), and flavanone (naringenin derivatives) as the major phenolic compounds in extracts of tomato waste. The results obtained by Aires et al. [136] showed that the major polyphenol found in tomato wastes were kaempferol-3-O-rutinoside and caffeic acid. Several papers [135–138] reported the amounts of caffeic, chlorogenic, p-coumaric acids, kaempferol and quercetin, among other phenolic compounds found in tomato by-products. In the tomato's wastes, Di Donato et al. [139] identified two main flavonoid compunds e.g., kaempferol rutinoside and quercetin rutinoside. Rutin and chlorogenic acid were the most abundant individual phenolics found by García–Valverde et al. [140] in all studied tomato varieties.

Table 10. Phytochemicals identified in tomato wastes.

Name	MW [g mol^{-1}]	Molecular Formula	References
Phenolic acids—hydroxycinnamic acids			
Chlorogenic acid	354.31	$C_{16}H_{18}O_9$	Bakic et al. [127]
Isochlorogenic acid	354.31	$C_{16}H_{18}O_9$	Szabo et al. [141]
p-Coumaric acid	164.16	$C_9H_8O_3$	Nour et al. [133]
Ferulic acid	194.18	$C_{10}H_{10}O_4$	Perea–Dominguez et al. [131]
Caffeic acid	180.16	$C_9H_8O_4$	Aires et al. [136]
3,4,5-tricaffeoylquinic acid	678.60	$C_{34}H_{30}O_{15}$	Szabo et al. [141]
Cinnamic acid	148.16	$C_9H_8O_2$	Kalogeropoulos et al. [138]
Phloretic acid	166.18	$C_9H_{10}O_3$	Kalogeropoulos et al. [138]
Sinapic acid	224.21	$C_{11}H_{12}O_5$	Kalogeropoulos et al. [138]
Rosmarinic acid	360.31	$C_{18}H_{16}O_8$	Ćetković et al. [135]
Phenolic acids—hydroxybenzoic acids			
Gallic acid	170.12	$C_7H_6O_5$	Nour et al. [133]
Ellagic acid	302.18	$C_{14}H_6O_8$	Nour et al. [133]
Vanillic acid	168.15	$C_8H_8O_4$	Nour et al. [133]
Syringic acid	198.17	$C_9H_{10}O_5$	Nour et al. [133]
Protocatechic acid	154.12	$C_7H_6O_4$	Elbadrawy and Sello [134]
p-Hydroxybenzoic acid	138.12	$C_7H_6O_3$	Kalogeropoulos et al. [138]
Flavonoids			
Quercetin	302.24	$C_{15}H_{10}O_7$	Elbadrawy and Sello [134]
Quercetin-3-β-O-glucoside	463.40	$C_{21}H_{19}O_{12}$	Valdez–Morales et al. [142]
Quercetin-3-O-sophorosid	626.50	$C_{27}H_{30}O_{17}$	Kumar et al. [143]
Apigenin-7-O-glucoside	432.40	$C_{21}H_{20}O_{10}$	Concha-Meyer et al. [144]
Isorhamnetin	316.26	$C_{16}H_{12}O_7$	Kumar et al. [143]
Isorhamnetin-3-O-gentiobioside	640.50	$C_{28}H_{32}O_{17}$	Kumar et al. [143]

Table 10. Cont.

Name	MW [g mol^{-1}]	Molecular Formula	References
Rutin	610.52	$C_{27}H_{30}O_{16}$	Aires et al. [136]
Kaempferol	286.23	$C_{15}H_{10}O_6$	Perea–Dominguez et al. [131]
Kaempferol-3-O-rutinoside	394.52	$C_{27}H_{30}O_{15}$	Aires et al. [136]
Kaempferol-3-O-glucoside	447.37	$C_{21}H_{19}O_{11}$	Kumar et al. [143]
Myricetin	318.24	$C_{15}H_{10}O_8$	Nour et al. [133]
Naringenin	272.26	$C_{15}H_{12}O_5$	Elbadrawy and Sello [134]
Catechin	290.26	$C_{15}H_{14}O_6$	Perea–Dominguez et al. [131]
Epicatechin	290.27	$C_{15}H_{14}O_6$	Kalogeropoulos et al. [138]
Chrysin	254.24	$C_{15}H_{10}O_4$	Kalogeropoulos et al. [138]
Luteolin	286.24	$C_{15}H_{10}O_6$	Kalogeropoulos et al. [138]
Luteolin-7-O-glucoside	448.37	$C_{21}H_{20}O_{11}$	Concha–Meyer et al. [144]
Isoflavones			
Daidzein	254.23	$C_{15}H_{10}O_4$	Kumar et al. [143]
Genistein	270.24	$C_{15}H_{10}O_5$	Kumar et al. [143]
Stilbenes			
Resveratrol	228.24	$C_{14}H_{12}O_3$	Kalogeropoulos et al. [138]
Carotenoids			
Lycopene	536.89	$C_{40}H_{56}$	Fritsch et al. [130]
β-Carotene	536.89	$C_{40}H_{56}$	Kalogeropoulos et al. [138]
Sterols			
β-Sitosterol	414.72	$C_{29}H_{50}O$	Kalogeropoulos et al. [138]
Δ^5-Avenasterol	412.70	$C_{29}H_{48}O$	Kalogeropoulos et al. [138]
Campesterol	400.69	$C_{28}H_{48}O$	Kalogeropoulos et al. [138]
Cholestanol	388.70	$C_{27}H_{48}O$	Kalogeropoulos et al. [138]
Cholesterol	386.65	$C_{27}H_{46}O$	Kalogeropoulos et al. [138]
24-Oxocholesterol	400.60	$C_{27}H_{44}O_2$	Kalogeropoulos et al. [138]
Stigmasterol	412.69	$C_{29}H_{48}O$	Kalogeropoulos et al. [138]
Tocopherols			
Tocopherol			Kalogeropoulos et al. [138]
Terpenes			
Squalene	410.73	$C_{30}H_{50}$	Kalogeropoulos et al. [138]
Cycloartenol	426.72	$C_{30}H_{50}O$	Kalogeropoulos et al. [138]
β-Amyrin	426.73	$C_{30}H_{50}O$	Kalogeropoulos et al. [138]
Oleanolic acid	456.71	$C_{30}H_{48}O_3$	Kalogeropoulos et al. [138]
Ursolic acid	456.70	$C_{30}H_{48}O_3$	Kalogeropoulos et al. [138]
Palmitic acid	256.43	$C_{16}H_{32}O_2$	Elbadrawy and Sello [134]
Palmitoleic acid	254.41	$C_{16}H_{30}O_2$	Elbadrawy and Sello [134]
Stearic acid	284.48	$C_{18}H_{36}O_2$	Elbadrawy and Sello [134]
Oleic acid	282.47	$C_{18}H_{34}O_2$	Elbadrawy and Sello [134]
Linolenic acid	278.43	$C_{18}H_{30}O_2$	Elbadrawy and Sello [134]
Linoleic acid	280.45	$C_{18}H_{32}O_2$	Elbadrawy and Sello [134]
Myristic acid	228.37	$C_{14}H_{28}O_2$	Elbadrawy and Sello [134]

Traditionally, the bioactivity of tomatoes and their products has been attributed to carotenoids (β-carotene and lycopene). The results of Nour et al. [133] confirmed that dried tomato wastes contain considerable amounts of lycopene (510.6 mg/kg) and β-carotene (95.6 mg/kg) and exhibited good antioxidant properties. The results obtained by Fărcaş et al. [145] confirmed lycopene as the main carotenoid of tomato waste in a concentration between 42.18 and 70.03 mg/100 g DW (dry weight). Simultaneously, peels contain around 5 times more lycopene compared to tomato pulp [146,147]. The lycopene content in peel was 734 μg/g DW, but significant amounts of β-carotene, cis-β-carotene and lutein were also determined. The study by Górecka et al. [148] showed that tomato waste could be considered a promising source of lycopene for the production of functional foods.

Peels, as one of the main residues of tomato, are a richer source of nutrients and biologically active compounds than the pulp [137,149]. Despite of high concentration of carotenoids, peels also contain a considerable amount of polyphenols. The results obtained by Hsieh et al. [97] showed that the main flavonoids detected in fresh tomato peel were quercetin, myricctin, apigenin, catechin, puerarin, fisetin, hesperidin, naringin, rutin and their levels were reported as 4.2, 2.9, 1.9, 0.9, 0.8, 0.5, 0.3, 0.2, and 0.2 mg/100 g, respectively. It has been proven that tomato peel extracts contain high amounts of kaemferol-3-O-rutinoside (from 8.5 to 142.5 mg/kg) [127], quercetin derivatives, *p*-coumaric acid and chlorogenic acid derivative [150,151]. The main phenolic acids identified in tomato peel are protocatechuic, vanillic, gallic, catechin and caffeic acid. Their corresponding concentrations were 5.52, 3.85, 3.31, 2.98, and 0.50 mg/100 g, respectively [134]. The results of Lucera et al. [152] showed that tomato peels contain 4.90 mg/g DW of total phenolic and 2.21 mg/g DW of total flavonoids. The total polyphenolic content in tomato peels and seeds was higher than in the pulp. On the other hand, tomato peel has a very small amount of anthocyanin [153].

Tomato seeds are considered a potential natural source of antioxidants due to their rich phytochemical profile. Many publications indicate that tomato seeds contain, e.g., carotenoids, proteins, polyphenols, phytosterols, minerals and vitamin E [154]. According to Eller et al. [155], the total content of phenolic compounds in the tomato seed extract was 20.66 mg/100 g. Quercetin-3-O-sophoroside, isorhamnetin-3-O-sophoroside, and kaempferol-3-O-sophoroside were present in the highest concentrations of the total phenolic compounds. Quercetin derivatives contributed approximately 37% of the total flavonoid content. Pellicanò et al. [156] found naringenin (84.04 mg/kg DW) as the most abundant flavonoid identified, followed by caffeic acid (26.60 mg/kg DW). Apart from phenolics, carotenoids are the next class of bioactive compounds present in tomato seeds. Qualitatively, the carotenoid composition (β-carotene and lycopene isoforms: lycopene all *trans*, lycopene *cis* 1, lycopene *cis* 2, lycopene *cis* 3) in tomato seeds is similar to that of the carotenoids in tomato fruit [157].

Tomato waste has attracted great interest due to its biological activity and potential applications of phytochemicals (Table 11).

Table 11. Biological activity and potential applications of phytochemicals obtained from tomato wastes.

Material	Extract/Compound	Biological Activity/Application	References
Tomato seeds	polyphenols oil	- antioxidant activity	Zuorro et al. [154]
Tomato by-products	extract	- high nutritional quality - natural antioxidants for the formulation of functional foods or to serve as additives in food systems to elongate their shelf-life - oxidative stability of dairy products - potential nutraceutical resource - animal feed	Eller et al. [155] Savatović et al. [158] Elbadrawy and Sello [134] Nour et al. [159] Abid et al. [160] Ćetković et al. [135] Trombino et al. [161]
Tomato peel	fiber	- food supplement, improving the different chemical, physical and nutritional properties of foods	Navarro–González et al. [137]
	lycopene carotenoids	- natural color or bioactive ingredient - natural antioxidants and colorants	Ho et al. [162] Horuz and Belibagli [163]

2.6. Banana Residues

Banana (*Musa* spp., Musaceae family) is one of the main fruit crops cultivated for its edible fruits in tropical and subtropical regions. The main by-product of bananas is its peels, which represent approx. 30% of the whole fruit [164]. Moreover, banana waste also includes small-sized, damaged, or rotting fruit, leaves, stems, and pseudoparts. Banana peels are sometimes used as feedstock for livestock, goats, monkeys, poultry, rabbits, fish, zebras, and many other species. They are rich in vitamin B6, manganese, vitamin C, fiber, potassium, biotin, and copper [165], but also in phytochemicals with high antioxidant capacity such as phenolics (flavonols, hydroxycinnamic acids, gallocatechin), anthocyanin (delphinidin, cyanidin), carotenoids (β-carotenoids, α-carotenoids, and xanthophylls), catecholamines, sterols and triterpenes (Table 12). Banana peels are natural antacids and are helpful in acid reflux, heartburn, and diarrhea [165].

Table 12. Phytochemicals identified in banana wastes and their concentration.

Name	Banana Residues	MW [g mol^{-1}]	C$_x$H$_y$O$_z$	Concentration	References
Total phenolics				53,800 [a]	Kabir et al. [166]
				15,180–31,450 [a,c]	Chaudhry et al. [167]
				29,200 [a]	Rebello et al. [168]
Total flavonoids				16,440 [b]	Kabir et al. [166]
				10,800–22,110 [b,c]	Chaudhry et al. [167]
Phenolic acids—benzoic acids					
Gallic acid	banana peel	170.12	C$_7$H$_6$O$_5$	77.3 [f]	Behiry et al. [169]
Ellagic acid	banana peel	302.20	C$_{14}$H$_6$O$_8$	161.9 [f]	Behiry et al. [169]
Salicylic acid	banana peel	138.121	C$_7$H$_6$O$_3$	2.7 [f]	Behiry et al. [169]
Phenolic acids—hydroxycinnamic acids					
Chlorogenic acid	banana pseudostem and rhizome	354.31	C$_{16}$H$_{18}$O$_9$		Kandasamy et al. [170]
Ferulic acid	red banana peel			63.55 [e]	Avram et al. [171]
	yellow banana peel	194.18	C$_{10}$H$_{10}$O$_4$	34.97 [e]	Avram et al. [171]
	banana peel			16.8 [f]	Behiry et al. [169]
Sinapic acid	red banana peel	224.21	C$_{11}$H$_{12}$O$_5$	35.17 [e]	Avram et al. [171]
	yellow banana peel			19.44 [e]	Avram et al. [171]
Cinnamic acid	banana peel	148.16	C$_9$H$_8$O$_2$	0.7 [f]	Behiry et al. [169]
o-coumaric acid	banana peel	164.158	C$_9$H$_8$O$_3$	11.2 [f]	Behiry et al. [169]
Flavonoids—flavonols					
Kaempferol	red banana peel	286.239	C$_{15}$H$_{10}$O$_6$	28.80 [e]	Avram et al. [171]
	yellow banana peel			9.30 [e]	Avram et al. [171]
Quercetin	red banana peel	302.236	C$_{15}$H$_{10}$O$_7$	6.14 [e]	Avram et al. [171]
	yellow banana peel			1.14 [e]	Avram et al. [171]
Isoqercitrin	red banana peel	464.096	C$_{21}$H$_{20}$O$_{12}$	10.47 [e]	Avram et al. [171]
	yellow banana peel			14.54 [e]	Avram et al. [171]
Rutin	banana peel	610.517	C$_{27}$H$_{30}$O$_{16}$	9730.8 [f]	Behiry et al. [169]
Myricetin	banana peel	318.235	C$_{15}$H$_{10}$O$_8$	115.2 [f]	Behiry et al. [169]
Myricetin-3-rutinoside	banana peel	626.51	C$_{27}$H$_{30}$O$_{17}$	22.50 [d]	Behiry et al. [169]
Quercetin-3-rutinoside-3-rhamnoside	banana peel	756.7	C$_{33}$H$_{40}$O$_{20}$	12.91 [d]	Rebello et al. [168]
Kaempherol-3-rutinoside-3-rhamnoside	banana peel	740.7	C$_{33}$H$_{40}$O$_{19}$	5.32 [d]	Rebello et al. [168]
Quercetin-7-rutinoside	banana peel	610.5	C$_{27}$H$_{30}$O$_{16}$	8.78 [d]	Rebello et al. [168]
Quercetin-3-rutinoside	banana peel	610.5	C$_{27}$H$_{30}$O$_{16}$	29.87 [d]	Rebello et al. [168]
Kaempferol-7-rutinoside	banana peel	594.52	C$_{27}$H$_{30}$O$_{15}$	4.12 [d]	Rebello et al. [168]
Laricitrin-3-rutinoside	banana peel	640.16	C$_{28}$H$_{32}$O$_{17}$	2.22 [d]	Rebello et al. [168]
Kaempferol-3-rutinoside	banana peel	594.52	C$_{27}$H$_{30}$O$_{15}$	12.35 [d]	Rebello et al. [168]
Isorhamnetin-3-rutinoside	banana peel	624.5	C$_{28}$H$_{32}$O$_{16}$	1.31 [d]	Rebello et al. [168]
Syringetin-3-rutinoside	banana peel	654.6	C$_{29}$H$_{34}$O$_{17}$	0.63 [d]	Rebello et al. [168]
Flavonoids—flavanones					
Naringenin	banana peel			84.7 [f]	Behiry et al. [169]
Flavonoids-flavanols					
Catechin	banana peel	290.27	C$_{15}$H$_{14}$O$_6$	1.34 [d]	Rebello et al. [168]
Epicatechin	banana peel	290.27	C$_{15}$H$_{14}$O$_6$	2.55 [d]	Rebello et al. [168]
Gallocatechin	banana peel	306.27	C$_{15}$H$_{14}$O$_7$	4.20 [d]	Rebello et al. [168]
Procyanidin B1	banana peel	578.14	C$_{30}$H$_{26}$O$_{12}$	1.27 [d]	Rebello et al. [168]
Procyanidin B2	banana peel	578.14	C$_{30}$H$_{26}$O$_{12}$	81.95 [d]	Rebello et al. [168]

Table 12. Cont.

Name	Banana Residues	MW [g mol^{-1}]	$C_xH_yO_z$	Concentration	References
Procyanidin B4	banana peel	578.14	$C_{30}H_{26}O_{12}$	7.90 [d]	Rebello et al. [168]
Other compounds					
Cycloeucalenol acetate	banana pseudostem and rhizome	468.77	$C_{32}H_{52}O_2$		Kandasamy et al. [170]
4-epicyclomusalenone	banana pseudostem and rhizome	424.71	$C_{30}H_{48}O$		Kandasamy et al. [170]

[a] expressed in mg GAE kg^{-1} DM, [b] expressed in mg QE kg^{-1} DM, [c] depending on the method of extraction, [d] expressed in molar proportion (%), [e] expressed in ug/mL of crude extract, [f] expressed in mg kg^{-1} of dry extract.

Previous studies reported that the banana peel is rich in chemical compounds as antioxidant and antimicrobial activities [167–169,171]. Moreover, ethanoic extract from banana peel exhibited the strongest antihyperglycemic activity in comparison with the extract from pulp, seed, and flower [172]. Phytochemicals derived from banana peel were tested as a biofungicide against *Fusarium culmorum* and *Rhizoctonia solani* and as a bactericide against *Agrobacterium tumefaciens* for the natural preservation of wood during handling or in service. Encapsulation is successfully investigated as the method for stabilizing the banana peel extract and its bioactive compounds during storage [173].

Other phytochemical components present in the banana peel extracts, such as ethanediol and butanediol, were determined as highly reducing agents to synthesize silver nanoparticles, which are significant to the medical and chemical industries [173].

The harvesting of the fruits in the plantation requires the decapitation of the whole; therefore, the valuable banana by-products, in addition to peels, are the pseudostem, leaves, inflorescence, and fruit stalk, but also rhizome, which can also be used as a raw material for the acquisition of phytochemicals [174]. Kandasamy et al. [170] isolated three compounds from the pseudostem and rhizome of bananas, including chlorogenic acids, cycloeucalenol acetate, and 4-epicyclomusalenone. Crude extract and isolated compounds are characterized by strong antibacterial, antifungal, antiplatelet aggregation, and anticancer activities.

Using the inflorescence of bananas, anthocyanins can be obtained as good biocolorants with attractive colors, moderate stability in food systems, water solubility, and benefits for health [175]. Cyanidin-3-rutinoside, as the main compound, could be exploited as a cheap source of natural food colorant.

The newest application and explored properties of biologically active compounds from banana residues are presented in Table 13.

Table 13. Biological activity and potential applications of phytochemicals obtained from banana residues.

Material	Extract/Compound	Biological Activity/Application	References
Banana peel	extract	- as additives for formulation of bioactive compounds-rich yogurts - antioxidants activity - DPPH• scavenging activity - ABTS+• scavenging activity - α-glucosidase inhibitory activity	Kabir et al. [166]
Banana peel	acetonic, ethanoic, and methanolic extracts	- antioxidant activity - antimicrobial activity against *Staphylococcus aureus, Pseudomonas aeruginosa, Escherichia Coli, Saccharomyces cerevisiae*	Chaudhry et al. [167]

Table 13. Cont.

Material	Extract/Compound	Biological Activity/Application	References
Banana peel	extract	- application as corrosion inhibitors	Vani et al. [176]
Banana pseudostem and rhizome	crude extracts (hexane, chloroform, ethyl acetate, and methanolic) Isolates: chlorogenic acid 4-epicyclomusalenone cycloeucalenol acetate	- antioxidant activity - platelet aggregation inhibitory activity - antimicrobial activity - cytotoxicity	Kandasamy et al. [170]
Banana peel	extract	- antioxidant activity	Rebello et al. [168]
Yellow and red banana peel	hydroalcoholic extracts	- the antioxidant, cytotoxic, and antimicrobial effects	Avram et al. [170]
Banana peel	Methanolic extract	- application as biofungicide against the growth of *Fusarium culmorum* and *Rhizoctonia solani*, and as a bactericide against *Agrobacterium tumefaciens* for natural wood preservation during handling or in service.	Behiry et al. [169]
Banana peel, pulp, seed, and flower	Ethanolic extract	- very strong antioxidant activity - antihyperglycemic activity at a dose of 350 mg/kg body weight	Nofianti et al. [172]
Banana peel	Water extract contained ethanediol and butanediol	- highly reducing agent for metals used for the synthesis of silver nanoparticles	Buendía-Otero et al. [174]
Banana inflorescence		- as good biocolorants with attractive colors, moderate stability in food systems, water-solubility, and benefits for health	Padam et al. [175]

2.7. Apple Residues

Poland is the main producer of apples in the world, with an annual production of over 4 million tons [177]. About 25% of apple biomass was wasted during crop and processing. Apple pomace as a waste from apple juice and cider processing consists mainly of apple skin/flesh, seeds, and stems [178]. Until recently, apple waste was used as livestock feed, bioenergy feedstock, as well as for food supplementation and pectin extraction, but still, it is far from being used at its full potential, particularly considering its application in the pharmaceuticals and cosmetics industry [179,180]. Nonetheless, apple pomace has the potential to become a source of valuable biomaterials for agriculture. It contains numerous phytochemicals in the form of pectin and dietary fibers, but also polyphenols, triterpenoids, and volatiles. Interestingly, apple pomace is a richer source of antioxidants than fresh fruits itself because it has a significantly lower content of water; moreover, many valuable bioactive compounds are found mainly in the peels and seeds [180].

Polyphenols are the main valuable constituents of apple pomace. Waldbauer et al. [181] reported that the total phenolic content in apple pomace is in the range of 262–856 mg of total phenols/100 g. This content differs between studies due to the use of different solvents, extraction conditions, and apple varieties [182,183].

Four major phenolic groups are hydroxycinnamic acids, dihydrochalcone derivatives (phloretin and its glycosides), flavan-3-ols (catechin and procyanidins), and flavonols (quercetin and its glycosides) [184,185].

Although the phytochemical composition of apple pomace has been studied for a long time, new compounds with beneficial properties are still being isolated and identified. Ramirez-Ambrosi et al. [186] identified 52 phenolic compounds using a newly developed, rapid, selective, and sensitive strategy of ultrahigh-performance liquid chromatography with diode array detection coupled to electrospray ionization and quadrupole time-of-flight mass spectrometry (UHPLC-DAD–ESI-Q-ToF-MS) with automatic and simultaneous acquisition of exact mass at high and low collision energy. Among new compounds, two dihydrochalcones (two isomers of phloretin-pentosyl-hexosides) and three flavonols (isorhamnetin-3-O-rutinoside, isorhamnetin-3-O-pentosides and isorhamnetin-3-O-arabinofuranoside) have been tentatively identified for the first time in apple pomace.

One of the compounds newly identified in the last few years in apple pomace is monoterpene–pinnatifidanoside D [185]. This compound has been isolated for the first time from *Crataegus pinnatifida* and exhibited small antiplatelet aggregation activity.

Mohammed and Mustafa [187] and Khalil and Mustafa [188] isolated and structurally elucidated novel furanocoumarins from apple seeds. Isolated compounds exhibited promising antimicrobial activity against *Pseudomonas aeruginosa, Klebsiella pneumonia, Haemophilus influenzae, Escherichia coli, Candida albicans,* and *Aspergillus niger*.

The main compounds determined in apple by-products with ranges of their concentrations are listed in Table 14.

Table 14. Total phenolic content (TPC), total flavonoid content (TFC), and main phytochemicals identified and quantified in apple pomace.

Name	MW [g mol^{-1}]	$C_xH_yO_z$	Concentration [mg/kg dm *]	References
Total phenolic content (TPC)			2620–8560 [a]	Waldbauer [181]
			1590–10,620 [a]	Li et al. [182]
			4399–8100 [a]	Gorjanović et al. [183]
Total flavonoid content (TFC)			18,600–27,400 [b]	Gorjanović et al. [183]
	Phenolic acids—hydroxybenzoic acids			
Gallic acid	170.12	$C_7H_6O_5$	2.22–4.80 [d]	Gorjanović et al. [183]
4-hydroxybenzoic acid	137.02	$C_7H_5O_3$	17.66–69.56 [c]	Li et al. [182]
Protocatechuic acid	154.12	$C_7H_6O_4$	2.78–30.50 [c]	Li et al. [182]
p-hudroxybenzoic acid	138.22	$C_7H_6O_3$	1.16–5.80 [d]	Gorjanović et al. [183]
	Cyclohexanecarboxylic acids			
Quinic acid	192.17	$C_7H_{12}O_6$	227.4–418 [c]	Uyttebroek et al. [179]
	Phenolic acids—hydroxycinnamic acids			
Chlorogenic acid	354.31	$C_{16}H_{18}O_9$	41.80–160.40 [c]	Li et al. [182]
			89.0–308.3 [d]	Gorjanović et al. [183]
			38.9–312.8	Uyttebroek et al. [179]
			960	Pingret et al. [189]
p-coumaroylquinic acid	338.31	$C_{16}H_{18}O_8$	94	Pingret et al. [189]
Sinapic acid	224.212	$C_{11}H_{12}O_5$	2.03–7.20 [d]	Gorjanović et al. [183]
Caffeic acid	180.16	$C_9H_8O_4$	0.12–0.35 [d]	Gorjanović et al. [183]
p-Coumaric acid	164.16	$C_9H_8O_3$	2.52–23.11 [c]	Li et al. [182]
			0.32–0.76 [d]	Gorjanović et al. [183]
Ferulic acid	194.18	$C_{10}H_{10}O_4$	1.70–4.21 [c]	Li et al. [182]
			13.24–23.80 [d]	Gorjanović et al. [183]
	Flavonoids—flavonols			
Rutin	610.52	$C_{27}H_{30}O_{16}$	7.99–46.93 [d]	Gorjanović et al. [183]
			19.32	Oleszek et al. [185]
			2.24–3.26 [c]	Uyttebroek et al. [179]
			10 [b]	Pingret et al. [189]
Quercetin	302.24	$C_{15}H_{10}O_7$	7.2–14.2 [d]	Gorjanović et al. [183]
			25.2 [e]	Oleszek et al. [185]
Quercetin-3-O-galactoside	464.38	$C_{21}H_{20}O_{12}$	80.8–165.2 [d]	Gorjanović et al. [183]
Quercetin-3-O-pentosyl	434.35	$C_{20}H_{18}O_{11}$	44.8 [e]	Oleszek et al. [185]
Hyperoside	464.38	$C_{21}H_{20}O_{12}$	434 [e]	Oleszek et al. [185]
			122 [b]	Pingret et al. [189]
Isoquercetin	464.38	$C_{21}H_{20}O_{12}$	70 [e]	Oleszek et al. [185]
			42	Pingret et al. [189]
Quercitrin	448.38	$C_{21}H_{20}O_{11}$	442.4 [e]	Oleszek et al. [185]
			70.14–109.5 [c]	Uyttebroek et al. [179]
			40 [b]	Pingret et al. [189]

Table 14. Cont.

Name	MW [g mol^{-1}]	C$_x$H$_y$O$_z$	Concentration [mg/kg dm *]	References
Isoquercitrin	464.0955	C$_{21}$H$_{20}$O$_{12}$	10.65–15.5 [c] 285.6 [e]	Uyttebroek et al. [179] Oleszek et al. [185]
Avicularin	434.35	C$_{20}$H$_{18}$O$_{11}$	81.6–125.7 24	Uyttebroek et al. [179] Pingret et al. [189]
Reynoutrin	434.35	C$_{20}$H$_{18}$O$_{11}$	145.6 [e] 54 [b]	Oleszek et al. [185] Pingret et al. [189]
Isorhamnetin			1.10–17.62 [d]	Gorjanović et al. [183]
Isorhamnetin-3-O-arabinofuranoside	478.41	C$_{22}$H$_{22}$O$_{12}$		Ramirez–Ambrosi et al. [186]
isorhamnetin-3-O-pentoside	478.41	C$_{22}$H$_{22}$O$_{12}$		Ramirez–Ambrosi et al. [186]
Isorhamnetin-3-O-rutinoside	624.55	C$_{28}$H$_{32}$O$_{16}$	0.10–1.11 [d]	Gorjanović et al. [183]
Isorhamnetin-3-O-rhamnoside	462.41	C$_{22}$H$_{22}$O$_{11}$		Ramirez–Ambrosi et al. [186]
Kaempferol	286.24	C$_{15}$H$_{10}$O$_{6}$	0.62–2.46 [d]	Gorjanović et al. [183]
Kaempferol-7-O-glucoside	448.38	C$_{21}$H$_{20}$O$_{11}$	0.03–1.19 [d]	Gorjanović et al. [183]
Quercetin-3-O-rhamnoside	448.38	C$_{21}$H$_{20}$O$_{11}$	34.1–121.9 [d]	Gorjanović et al. [183]
Guajavarin	434.353	C$_{20}$H$_{18}$O$_{11}$	161 [b]	Pingret et al. [189]
Hyperin	463.371	C$_{21}$H$_{19}$O$_{12}$	64.02–92.4 [c]	Uyttebroek et al. [179]
Flavonoids—flavanonols				
Taxifolin	304.254	C$_{15}$H$_{12}$O$_{7}$	0.16–0.46 [d]	Gorjanović et al. [183]
Flavonoids—flavanols				
Catechin	290.27	C$_{15}$H$_{14}$O$_{6}$	1.50–31.70 [c] 1.05–7.45 [c] 52	Li et al. [182] Uyttebroek et al. [179] Pingret et al. [189]
Epicatechin	290.27	C$_{15}$H$_{14}$O$_{6}$	34.4–166.3 [c] 244	Uyttebroek et al. [179] Pingret et al. [189]
Procyanidin	594.53	C$_{30}$H$_{26}$O$_{13}$	2900 3408	Fernandes et al. [178] Pingret et al. [189]
Procyanidin B2	578.52	C$_{30}$H$_{26}$O$_{12}$	42.8–208.1	Uyttebroek et al. [179]
Naringenin	272.26	C$_{15}$H$_{12}$O$_{5}$	0.11–0.24 [d]	Gorjanović et al. [183]
Eriodictyol	288.26	C$_{15}$H$_{12}$O$_{6}$	0.11–0.21 [d]	Gorjanović et al. [183]
Naringin	580.541	C$_{27}$H$_{32}$O$_{14}$	0.22–0.60 [d]	Gorjanović et al. [183]
Flavonoids—flavones				
Apigenin	270.24	C$_{15}$H$_{10}$O$_{5}$	0.31–0.48 [d]	Gorjanović et al. [183]
Apigenin-7-O-glucoside	432.38	C$_{21}$H$_{20}$O$_{10}$	0.47–1.01 [d]	Gorjanović et al. [183]
Chrysin	254.25	C$_{15}$H$_{10}$O$_{4}$	0.11–0.22 [d]	Gorjanović et al. [183]
Luteolin	286.24	C$_{15}$H$_{10}$O$_{6}$	0.10–0.26 [d]	Gorjanović et al. [183]
Flavonoids—dihydrochalcones				
Phloretin	274.26	C$_{15}$H$_{14}$O$_{5}$	0.29–0.98 [d]	Gorjanović et al. [183]
Phlorizin	436.4	C$_{21}$H$_{24}$O$_{10}$	112–215 [d] 361.2 [f] 56.8–198.6 [c] 1008	Gorjanović et al. [183] Oleszek et al. [185] Uyttebroek et al. [179] Pingret et al. [189]
Phloretin 2-O-glucoside	452.41	C$_{21}$H$_{24}$O$_{11}$		Ramirez–Ambrosi et al. [186]
Phloretin -xylosyl-glucoside	568.52	C$_{26}$H$_{32}$O$_{14}$	142	Pingret et al. [189]
3-hydroxyphloretin-2'-O-xylosylglucoside	584.52	C$_{26}$H$_{32}$O$_{15}$		Ramirez–Ambrosi et al. [186]
3-hydroxyphloretin-2'-O-glucoside	452	C$_{21}$H$_{24}$O$_{11}$		Ramirez–Ambrosi et al. [186]
Coumarins **				
Aesculin	340.282	C$_{15}$H$_{16}$O$_{9}$	5.53–10.67	Gorjanović et al. [183]
(E)-12-(2'-Chlorovinyl) bergapten	277.5	C$_{14}$H$_{10}$O$_{4}$Cl		Mohammed and Mustafa [187]

Table 14. Cont.

Name	MW [g mol^{-1}]	C$_x$H$_y$O$_z$	Concentration [mg/kg dm *]	References
		Flavonoids—flavanones		
12-(1′,1′-dihydroxyethyl) bergapten	276	C$_{14}$H$_{12}$O$_6$		Mohammed and Mustafa [187]
12-(2′-chloropropan-2′-yl)-8-hydroxybergapten	308.5	C$_{15}$H$_{13}$O$_5$Cl		Mohammed and Mustafa [187]
12-Hydroxy-11-chloromethylbergapten	332.5	C$_{13}$H$_9$O$_5$Cl		Mohammed and Mustafa [187]
officinalin	220	C$_{11}$H$_8$O$_5$		Khalil and Mustafa [188]
8-(tert-butyl)officinalin	276	C$_{15}$H$_{16}$O$_5$		Khalil and Mustafa [188]
8-Hydroxyofficinalin	236	C$_{11}$H$_8$O$_6$		Khalil and Mustafa [188]
Officinalin-8-acetic acid	278	C$_{13}$H$_{10}$O$_7$		Khalil and Mustafa [188]
8-(2′-hydroxypropan-2′-yl) officinalin	289	C$_{15}$H$_{16}$O$_6$		Khalil and Mustafa [188]
		Triterpenoids		
α-amyrin	426.72	C$_{30}$H$_{50}$O	94.0	Woźniak et al. [190]
β-amyrin	426.72	C$_{30}$H$_{50}$O	41.4	Woźniak et al. [190]
Uvaol	442.72	C$_{30}$H$_{50}$O$_2$	53.9	Woźniak et al. [190]
Erythtodiol	442.72	C$_{30}$H$_{50}$O$_2$	18.0	Woźniak et al. [190]
Ursolic aldehyde	440.70	C$_{30}$H$_{48}$O$_2$	73.9	Woźniak et al. [190]
Ursolic acid	456.70	C$_{30}$H$_{48}$O$_3$	7125.1	Woźniak et al. [190]
Oleanolic acid	456.70	C$_{30}$H$_{48}$O$_3$	1591.4	Woźniak et al. [190]
Pomolic acid	472.70	C$_{30}$H$_{48}$O$_4$	870.3	Woźniak et al. [190]
		Pigments ***		
all-trans-neoxanthin	600.884	C$_{40}$H$_{56}$O$_4$	1.14–7.11 [d]	Delgado–Pelayo [191]
all-trans-violaxanthin	600.870	C$_{40}$H$_{56}$O$_4$	1.70–18.26 [d]	Delgado–Pelayo [191]
9-cis-violaxanthin	600.870	C$_{40}$H$_{56}$O$_4$	0.23–2.37 [d]	Delgado–Pelayo [191]
9-cis-Neoxanthin	600.884	C$_{40}$H$_{56}$O$_4$	0.56–21.92 [d]	Delgado–Pelayo [191]
13-cis-violaxanthin	600.884	C$_{40}$H$_{56}$O$_4$	0.10–0.29 [d]	Delgado–Pelayo [191]
all-trans-antheraxanthin	584.885	C$_{40}$H$_{56}$O$_3$	0.09–0.57 [d]	Delgado–Pelayo [191]
all-trans-zeaxanthin	568.886	C$_{40}$H$_{56}$O$_2$	0.08–0.52 [d]	Delgado–Pelayo [191]
all-trans-lutein	568.871	C$_{40}$H$_{56}$O$_2$	1.32–61.53 [d]	Delgado–Pelayo [191]
9-cis-lutein	568.871	C$_{40}$H$_{56}$O$_2$	0.06–1.61 [d]	Delgado–Pelayo [191]
13-cis-lutein	568.871	C$_{40}$H$_{56}$O$_2$	0.10–2.76 [d]	Delgado–Pelayo [191]
all-trans-β-carotene	536.8726	C$_{40}$H$_{56}$	1.49–30.31 [d]	Delgado–Pelayo [191]
Monoestrified xanthophylls			3.01–10.18 [d]	Delgado–Pelayo [191]
Diesterified xanthophylls			4.93–38.39 [d]	Delgado–Pelayo [191]
Chlorophyll a	893.509	C$_{55}$H$_{72}$MgN$_4$O$_5$	18.39–1049.26 [d]	Delgado–Pelayo [191]
Chlorophyll b	907.492	C$_{55}$H$_{70}$MgN$_4$O$_6$	4.78–309.86 [d]	Delgado–Pelayo [191]
		Other compounds		
Resveratrol	228.24	C$_{14}$H$_{12}$O$_3$	0.16–0.89	Gorjanović et al. [183]
Pterostilbene	256.296	C$_{16}$H$_{16}$O$_3$	0.19–0.90	Gorjanović et al. [183]
Pinocembrin	256.25	C$_{15}$H$_{12}$O$_4$	0.22–0.39	Gorjanović et al. [183]
Palmitic acid	256.4	C$_{16}$H$_{32}$O$_2$	7.25 [f]	Walia [192]
Linoleic acid	280.45	C$_{18}$H$_{32}$O$_2$	43.81 [f]	Walia [192]
Oleic acid	282.47	C$_{18}$H$_{34}$O$_2$	46.50 [f]	Walia [192]
Stearic acid	284.48	C$_{18}$H$_{36}$O$_2$	1.72 [f]	Walia [192]
Arachidic acid	312.54	C$_{20}$H$_{40}$O$_2$	0.72 [f]	Walia [192]
Pinnatifidanoside D	518	C$_{24}$H$_{38}$O$_{12}$	344.4	Oleszek et al. [185]

* dm—dry matter, [a] expressed as mg gallic acid equivalent, [b] expressed as quercetin equivalent, [c] depending on the methods of extraction or apple pressing, [d] depending on apple varieties, [e] expressed as rutin equivalent, [f] expressed in % of the oil extracted from apple seeds, ** determined in seeds, *** determined in peels.

Many have been written about the application of apple pomace itself. However, the present work concerns the properties and application of bioactive compounds derived from apple pomace. The newest studies reported valuable activities and interesting applications of phytochemicals from apple pomace are listed in Table 15. Preclinical studies have found apple pomace extracts and isolated compounds improved lipid metabolism, antioxidant status, and gastrointestinal function and had a positive effect on metabolic disorders (e.g., hyperglycemia, insulin resistance, etc.) [193]. As was reported by Gołębiewska et al. [194], despite medicine and cosmetics, apple pomace phytochemicals found recent applications in building and construction industries as green corrosion inhibitors and wood protectors [194].

Table 15. Biological activity and potential applications of phytochemicals obtained from apple residues.

Material	Extract/Compound	Biological Activity/Application	References
Apple seeds	coumarins	- antioxidant activity - antitumor activity	Khalil and Mustafa [188]
Apple pomace	phenolic-rich fractions: phloridzin, phloretin, quercitrin, and quercetin as major constituents	- anti-inflammatory, cytotoxic activity, anticancer activity (SiHa, KB, and HT-29 cell lines)	Rana et al. [195]
Apple pomace	crude extract and four fractions	- antioxidant activity - antifungal activity against crop pathogens: *Neosartorya fischeri*, *Fusarium oxysporum*, *Botrytis* sp. *Petriella setifera*	Oleszek et al. [185]
Flour from apple pomace	ethanolic extract	antioxidant, antidiabetic, and antiobesity effects	Gorjanović et al. [183]
Apple pomace	Ursolic acid	antimicrobial, anti-inflammatory, and antitumor activities	Cargnin et al. [196]
Apple peel	ursolic acid	antimalarial activity	Silva et al. [197]
Apple pomace	ethanolic extract: 5-O-caffeoylquinic acid as the major compound	- antioxidant and antimicrobial activity (against *Propionibacterium acnes*) - application in dermal formulations	Arraibi et al. [198]
Apple pomace	Extracts (boiling water with 1% acetic acid) and fractions (polyphenols and carbohydrates)	- antioxidant activity - anti-inflammatory activity - application as a food ingredient in yogurt formulation	Fernandes et al. [178]
Apple pomace	phloretin, phloridzin	antioxidant and antibacterial activity (*Staphylococcus aureus*, *Escherichia coli*)	Zhang et al. [199]
Apple pomace	Phloridzin oxidation products (POP)	application as natural yellow pigments in gelled desserts	Haghighi and Rezaei [200]
Apple pomace	Phloridzin oxidation products (POP)	- strong antioxidant activity - application as a yellow pigment	Liu et al. [201]
Apple peel	extract	- application as corrosion inhibitor for carbon steel	Vera et al. [202]

Phenolic content is related to the antioxidant properties of apple pomace, and procyanidins are considered the major contributors to the antioxidant capacity of apples. Despite high concentrations in apples, catechins and procyanidins are very often absent in the extract from apple pomace. The exposure of polyphenols to polyphenoloxidase during apple processing caused, in addition to native apple phytochemicals, their oxidation products also represent a significant part of the overall polyphenolic fraction. Moreover, the polyphenols can interact non-covalently with polysaccharides; thus, they become non-extractable. Fernandes et al. [178] reported that such complexes represented up to 40% of the available polyphenols from apple pomace, potentially relevant for agro-food waste valuation. Moreover, it has been revealed that the use of appropriate extraction procedures, such as microwave-superheated water extraction (MWE) of the hot water/acetone, as well as additional hydrolysis, made it possible to recover these valuable compounds from apple pomace. This knowledge will allow for designing more diversified solutions for agro-food waste valuation [178]. The strong antioxidant in apple pomace is quercetin, which has protective effects against breast and colon cancer, as well as heart and liver diseases [203].

Apple is a unique plant in the *Rosaceae* family due to the high content of phloridzin, a major phenolic compound in commercial varieties of apples [203]. Phloridzin has antidiabetic potential and could be applied as a natural sweetening agent [200]. Phloridzin from apple waste was also tested as the substrate for the production of food dye through its enzymatic oxidation. The yellow product, so-called phloridzin oxidation products (POP), turned out to be a good alternative to tartrazine and other potentially toxic food yellow pigments [200,201].

Interesting phytochemicals of apple pomace are triterpenoids, particularly ursolic acid. It has attracted attention because of its therapeutic potential associated with several functional properties such as antibacterial, antiprotozoal, anti-inflammatory, and antitumor [196]. Woźniak et al. [190] optimized the method of its extraction using supercritical carbon dioxide. The data obtained allowed the prediction of the extraction curve for the process conducted on a larger scale.

As has been mentioned previously, apple pomace contains some amount of seeds. Walia et al. [192] proved that also apple seed oil could be a promising raw material for the production of natural antioxidants and anticancer agents. The authors tested the fatty acid composition and physicochemical and antioxidant properties of oil extracted from apple seeds separated from industrial pomace. The dominant fatty acids were oleic acid (46.50%) and linoleic acid (43.81%).

The major constituent in apple seed is also amygdalin, which may be metabolized to toxic hydrogen cyanide [203,204]. However, in the literature, there are also several reports of the positive pharmacological activity of amygdalin. Luo et al. [205] showed its antifibrotic properties in the case of liver fibrosis. Song and Xu [206] proved that amygdalin exhibits analgesic effects in mice, probably by inhibiting prostaglandins E2 and nitric oxide synthesis. Despite so many above reports, there is still a need for human and animal studies to confirm the protection against the disease's effects of apple pomace.

2.8. Winery Waste

The major winery by-products are grape pomace and marc, including seeds, pulp, skins, stems, and leaves. Bioactive phytochemicals present in residues from wine-making are mainly represented by polyphenols belonging to various groups of compounds, such as phenolic acids (hydroxybenzoic acids and hydroxycinnamic acids), flavonoids (flavanols or flavan-3-ols, anthocyanins, proanthocyanidins, flavones, and flavonols), and stilbenes and anthocyanins. The relative concentrations of the different phenolic compounds are influenced by genotype (red or white grapes), a distinct fraction of residues, as well as agro-climatic conditions [207]. The presence of polyphenolic compounds in grape residues supports the potential of the investigation and valorization of this agro-industrial waste. The compounds identified in grapes by-products with their concentrations are listed in Table 16.

Table 16. Phytochemicals identified and quantified in grape residues.

Name	MW [g mol^{-1}]	$C_xH_yO_z$	Concentration [mg/kg dm]	References
Total phenolic content (TPC)			280–7770 [b,e,f]	Pintać et al. [208]
			14,200–26,700 [a,e]	Eyiz et al. [209]
Total flavonoid content (TFC)			40–1150 [b,e,f]	Pintać et al. [208]
			2403–4178 [a,e]	Eyiz et al. [209]
Total monomeric anthocyanins			539–1598 [a,e]	Eyiz et al. [209]
Total proanthocyanidin			3.23–6.32 [a,e]	Eyiz et al. [209]
Phenolic acids—hydroxybenzoic acid				

Table 16. Cont.

Name	MW [g mol^{-1}]	C$_x$H$_y$O$_z$	Concentration [mg/kg dm]	References
Gallic acid	170.12	C$_7$H$_6$O$_5$	24–246 [a,e] 250 [a] 4.86–70 [a,e,f] 75.5 [a] 596.36 [a] 3030 [c]	Farías–Campomanes et al. [210] Wang et al. [211] Pintać et al. [208] Daniel et al. [212] Wittenauer et al. [213] Jara-Palacios et al. [214]
Digalloylquinic acid	496.4	C$_{21}$H$_{20}$O$_{14}$	299 [a]	Gonçalves et al. [215]
Ellagic acid	302.197	C$_{14}$H$_6$O$_8$	620 [a] 8.37–64.1 [b,e,f] 4.315 [a]	Wang et al. [211] Pintać et al. [208] Daniel et al. [212]
Protocatechuic acid	154.12	C$_7$H$_6$O$_4$	9–63 [a,e] 940 [c]	Farías–Campomanes et al. [210] Jara–Palacios et al. [214]
Vanillic acid	168.15	C$_8$H$_8$O$_4$	24–237 [a,e] 0.53–13.0 [b,e,f] 10 [a]	Farías–Campomanes et al. [210] Pintać et al. [208] Daniel et al. [212]
4-hydroxybenzoic acid	138.122	C$_7$H$_6$O$_3$	9–63 [a,e] 0.16–1.71 [b,e,f]	Farías–Campomanes et al. [210] Pintać et al. [208]
Syringic acid	198.17	C$_9$H$_{10}$O$_5$	48–593 [a,e] 0.13–20.6 [b,e,f]	Farías–Campomanes et al. [210] Pintać et al. [208]
Galloylshikimic acid	326.25	C$_{14}$H$_{14}$O$_9$	438.1 [a]	Gonçalves et al. [215]
Phenolic acids—hydroxycinnamic acid				
Chlorogenic acid	354.31	C$_{16}$H$_{18}$O$_9$	0.14–11.50 [b,e,f] 4.715 [a]	Pintać et al. [208] Daniel et al. [212]
Caffeic acid	180.16	C$_9$H$_8$O$_4$	0.41–1.68 [b,e,f] 9.735 [a] 630 [c] 735.32 [a]	Pintać et al. [208] Daniel et al. [212] Jara-Palacios et al. [214] Wittenauer et al. [213]
Caftaric acid	312.23	C$_{13}$H$_{12}$O$_9$	880 [c] 11–168 [a,g]	Jara-Palacios et al. [214] Jara-Palacios et al. [216]
cis-Coutaric acid	296.23	C$_{13}$H$_{12}$O$_8$	5.3–11.8 [a,g]	Jara-Palacios et al. [216]
trans-coutaric	296.23	C$_{13}$H$_{12}$O$_8$	5.5–20.7 [a,g]	Jara-Palacios et al. [216]
p-Coumaric acid	164.16	C$_9$H$_8$O$_3$	6–39 [a,e] 0.13–1.49 [b,e,f] 8.175 [a] 510 [c]	Farías–Campomanes et al. [210] Pintać et al. [208] Daniel et al. [212] Jara-Palacios et al. [214]
Flavonoids—flavonols				
Quercetin	302.236	C$_{15}$H$_{10}$O$_7$	3–15 [a,e] 11.3–78.9 [b,e,f] 200 [a] 2.473–15.637 [c] 4.7 [a] 2870 [c] 344–403 [c,f]	Farías–Campomanes et al. [210] Pintać et al. [208] Wang et al. [211] Balea et al. [217] Daniel et al. [212] Jara-Palacios et al. [214] Drosou et al. [218]
Quercetin-3-O-glucoside	463.371	C$_{21}$H$_{19}$O$_{12}$	0.39–38.0 [b,e,f] 67.6 [a] 2374.32 [a] 16,900 [c] 475–609 [c,f]	Pintać et al. [208] Gonçalves et al. [215] Wittenauer et al. [213] Jara-Palacios et al. [214] Drosou et al. [218]
Quercetin-3-O-glucuronide	478.362	C$_{21}$H$_{18}$O$_{13}$	13.4 [a] 2432.29 [a] 15,800 [c] 990–1285 [c,f]	Gonçalves et al. [215] Wittenauer et al. [213] Jara-Palacios et al. [214] Drosou et al. [218]
Quercetin-3-O-pentoside	434.35	C$_{20}$H$_{18}$O$_{11}$	52.0 [a]	Gonçalves et al. [215]
Quercetin-3-O-rhamnoside	448.4	C$_{21}$H$_{20}$O$_{11}$	49.4 [a]	Gonçalves et al. [215]
Quercetin-3-O-galactoside			2120 [c]	Jara-Palacios et al. [214]
Hyperoside	464.38	C$_{21}$H$_{20}$O$_{12}$	0.17–5.67 [b,e,f]	Pintać et al. [208]

Table 16. Cont.

Name	MW [g mol^{-1}]	$C_xH_yO_z$	Concentration [mg/kg dm]	References
Rutin	610.52	$C_{27}H_{30}O_{16}$	0.11–8.19 [b,e,f] 2.136 [c] 5.3 [a] 690 [c]	Pintać et al. [208] Balea et al. [217] Daniel et al. [212] Jara–Palacios et al. [214]
Isorhamnetin	316.265	$C_{16}H_{12}O_7$	6.42–72.9 [b,e,f]	Pintać et al. [208]
Isorhamnetin 3-O-glucoside	478.406	$C_{22}H_{22}O_{12}$	66.3 [a] 145–175 [c,f]	Gonçalves et al. [215] Drosou et al. [218]
Myricetin	318.24	$C_{15}H_{10}O_8$	170 [a] 0.21–2.31 [b,e,f] 0.341–1.029 [c] 452–711 [c,f]	Wang et al. [211] Pintać et al. [208] Balea et al. [217] Drosou et al. [218]
Myricetin-3-O-hexoside	480.38	$C_{21}H_{20}O_{13}$	184.6 [a]	Gonçalves et al. [215]
Myricetin-3-O-glucoside	480.38	$C_{21}H_{20}O_{13}$	781–1044 [c]	Drosou et al. [218]
Quercitrin	448.38	$C_{21}H_{20}O_{11}$	0.21–3.99 [b,e,f]	Pintać et al. [208]
Laricitrin-O-hexoside	494.405	$C_{22}H_{22}O_{13}$	46.8 [a] 216–434 [c,f]	Gonçalves et al. [215] Drosou et al. [218]
Kaemferol	286.239	$C_{15}H_{10}O_6$	80 [a] 2.45–53.1 [b,e,f] 3.38–5.74 [c] 150 [c]	Wang et al. [211] Pintać et al. [208] Balea et al. [217] Jara–Palacios et al. [214]
Kaempferol 3-O-glucoside	448.38	$C_{21}H_{20}O_{11}$	0.05–23.0 [b,e,f] 3670 [c]	Pintać et al. [208] Jara–Palacios et al. [214]
Kaempferol 3-glucuronide	462.4	$C_{21}H_{18}O_{12}$	310 [c]	Jara–Palacios et al. [214]
Syringetin 3-glucoside	508.432	$C_{23}H_{24}O_{13}$	168–200 [c,f]	Drosou et al. [218]
Quercitrin	448.38	$C_{21}H_{20}O_{11}$	3.272–14.952 [c]	Balea et al. [217]
Isoquercitrin	464.0955	$C_{21}H_{20}O_{12}$	2.429–65.698 [c]	Balea et al. [217]
Flavonoids—flavanols				
Catechin	290.27	$C_{15}H_{14}O_6$	1460 [a] 5.01–193 [b,e,f] 945 [a] 1101.7 [a] 10,496.63 [a] 12,200 [c]	Wang et al. [211] Pintać et al. [208] Gonçalves et al. [215] Daniel et al. [212] Wittenauer et al. [213] Jara–Palacios et al. [214]
Epicatechin	290.271	$C_{15}H_{14}O_6$	1280 [a] 5.80–309 [b,e,f] 949 [a] 322.5 [a] 8994.93 [a] 6340 [c]	Wang et al. [211] Pintać et al. [208] Gonçalves et al. [215] Daniel et al. [212] Wittenauer et al. [213] Jara–Palacios et al. [214]
Epigallocatechin	306.27	$C_{15}H_{14}O_7$	900 [a]	Wang et al. [211]
Procyanidin dimers	578.1424	$C_{30}H_{26}O_{12}$	3306 [a]	Gonçalves et al. [215]
Procyanidin trimers	866.77	$C_{45}H_{38}O_{18}$	1105 [a] 12,920 [c]	Gonçalves et al. [215] Jara–Palacios et al. [214]
Procyanidin tetramer	1155.0	$C_{60}H_{50}O_{24}$	806 [a] 16,540 [c]	Gonçalves et al. [215] Jara–Palacios et al. [214]
Procyanidin B1	578.1424	$C_{30}H_{26}O_{12}$	4858.58 [c] 15,500 [c]	Wittenauer et al. [213] Jara–Palacios et al. [214]
Procyanidin B2	578.1424	$C_{30}H_{26}O_{12}$	4277.04 [c] 4940 [c]	Wittenauer et al. [213] Jara–Palacios et al. [214]
Procyanidin B3	578.1424	$C_{30}H_{26}O_{12}$	4350 [c]	Jara–Palacios et al. [214]
Procyanidin B4	578.1424	$C_{30}H_{26}O_{12}$		Jara–Palacios et al. [216]
Flavonoids—flavones				
Apigenin	270.24	$C_{15}H_{10}O_5$	0.58 [b]	Pintać et al. [208]
Apigenin 7-O-glucoside	432.38	$C_{21}H_{20}O_{10}$	0.02–12.7 [b,e,f]	Pintać et al. [208]
Luteolin	286.24	$C_{15}H_{10}O_6$	0.23–1.07 [b,e,f]	Pintać et al. [208]
Luteolin-7-O-glucoside	448.38	$C_{21}H_{20}O_{11}$	0.36–4.46 [b,e,f]	Pintać et al. [208]

Table 16. Cont.

Name	MW [g mol^{-1}]	C$_x$H$_y$O$_z$	Concentration [mg/kg dm]	References
		Flavonoids—flavanones		
Chrysoeriol	300.27	C$_{16}$H$_{12}$O$_6$	0.04–0.51 [b,e,f]	Pintać et al. [208]
Naringenin	272.26	C$_{15}$H$_{12}$O$_5$	0.11–0.83 [b,e,f]	Pintać et al. [208]
		Flavonoids-flavanonols		
Astilbin	450.396	C$_{21}$H$_{22}$O$_{11}$	3120–4200 [b,e]	Negro et al. [219]
		Flavonoids—anthocyanins		
Delphinidin 3-O-glucoside	465.387	C$_{21}$H$_{21}$O$_{12}$	4.68–54.7 [b,e,f]	Pintać et al. [208]
			775–936 [c,f]	Drosou et al. [218]
			7–57 [a,e]	Negro et al. [219]
Cyanidin 3-O-glucoside	449.388	C$_{21}$H$_{21}$O$_{11}$	2.21–11.3 [b,e,f]	Pintać et al. [208]
			3–37 [b,e]	Negro et al. [219]
Petunidin-3-O-glucoside	479.41	C$_{22}$H$_{23}$O$_{12}$	1.28–35.4 [b,e,f]	Pintać et al. [208]
			77.0 [a]	Gonçalves et al. [215]
			1295–1618 [c,f]	Drosou et al. [218]
Peonidin-3-O-glucoside	463.41	C$_{22}$H$_{23}$O$_{11}$	1.51–64.7 [b,e,f]	Pintać et al. [208]
			202.2 [a]	Gonçalves et al. [215]
			1591–2044 [c,f]	Drosou et al. [218]
Malvidin 3-glucoside	493.441	C$_{23}$H$_{25}$O$_{12}$	0.80–384 [b,e,f]	Pintać et al. [208]
			443.0 [a]	Gonçalves et al. [215]
			12,182–17,687 [c,f]	Drosou et al. [218]
Peonidin-3-O-acetyl glucoside	505.4	C$_{24}$H$_{25}$O$_{12}^+$	90.2 [a]	Gonçalves et al. [215]
Malvidin 3-O-acetyl glucoside	535.5	C$_{25}$H$_{27}$O$_{13}^+$	96.2 [a]	Gonçalves et al. [215]
			937–1182 [c,f]	Drosou et al. [218]
Malvidin 3-caffeoyl glucoside	655.6	C$_{32}$H$_{31}$O$_{15}$	1079–1450 [c,f]	Drosou et al. [218]
Petunidin 3-coumaroyl glucoside	625.5536	C$_{31}$H$_{29}$O$_{14}$	735–806 [c,f]	Drosou et al. [218]
Peonidin 3-coumaroyl glucoside	609.5542	C$_{31}$H$_{29}$O$_{13}$	796–1231 [c,f]	Drosou et al. [218]
Malvidin-3-coumaroyl glucoside	639.58	C$_{32}$H$_{31}$O$_{14}$	4700–7232 [c,f]	Drosou et al. [218]
Delphinidin	303.24	C$_{15}$H$_{11}$O$_7$	5570 [a]	Wang et al. [211]
Cyanidin	287.24	C$_{15}$H$_{11}$O$_6$	3620 [a]	Wang et al. [211]
Petunidin	317.27	C$_{16}$H$_{13}$O$_7$	15,500 [a]	Wang et al. [211]
Peonidin	301.27	C$_{16}$H$_{13}$O$_6$	25,320 [a]	Wang et al. [211]
Malvidin	331.30	C$_{17}$H$_{15}$O$_7$	10,390 [a]	Wang et al. [211]
		Terpenoids		
Ursolic acid	456.70	C$_{30}$H$_{48}$O$_3$	0.96–606 [b,e,f]	Pintać et al. [208]
		Coumarins		
Esculetin	178.14	C$_9$H$_6$O$_4$	0.23–0.66 [b,e,f]	Pintać et al. [208]
		Stilbenes		
resveratrol	228.243	C$_{14}$H$_{12}$O$_3$	0.07–3.37 [b,e,f]	Pintać et al. [208]
			5.3–6.2 [a,e]	Iora et al. [220]
		Fatty acids		
Palmitic acid (16:1)	256.4	C$_{16}$H$_{32}$O$_2$	85.43–110.97 [d]	Iora et al. [220]
Palmitoleic acid (16:1 n-7)	254.414	C$_{16}$H$_{30}$O$_2$	7.04–13.21 [d]	Iora et al. [220]
Stearic acid (18:0)	284.48	C$_{18}$H$_{36}$O$_2$	26.75–38.77 [d]	Iora et al. [220]
Oleic acid (18:1 n-9)	282.47	C$_{18}$H$_{34}$O$_2$	118.15–141.54 [d]	Iora et al. [220]
Linoleic acid (18:2 n-6)	280.4472	C$_{18}$H$_{32}$O$_2$	627.21–684.47 [d]	Iora et al. [220]
Linolenic acid (18:3 n-3)	278.43	C$_{18}$H$_{30}$O$_2$	11.26–19.97 [d]	Iora et al. [220]
Arachidic acid (20:0)	312.5304	C$_{20}$H$_{40}$O$_2$	3.12–3.45 [d]	Iora et al. [220]
Eicosenoic acid 20:1 n-9	310.51	C$_{20}$H$_{38}$O$_2$	0.89–2.57 [d]	Iora et al. [220]
Behenic acid 22:0	340.58	C$_{22}$H$_{44}$O$_2$	1.47–2.42 [d]	Iora et al. [220]
Lignoceric acid 24:0	368.63	C$_{24}$H$_{48}$O$_2$	1.03–1.67 [d]	Iora et al. [220]
SFA			117.79–157.07 [d]	Iora et al. [220]
MUFA			131.56–156.95 [d]	Iora et al. [220]
PUFA			647.17–695.73 [d]	Iora et al. [220]
n-6/n-3			31.43–60.80 [d]	Iora et al. [220]
SFA/PUFA			0.17–0.24 [d]	Iora et al. [220]
TFA			938.41–945.08 [d]	Iora et al. [220]

Table 16. Cont.

Name	MW [g mol^{-1}]	C$_x$H$_y$O$_z$	Concentration [mg/kg dm]	References
		Other compounds		
Vanillin	152.15	C$_8$H$_8$O$_3$	25.5 [a]	Daniel et al. [212]
trans-piceid	390.388	C$_{20}$H$_{22}$O$_8$	7.75 [a]	Daniel et al. [212]

[a] expressed in mg per kg of dry matter (DM), [b] expressed in mg per kg of fresh weight, [c] expressed in mg per kg of the extract, [d] expressed in mg per g of total lipids extracted from grape pomace, [e] depending on methods of extraction, [f] depending on varieties of grapes, [g] depending on the part of the pomace: seeds, skins, stems.

The residues derived from the grape processing contain phytochemicals of interest for the production of preservatives, dyes, enriched foods, medicines, and products aimed at personal care, pharmaceutical, and cosmetic industries. The presence of bioactive compounds with antioxidant, antimicrobial, anti-inflammatory, anti-tumor, and protective activity of the cardiovascular system provides possibilities for many applications [221]. The potential beneficial role of phytochemicals of grape pomace in the prevention of disorders associated with oxidative stress and inflammation, such as endothelial dysfunction, hypertension, hyperglycemia, diabetes, and obesity, is due to the mechanisms concerned especially modulation of antioxidant/prooxidant activity, improvement of nitric oxide bioavailability, reduction of pro-inflammatory cytokines and modulation of antioxidant/inflammatory signal pathways [222].

It has been proven that the antioxidant properties of polyphenols in grape pomace help to prevent radical oxidation of the polyunsaturated fatty acids of low-density lipoproteins (LDL) and hence, are conducive to the prevention of cardiovascular diseases [223]. The compounds derived from grape pomace were also tested for their anti-inflammatory and anti-carcinogenic effect [224]. Álvarez et al. [225] studied the impact of procyanidins from grape pomace as inhibitors of human endothelial NADPH oxidase and stated the decrease in the production of reactive oxygen species. A rich source of procyanidins is grape seeds. They are widely consumed in some countries in the form of powder as a dietary supplement because of several related health benefits associated with procyanidins. They present antitumor-promoting activity, inhibit growth and induce apoptosis in human prostate cancer cells, as well as significantly reducing atherosclerosis in the aorta.

Seeds contain a very broad spectrum of procyanidins, with the dominant compounds being the dimers, trimers, and tetramers of catechin or epicatechin. Higher polymers are also present but at much lower abundance. Besides, every polymer can also be found as a gallic acid ester.

Very important is the anti-microbial activity of bioactive compounds included in grapes wastes. Mendoza et al. [226] demonstrated the antifungal properties of extracts from winery by-products against *Botrytis cinerea*, the causal agent of gray mold, considered the most important pathogen responsible for postharvest decay of fresh fruit and vegetables. Moreover, a few reports are available in the literature about the effective action of polyphenol-rich extracts from vinification by-products against various pathogenic bacteria and insects, e.g., *Listeria monocytogenes*, *Leptinotarsa decemlineata*, and *Spodoptera littoralis* [1]. The potential health benefits of plant phenolics cause much interest and consideration in a lot of agri-food applications for phenolics extracted from grape wastes [16]. There are a lot of studies on the application of phytochemicals from grape pomace in the meat industry [221].

To facilitate the industrial application of wine waste polyphenols, encapsulation was recently developed to improve the stability of valuable compounds in different conditions of light and temperature [227,228].

The examples of the newest potential applications and valuable properties of phytochemicals derived from winery waste are listed in Table 17.

Table 17. Biological activity and potential applications of phytochemicals obtained from grape residues.

Material	Extract/Compound	Biological Activity/Application	References
Fresh and fermented grape pomace	Extract	- antioxidant, anti-inflammatory, and antiproliferative activity	Balea et al. [217]
Grape pomace	Hydroalcoholic extract (saponins, tannins, and flavonoids as active constituents)	- anthelmintic activity	Soares et al. [229]
Grape pomace	Whole apple pomace (phenolic compounds as main constituents)	- reduction of the severity of non-alcoholic hepatic steatosis - inhibition of steatohepatitis - improvement in insulin sensitivity - reduction of ectopic fat deposition in mice	Daniel et al. [212]
Grape pomace	crude extract and four fractions: the most active free phenolic acids fraction	- inhibitory effect on collagenase and elastase	Wittenauer et al. [213]
White grape pomace	extract: catechin, epicatechin, quercetin, and gallic acid as the main active constituents	- antiproliferative activity against adenocarcinoma cell	Jara–Palacios et al. [214]
Grape pomace	Ethanolic extract	- antioxidant activity - potential application as additives to food enhancing nutritional value and improving storability	Iora et al. [220]
Grape stem	extracts	- prevention of radical oxidation of the polyunsaturated fatty acids of low-density lipoproteins (LDL) - reduction of intracellular reactive oxygen species (ROS) - prevention of cardiovascular diseases	Anastasiadi et al. [223]
Grape seeds	procyanidin-rich extract	- antibacterial activity against *Helicobacter pylori* (H. pylori)	Silvan et al. [230]
Grape seeds	procyanidin-rich extract	- antihypertensive activity	Quiñones et al. [231]
Grape pomace	phenolics	- antioxidant properties	Tournour et al. [232]
Grape pomace	"Enocianina"—anthocyanin-rich extract	- radical scavenging, enzymatic, antioxidant and anti-inflammatory activity - application as a colorant in the food industry	Della Vedova et al. [233]
Grape pomace	phenolics	- photoprotective activity - reduction of the negative effects of UV radiation on the skin, such as erythema and photoaging	Hübner et al. [234]
Grape pomace	extracts	- wastewater remediation	Gavrilas et al. [235]
Grape pomace	ethanolic extract	- application as additives to yogurt	Olt et al. [236]
Grape pomace	alcoholic extract	- application as a reducing agent of the precursor silver nitrate, a process that has led to the obtaining of silver nanoparticles (NP Ag) by reducing the ions.	Asmat–Campos et al. [237]
Grape skin	resveratrol	- as an antioxidant in the meat industry	Andrés et al. [238]
Grape seeds	flavonoids	- antimicrobial activity in meat	Biniari et al. [239]
Grape steam	procyanidins	- inhibition of toxic compounds	Bordiga et al. [240]

Table 17. Cont.

Material	Extract/Compound	Biological Activity/Application	References
Grape pulp	phenolic compounds	- pigment protection in meat	Chen et al. [241]
Grape pomace	anthocyanins	- modulation of the sensory characteristic of meat	Crupi et al. [242]
Grape pomace	stilbenes	- modulation of the sensory characteristic of meat	Mainente et al. [243]
Grape seeds	Unsaturated fatty acids (linoleic and oleic acid)	- substitution nitrate and nitrite	Gárcia–Lomillo and González-San José [244]

2.9. Citrus Residues

Citrus fruits from the family *Rutaceae* include oranges, lemons, limes, grapefruits, mandarins, and tangerines. They are well known for their nutritional value, as they are good sources of dietary fiber, pectin, vitamin C, vitamin B group, carotenoids, flavonoids, and limonoids (Table 18). It is estimated that approximately 140 chemical components have been isolated and identified from citrus peels, and flavonoids are the main group of phytochemicals with biological activity [245]. Afsharnezhad et al. [165] evaluated the antioxidant potential of extract from various fruit peels and stated that the maximum DPPH radical scavenging activity, total phenols, and total anthocyanins were observed in orange peels.

Table 18. Phytochemicals identified and quantified in citrus residues.

Name	Citrus Residues	MW [g mol^{-1}]	$C_xH_yO_z$	Concentration [mg/kg dm]	References
Total phenols	kinnow peel			13,840–27,910 [a,c]	Yaqoob et al. [246]
	lime peel			5.2 [b]	Karetha et al. [247]
	mandarin peel			4.0 [b]	Karetha et al. [247]
	lemon peel			4.7 [b]	Karetha et al. [247]
	pomelo peel			6.4 [b]	Karetha et al. [247]
	rough lemon peel			4.1 [b]	Karetha et al. [247]
	citron peel			6.8 [b]	Karetha et al. [247]
	sour orange peel			30.4–1354.4 [a]	Benayad et al. [248]
	lime and orange peel			3860	Barbosa et al. [249]
	orange peel			7055–19,885 [a]	Liew et al. [250]
	orange seeds oil			4430	Jorge et al. [251]
Total flavonoids	kinnow peel			610–11,770 [a]	Yaqoob et al. [246]
	sour orange peel			2.3–603.6 [a]	Benayad et al. [248]
	orange peel			854.7–2975.4 [a]	Liew et al. [250]
	sour orange peel			589.4	Olfa et al. [252]
	lime peel			95.3	Olfa et al. [252]
	orange peel			132.2	Olfa et al. [252]
	lemon peel			610.5	Olfa et al. [252]
	mandarin peel			275.9	Olfa et al. [252]
Total carotenoids	orange seeds oil			19	Jorge et al. [251]
Organic acids					
Lactic acid	orange peel	90.08	$C_3H_6O_3$	5463–9861 [a]	Liew et al. [250]
Citric acid	orange peel	192.1	$C_6H_8O_7$	19,587–27,910 [a]	Liew et al. [250]
L-mallic acid	orange peel	134.1	$C_4H_6O_5$	3056–5064 [a]	Liew et al. [250]
Kojic acid	orange peel	141.1	$C_6H_6O_4$	111.2–116.4 [a]	Liew et al. [250]
Ascorbic acid	orange peel	176.1	$C_6H_8O_6$	1.12–7.32 [d]	Liew et al. [250]
Phenolic acids—hydroxybenzoic acids					
Ellagic acid	lime and orange peel	302.20	$C_{14}H_6O_8$	109.7	Barbosa et al. [249]
	lime and orange peel			5.7	Barbosa et al. [249]
Gallic acid	sour orange peel	170.12	$C_7H_6O_5$	111.3–866.7 [a]	Benayad et al. [249]
	orange peel			8.84–17.81 [a]	Liew et al. [250]
Protocatechuic acid	orange peel	154.12	$C_7H_6O_4$	24.55–65.92 [a]	Liew et al. [250]

Table 18. Cont.

Name	Citrus Residues	MW [g mol^{-1}]	C$_x$H$_y$O$_z$	Concentration [mg/kg dm]	References
4-hydroxybenzoic acid	orange peel	138.12	C$_7$H$_6$O$_3$	26.27–42.50 [a]	Liew et al. [250]
	Phenolic acids—hydroxycinnamic acids				
Ferulic acid	sour orange peel			360.0–17,237.7 [a]	Benayad et al. [248]
	orange peel			154.8–477.3 [a]	Liew et al. [250]
	yuzu peel			135	Lee et al. [253]
	sour orange peel			139	Lee et al. [253]
	mandarin peel	194.18	C$_{10}$H$_{10}$O$_4$	101	Lee et al. [253]
	lime peel			18	Lee et al. [253]
	grapefruit peel			29	Lee et al. [253]
	lemon peel			18	Lee et al. [253]
	orange peel			19	Lee et al. [253]
p-coumaric acid	sour orange peel			242.4	Benayad et al. [248]
	yuzu peel			101	Lee et al. [253]
	sour orange peel			123	Lee et al. [253]
	mandarin peel	164.16	C$_9$H$_8$O$_3$	52	Lee et al. [253]
	lime peel			76	Lee et al. [253]
	grapefruit peel			16	Lee et al. [253]
	lemon peel			48	Lee et al. [253]
	orange peel			18	Lee et al. [253]
Chlorogenic acid	mandarin peel			0.08–68.58 [a]	Šafranko et al. [254]
	sour orange peel			4.494	Benayad et al. [248]
	yuzu peel	354.31	C$_{16}$H$_{18}$O$_9$	39	Lee et al. [253]
	sour orange peel			96	Lee et al. [253]
	mandarin peel			40	Lee et al. [253]
Caffeic acid	sour orange peel			384.0–1326.1 [a]	Benayad et al. [248]
	orange peel			54.5–210.1 [a]	Liew et al. [250]
	yuzu peel			55	Lee et al. [253]
	sour orange peel	180.16	C$_9$H$_8$O$_4$	27	Lee et al. [253]
	mandarin peel			15	Lee et al. [253]
	lime peel			4	Lee et al. [253]
	lemon peel			12	Lee et al. [253]
	Flavonoids—flavonols				
Rutin	mandarin peel			0.18–4.27 [a]	Šafranko et al. [254]
	orange peel	610.52	C$_{27}$H$_{30}$O$_{16}$	9.56–10.11 [a]	Liew et al. [250]
	mandarin peel			177	Lee et al. [253]
	Flavonoids—flavanols				
Catechin	sour orange peel	290.26	C$_{15}$H$_{14}$O$_6$	378.3–1296 [a]	Benayad et al. [248]
	orange peel			40.92–366.8 [a]	Liew et al. [250]
Epigallocatechin	orange peel			84.23–317.14 [a]	Liew et al. [250]
	Flavonoids-flavones				
Apigenin	sour orange peel	270.24	C$_{15}$H$_{10}$O$_5$	38,552.1	Benayad et al. [248]
	orange peel			57.91–159.67	Liew et al. [250]
Diosmetin	lime and orange peel	300.26	C$_{16}$H$_{12}$O$_6$	3.2	Barbosa et al. [249]
Vitexin	orange peel	432.38	C$_{21}$H$_{20}$O$_{10}$	30.73–117.27 [a]	Liew et al. [250]
Luteolin	orange peel	286.24	C$_{15}$H$_{10}$O$_6$	93.47–275.14 [a]	Liew et al. [250]
Tangeretin	lime and orange peel	372.37	C$_{20}$H$_{20}$O$_7$	14.1	Barbosa et al. [249]
	Flavonoids-flavanones				
Naringenin	lime and orange peel	272.25	C$_{15}$H$_{12}$O$_5$	4.7	Barbosa et al. [249]
	sour orange peel			5745.6–96,942 [a]	Benayad et al. [248]
Hesperetin	lime and orange peel	302.28	C$_{16}$H$_{14}$O$_6$	10.5	Barbosa et al. [249]

Table 18. Cont.

Name	Citrus Residues	MW [g mol^{-1}]	$C_xH_yO_z$	Concentration [mg/kg dm]	References
	lime and orange peel			2326.5	Barbosa et al. [249]
	mandarin peel			0.16–15.07 [a]	Šafranko et al. [254]
	yuzu peel			5367	Lee et al. [253]
Hesperidin	mandarin peel	610.57	$C_{28}H_{34}O_{15}$	21,496	Lee et al. [253]
	lime peel			4862	Lee et al. [253]
	lemon peel			6400	Lee et al. [253]
	orange peel			16,299	Lee et al. [253]
	lime and orange peel			10.2	Barbosa et al. [249]
	yuzu peel			5255	Lee et al. [253]
	sour orange peel			19,750	Lee et al. [253]
Naringin	mandarin peel	580.54	$C_{27}H_{32}O_{14}$	146	Lee et al. [253]
	lime peel			36	Lee et al. [253]
	grapefruit peel			31,314	Lee et al. [253]
	lemon peel			41	Lee et al. [253]
	lime and orange peel			293.4	Barbosa et al. [249]
	mandarin peel			0.03–5.11 [a]	Šafranko et al. [254]
	yuzu peel			4734	Lee et al. [253]
	sour orange peel			64	Lee et al. [253]
Narirutin	mandarin peel	580.54	$C_{27}H_{32}O_{14}$	10,642	Lee et al. [253]
	lime peel			559	Lee et al. [253]
	grapefruit peel			2827	Lee et al. [253]
	lemon peel			185	Lee et al. [253]
	orange peel			1342	Lee et al. [253]
		Furanocumarins			
	sour orange peel			64	Lee et al. [253]
Bergapten	lime peel	216.19	$C_{12}H_8O_4$	196	Lee et al. [253]
	lemon peel			3	Lee et al. [253]
	lime peel			81	Lee et al. [253]
Bergamottin	grapefruit peel	338.40	$C_{21}H_{22}O_4$	25	Lee et al. [253]
	lemon peel			16	Lee et al. [253]
		Volatile compounds			
Caprylaldehyde	sour orange peel	128.21	$C_8H_{16}O$	180.5 [b]	Benayad et al. [248]
Decanal	sour orange peel	156.27	$C_{10}H_{20}O$	167.2 [b]	Benayad et al. [248]
Decanol	sour orange peel	158.28	$C_{10}H_{22}O$	129.8 [b]	Benayad et al. [248]
Geranyl Acetate	sour orange peel	196.29	$C_{12}H_{20}O_2$	172.7 [b]	Benayad et al. [248]
D-limonene	sour orange peel	136.24	$C_{10}H_{16}$	3939.4 [b]	Benayad et al. [248]
β-linalool	sour orange peel	154.25	$C_{10}H_{18}O$	2038.7 [b]	Benayad et al. [248]
Linalool oxide	sour orange peel	170.25	$C_{10}H_{18}O_2$	282.0 [b]	Benayad et al. [248]
Linalyl acetate	sour orange peel	196.29	$C_{12}H_{20}O_2$	589.1 [b]	Benayad et al. [248]
β-myrcene	sour orange peel	136.23	$C_{10}H_{16}$	1972.8 [b]	Benayad et al. [248]
Nerol	sour orange peel	154.25	$C_{10}H_{18}O$	106.2 [b]	Benayad et al. [248]
β-ocimene	sour orange peel	136.23	$C_{10}H_{16}$	465.2 [b]	Benayad et al. [248]
α-pinene	sour orange peel	136.23	$C_{10}H_{16}$	350.1 [b]	Benayad et al. [248]
β-pinene	sour orange peel	136.23	$C_{10}H_{16}$	417.6 [b]	Benayad et al. [248]
α-terpineol	sour orange peel	154.25	$C_{10}H_{18}O$	389.5 [b]	Benayad et al. [248]
		Carotenoids			
Violaxantin dilaurate	mandarin peel	965.44	$C_{64}H_{100}O_6$	1.33	Huang et al. [255]
Violaxanthin dipalmitate	mandarin peel	1077.7	$C_{72}H_{116}O_6$	2.07	Huang et al. [255]
Zeaxanthin	mandarin peel	568.88	$C_{40}H_{56}O_2$	1.31	Huang et al. [255]
α-cryptoxanthin	mandarin peel	552.85	$C_{40}H_{56}O$	0.10	Huang et al. [255]
β-cryptoxanthin	mandarin peel	552.85	$C_{40}H_{56}O$	4.96	Huang et al. [255]
Lutein	kinnow peel	568.87	$C_{40}H_{56}O_2$	9.26–28.89 [a]	Saini et al. [256]
	mandarin peel			0.88	Huang et al. [255]
β-carotene	mandarin peel	536.87	$C_{40}H_{56}$	5.87	Huang et al. [255]
(E/Z)-phytoene	mandarin peel	544.94	$C_{40}H_{64}$	25.07	Huang et al. [255]
β-citraurin	mandarin peel	432.6	$C_{30}H_{40}O_2$	1.57	Huang et al. [255]

Table 18. Cont.

Name	Citrus Residues	MW [g mol^{-1}]	C$_x$H$_y$O$_z$	Concentration [mg/kg dm]	References
α-tocopherol	orange seeds oil	430.71	C$_{29}$H$_{50}$O$_2$	135.7	Jorge et al. [251]
phytosterol	orange seeds oil	414.72	C$_{29}$H$_{50}$O	1304.2	Jorge et al. [251]
malic acid	sour orange peel	134.09	C$_4$H$_6$O$_5$	122.4–2247 [a]	Benayad et al. [248]

[a] depending on methods of extraction, [b] expressed in mg kg^{-1} of fresh matter of peel, [c] expressed in mg kg of the extract.

Citrus peels are widely used by-products for the production of essential oils, which have great commercial importance due to their aroma, antifungal and antimicrobial properties. Citrus essential oil is employed in the food industry, perfumes, cosmetics, domestic household products, and pharmaceuticals [257]. The main ingredient is limonene, accounting for more than 94% of citrus essential oil [258]. It is used as an insect-killing agent in pesticides and a good biodegradable and non-toxic solvent [257]. Furthermore, limonene has shown regulatory effects on neurotransmitters and stimulant-induced changes in dopamine neurotransmission [258].

The citrus waste contained high amounts of organic and phenolic acids, as well as flavonoids. Among flavonoids, the main compounds are flavanones and flavones (such as naringenin, hesperetin, and apigenin glycosides) as well as polymethoxylated flavones (PMFs), not found in other fruit species [259,260]. Okino Delgado and Feuri [258] indicated that polymethoxylated flavones, at a dosage of 250 mg/kg, exhibit an anti-inflammatory effect comparable to ibuprofen. The most widely studied PMFs are tangeretin and nobiletin. They are exclusively derived from citrus peels. Lv et al. [261] stated that nobiletin and its derivatives showed anti-cancer activity. Generally, anticancer activity increases with the increasing number of methoxy groups because PMFs have then higher hydrophobicity for approaching and penetrating cancer cells [244]. Moreover, PMFs exhibit a broad spectrum of other biological activities such as anti-obesity, anti-atherosclerosis, antiviral and antioxidant properties [262,263].

Among flavanones, citrus peel is rich in eriocitrin, hesperidin, diosmin, neohesperidin, didymin, and naringin. Chiechio et al. [264] used red orange and lemon extract rich in flavanones for in vivo assays on male CD1 mice fed with a high-fat diet. The results showed that an 8-week treatment with the extract was able to induce a significant reduction in glucose, cholesterol, and triglyceride levels in the blood, with positive effects on the regulation of hyperglycemia and lipid metabolism. Barbosa et al. [265] tested flavanones obtained from citrus pomace by enzyme-assisted and conventional hydroalcoholic extraction as an agent against *Salmonella enterica* subsp. *enterica*. Tested extracts decreased the expression of genes associated with cell invasion. Moreover, the results suggest that extracts and flavanones inhibit *Salmonella Typhimurium* adhesion by interacting with fimbriae and flagella structures and downregulating fimbrial and virulence genes.

Citrus peels also contained some flavonols, such as rutin, isorhamnetin 3-O-rutinoside, quercetin-O-glucoside, and myricetin, as well as phenolic acids, but at a much lower concentration. It has been proven that *Citrus reticulata* waste extract, mainly including rutin, was the most effective against gram-negative bacteria and the three pathogenesis fungi: *Bacillus subtilis*, *Candida albicans* and *Aspergillus flavus* [266].

Citrus seeds are also a good source of valuable components, particularly oil rich in carotenoids (19.01 mg/kg), phenolic compounds (4.43 g/kg), tocopherols (135.65 mg/kg) and phytosterols (1304.2 mg/kg) [251]. This oil was characterized by high antioxidant activity ranging from 56.0% to 70.2%.

A summary of the main phytochemical constituents, together with their concentrations in citrus residues, as well as their newest applications and properties, is presented in Tables 18 and 19, respectively.

Table 19. Biological activity and potential applications of phytochemicals obtained from citrus residues.

Material	Extract/Compound	Biological Activity/Application	References
sour orange peel	acetone extract chloroform extract ethanol-water extract naringenin gallic acid	- hypoglycaemic and antidiabetic actions - α-glucosidase inhibition - α-amylase inhibition	Benayad et al. [248]
orange peel	ethanol and methanol extract	- antimicrobial activity against *Xanthomonas*, *Bacillus subtilis*, *Azotobacter*, *Pseudomonas*, *Klebsiella*	Gunwantrao et al. [267]
pomelo peel	extract	- antimicrobial and antioxidants activity	Khan et al. [268]
lemon peel	eriodictoyl, quercetin, and diosmetin	- antiviral activity against SARS-CoV-2	Khan et al. [269]
orange peel	extracts: methanol/water, ethanol/water and acetone/water	- antioxidant activity	Liew et al. [250]
sour orange lime orange lemon mandarin	ethanol/water extracts	- antioxidant activity	Olfa et al. [252]
kinnow peel and pomace	extract (supercritical CO_2 extraction)	- antioxidant activity - for making functional cookies	Yaqoob et al. [246]
citrus pomace (Persian lime and orange)	extract rich in aglycones of flavanones, mainly naringenin and hesperetin	- activity against *Salmonella enterica* subsp. *enterica* serovar Typhimurium	Barbosa et al. [265]
lemon, orange andgrapefruit peel	essential oils (EOs)	- antifungal activity against *Rhizoctonia solanii* and *Sclerotium rolfsii* - insecticidal activity against *Rhyzopertha dominica*, *Oryzaephilus* sp., and *Sitophilus granarius*	Achimón et al. [270]
mandarin peel	Extract rich in polyphenols, mainly narirutin and hesperidin	- inhibition of the growth of *Aspergillus flavus*	Liu et al. [271]
citrus peel	nobiletin	- activity against pancreatic cancer through cell cycle arrest	Jiang et al. [272]
citrus peel	nobiletin	- activity against prostate cancer thanks to its anti-inflammation properties	Ozkan et al. [273]
mandarin peel	polymethoxyflavone-rich extract (PMFE)	- alleviating the metabolic syndrome by regulating the gut microbiome and amino acid metabolism	Zeng et al. [263]
Mandarin peel	polymethoxyflavone-rich extract (PMFE)	- alleviating high-fat diet-induced hyperlipidemia	Gao et al. [262]
Orange and lemon peel	Extract rich in flavanones	- reduction in glucose, cholesterol and triglycerides levels in the blood, with positive effects on the regulation of hyperglycemia and lipid metabolism	Chiechio et al. [264]
Lime and orange peel	Extract rich in flavanones, mainly hesperetin, hesperidin, narirutin, and naringin	- antibacterial activity against *Salmonella enterica*	Barbosa et al. [265]
Bitter orange peel	Extract rich in luteolin 7-O glucoside	- antioxidant activity - activity against gram-positive bacteria and *Fusarium oxysporum*	Lamine et al. [266]

Table 19. Cont.

Material	Extract/Compound	Biological Activity/Application	References
Mandarin peel	Extract rich in rutin	- activity against gram-negative bacteria and the three pathogenesis fungi: Bacillus subtilis, Candida albicans and Aspergillus flavus.	Lamine et al. [266]
Orange peel	Extract rich in polymethoxyflavones	- antifungal activity against Aspergillus niger.	Lamine et al. [266]
Pomegranate peel	Ethanolic and methanolic extract	- activity against gram-positive, gram-negative, and two fungal pathogenic strains - used as a natural food preserver	Hanafy et al. [274]

2.10. Olive Waste

The cultivation of olive trees is a widespread practice in the Mediterranean region, accounting for about 98% of the world's olive cultivation. A large number of phenolic compounds occur in both olive oil and olive waste that includes both leaves and the residues of oil production [275,276]. Their chemical characterization was reported by Dermeche et al. [277]. The main groups of phenolic compounds in olive mill wastes are phenolic acids, secoiridoids, and flavonoids, and the most abundant polyphenols are oleuropein, hydroxytyrosol, verbascoside, apigenin-7-glucoside, and luteolin-7-glucoside [278] (Table 20). Olive mill wastewater obtained during oil production is a complex mixture of vegetation waters and processing waste of the olive fruit; it is characterized by a dark color, strong odor, a mildly acidic pH, and a very high inorganic and organic load [279]. The organic fraction consists essentially of sugars, tannins, polyphenols, polyalcohols, proteins, organic acids, pectins and lipids [277]. About 30 million m^3 of olive mill wastewater are produced annually in the world as a by-product of the olive oil extraction process; because of the high polyphenolic content (0.5–24 g/L), this by-product is difficult to biodegrade and a relevant environmental and economic issue [280].

Table 20. Phytochemicals identified and quantified in olive waste.

Name	Olive Residue	MW [g mol^{-1}]	C$_x$H$_y$O$_z$	Concentration	References
		Phenolic acids			
Cinnamic acid	deffated olives	148.16	C$_9$H$_8$O$_2$	2.3 [a] 12–205 [b,c]	Alu'datt et al. [281] Zhao et al. [282]
p-coumaric acid	deffated olives olive pomace	164.04	C$_9$H$_8$O$_3$	10.3 [a] 84–884 [b,c] 5.01 [b]	Alu'datt et al. [281] Zhao et al. [282] Benincasa et al. [283]
o-coumaric acid	olive pomace	164.04	C$_9$H$_8$O$_3$	70–1562 [b,c]	Zhao et al. [282]
Caffeic acid	deffated olives leaves OMWW * olive pomace	180.16	C$_9$H$_8$O$_4$	3.1 [a] 150 [b] 270 [b] 39–420 [b,c]	Alu'datt et al. [281] Ladhari et al. [284] Ladhari et al. [284] Zhao et al. [282]
Protocatechuic acid	deffated olives	154.12	C$_7$H$_6$O$_4$	22.2 [a]	Alu'datt et al. [281]
Hydroxybenzoic acid	deffated olives	138.12	C$_7$H$_6$O$_3$	4.2 [a]	Alu'datt et al. [281]
Vanillic acid	deffated olives olive pomace	168.14	C$_8$H$_8$O$_4$	9.0 [a] 203–2530 [b,c]	Alu'datt et al. [281] Zhao et al. [282]
Ferulic acid	deffated olives olive pomace	194.18	C$_{10}$H$_{10}$O$_4$	6.9 [a] 23–326 [b,c]	Alu'datt et al. [281] Zhao et al. [282]
Gallic acid	deffated olives olive pomace	170.12	C$_7$H$_6$O$_5$	7.1 [a] 7–223 [b,c]	Alu'datt et al. [281] Zhao et al. [282]
Syringic acid	deffated olives	198.17	C$_9$H$_{10}$O$_5$	4.1 [a]	Alu'datt et al. [281]
Sinapic acid	deffated olives	224.21	C$_{11}$H$_{12}$O$_5$	14.4 [a]	Alu'datt et al. [281]

Table 20. Cont.

Name	Olive Residue	MW [g mol^{-1}]	C$_x$H$_y$O$_z$	Concentration	References
4-hydroxyphenyl acetic acid	olive pomace	152.15	C$_8$H$_8$O$_3$	660–4450 [b,c]	Zhao et al. [282]
		Secoiridoids and derivatives			
Oleuropein	leaves	540.54	C$_{25}$H$_{32}$O$_{13}$	13,050 [b]	Ladhari et al. [284]
	OMWW			9 [b]	
	OMWW			103 [b]	Benincasa et al. [283]
	olive pomace			811–12,231 [b,c]	Zhao et al. [282]
Oleuropein aglycone	leaves	378.4	C$_{19}$H$_{22}$O$_8$	3410 [b]	Ladhari et al. [284]
	OMWW			6 [b]	
Verbascoside	leaves	624.59	C$_{29}$H$_{36}$O$_{15}$	1160 [b]	Ladhari et al. [284]
	OMWW			6 [b]	
	OMSW **			5 [b]	
	olive pomace			833–10,159 [b,c]	Zhao et al. [282]
				700 [b]	Benincasa et al. [283]
Ligstroside	leaves	524.51	C$_{25}$H$_{32}$O$_{12}$	360 [b]	Ladhari et al. [284]
	OMWW			21 [b]	
	OMSW			56 [b]	
Tyrosol	leaves	138.16	C$_8$H$_{10}$O$_2$	450 [b]	Ladhari et al. [284]
	OMWW			1870 [b]	
	OMSW			4 [b]	
	OMWW			182 [b]	Poerschmann et al. [285]
	OMWW			2043 [b]	Benincasa et al. [283]
	olive pomace			162–3514 [a,c]	Zhao et al. [282]
Hydroxytyrosol	leaves	154.16	C$_8$H$_{10}$O$_3$	130 [b]	Ladhari et al. [284]
	OMWW			4450 [b]	
	OMWW			225 [b]	Poerschmann et al. [285]
	OMWW			1481 [b]	Benincasa et al. [283]
	olive pomace			1356–17,298 [a,c]	Zhao et al. [282]
		Flavonoids			
Luteolin	leaves	286.24	C$_{15}$H$_{10}$O$_6$	2970 [b]	Ladhari et al. [284]
	OMWW			1010 [b]	
	OMSW			4 [b]	
	olive pomace			10–3515 [b,c]	Zhao et al. [282]
	OMWW			62.38 [b]	Benincasa et al. [283]
Luteolin 7-O-glucoside	leaves	448.37	C$_{21}$H$_{20}$O$_{11}$	7620 [b]	Ladhari et al. [284]
	OMWW			150 [b]	
	olive pomace			42–4086 [b,c]	Zhao et al. [282]
				88.55 [b]	Benincasa et al. [283]
Luteolin 7-O-rutinoside		594.51	C$_{27}$H$_{30}$O$_{15}$		
Luteolin 4'-O-glucoside	OMWW	448.37	C$_{21}$H$_{20}$O$_{11}$	11.48 [b]	Benincasa et al. [283]
Rutin	leaves	610.52	C$_{27}$H$_{30}$O$_{16}$	110 [b]	Ladhari et al. [284]
	OMWW			110 [b]	
	deffated olives			3.3 [a]	Alu'datt et al. [281]
				770–11,048 [b,c]	Uribe et al. [286]
	olive pomace				Zhao et al. [282]
				48.52 [b]	Benincasa et al. [283]
Hesperidin	deffated olives	610.56	C$_{28}$H$_{34}$O$_{15}$	7.4 [a]	Alu'datt et al. [281]
Quercetin	leaves	302.24	C$_{15}$H$_{10}$O$_7$	4390 [b]	Ladhari et al. [284]
	OMWW			1060 [b]	
	OMSW			37 [b]	
	deffated olives			5.7 [a]	Alu'datt et al. [281]
Apigenin		270.24	C$_{15}$H$_{10}$O$_5$	7–469 [b,c]	Benincasa et al. [283] Zhao et al. [282]
Apigenin 7-O-glucoside		432.38	C$_{21}$H$_{20}$O$_{10}$	55–1345 [b,c]	Zhao et al. [282]

* OMWW—olive mill wastewater, ** olive mill solid waste, [a] percentage of total phenolic content based on peak areas, [b] expressed in mg/g dry weight, [c] depending on the methods of extraction.

Polyphenols also occur in the leaves [287]. These compounds confer bioactive properties on olive leaf extracts, such as antioxidant, antimicrobial, and antitumor activity; the capacity to reduce the risk of coronary heart disease was also reported [288]. Olive leaves can be collected as a by-product during oil processing (about 10% of the total weight of the olives) but can also be a residue of olive tree pruning. Some authors estimated that about 25 kg of by-products (twigs and leaves) could be obtained annually by pruning per tree [289]. To date, this by-product is often used as animal feed, even if this natural resource rich in antioxidant phenolic compounds should be valorized [290].

The qualitative and quantitative content of phenolic compounds is often heterogeneous in olive by-products; however, several studies reported the bioactive properties of these phenolic compounds, promising potential as antioxidant, anti-inflammatory, and antimicrobial agents. The antioxidant activities of olive mill wastewater and olive pomace have been demonstrated by different antioxidant assays as DPPH radical-scavenging activity, superoxide anion scavenging, LDL oxidation, and the protection of catalase against hypochlorous acid [281,291,292]. An overview of the pharmacology of olive oil and its active ingredients has been reported by Visioli et al. [293]. Recently, a novel stable ophthalmic hydrogel containing a polyphenolic fraction obtained from olive mill wastewater was formulated [294]. Among olive polyphenols, hydroxytyrosol is one of the main phenolic compounds; it can occur in its free form or as secoiridoids (oleuropein and its aglycone). For its polarity, it is more abundant in olive mill wastewater and pomace rather than in olive oil. Anticancer, antioxidant, and anti-inflammatory properties have been reported for hydroxytyrosol [295,296]. In vitro antioxidant and skin regenerative properties have been reported by Benincasa et al. [297].

Moreover, the polyphenol fraction obtained from olive mill wastewater showed activities against bacteria, fungi, plants, animals, and human cells; antibacterial activities against several bacterial species (*Staphylococcus aureus*, *Bacillus subtilis*, *Escherichia coli* and *Pseudomonas aeruginosa*) have been reported by Obied et al. [298]. Fungicidal activities have also been reported [299]. Moreover, the effects of phenolic compounds from olive waste on *Aspergillus flavus* growth and aflatoxin B_1 production were investigated [300,301]. The olive mill wastewater polyphenols did not inhibit the *Aspergillus flavus* fungal growth rate but significantly reduced the aflatoxin B_1 production (ranging from 88 to 100%) at 15% concentration [302].

Finally, cytoprotection of brain cells by olive mill wastewater has been studied by Schaffer et al. [303]. The cytoprotective effects were correlated to the content of hydroxytyrosol.

These studies showed the numerous beneficial and bioactive activities of polyphenols fraction obtained by olive by-products; for their use, it is often carried out an appropriate fractionation and/or purification to control their concentration and to avoid some antagonist effects.

Various valuable properties and the newest studies on the application of biologically active compounds derived form olive waste are presented in Table 21.

Table 21. Biological activity and potential applications of phytochemicals obtained from olive waste.

Material	Extract/Compound	Biological Activity/Application	References
olive leave	extract	- antioxidant, antimicrobial - antitumor activity - reduction of the risk of coronary heart disease	Taamalli et al. [288]
OMWW *	phenolic extract	- antioxidant activity - DPPH radical-scavenging activity - superoxide anion scavenging	Kreatsouli et al. [291]
pressed olive cake	phenolic compounds	- LDL oxidation - the protection of catalase against hypochlorous acid	Alu'datt et al. [281]

Table 21. Cont.

Material	Extract/Compound	Biological Activity/Application	References
Olive oil mill waste	SFE extract and ethanol extract (hydroxytyrosol as the main compound)	- antioxidant activity - DPPH radical-scavenging activity - application as an antioxidant act against peroxidation of virgin olive and sunflower oils	Lafka et al. [292]
OMWW	polyphenolic fraction	- formulation of ophthalmic hydrogel containing a polyphenolic fraction	Di Mauro et al. [294]
dried olive mill wastewater	polyphenols	- application as ingredients in the food industry for obtaining functional and nutraceutical foods, as well as in the pharmaceutical industry	Benincasa et al. [297]
OMWW	polyphenol fraction	- antibacterial activities against *Staphylococcus aureus*, *Bacillus subtilis*, *Escherichia coli*, and *Pseudomonas aeruginosa*	Obied et al. [298]
olive leaves and olive pomace	phenolic compounds	- fungicidal activities - ability as antimicrobial, antifungal, antitoxigenic to reduce aflatoxigenic fungi hazard and its aflatoxins - application as a manufacturing process, like, food supplement or preservatives	Yangui et al. [299] Abdel–Razek et al. [300]
olive leaves	IR extract	- antiradical activity - antioxidant activity - inhibition of the growth of *Aspergillus flavus* and production of aflatoxin B_1 - inhibition of 20 strains of *Staphylococcus aureus*	Abi–Khattar et al. [302]
OMWW	hydroxytyrosol	cytoprotection of brain cell	Schaffer et al. [303]

* OMWW—olive mill wastewater.

3. Conclusions

The ever-increasing amount of processed food raw materials entails an increasing amount of biowaste. Their management has become a growing problem. The consulted literature shows that discussed waste still contains valuable ingredients, medicinally important phytochemicals, and good antioxidants, so it is very important to valorize them. Currently, the recovery of different valuable phytochemicals from agro-industrial waste has become an imperative research area among the scientific community because agro-industrial residues of plant materials are a cheap and natural source of bioactive compounds, which can be used in the prevention and treatment of various diseases. Despite many studies on the valuable properties and potential applications, still, not many solutions are implemented in the industry. This is probably caused by legislation that can affect the valorization of such waste biomass. There are not many regulatory and legal provisions for their use. In the European Union, the use of agricultural residues as food ingredients is regulated by the European Community Regulation (EC) No 178/2002. However, in order to use them as natural additives, proper authorization as a novel food is necessary (Regulation (EC) No 2015/2283) [304]. There is no doubt that the industrial application of the extracts needs to be regulated.

According to the circular bioeconomy and biorefinery concept, food waste should be recycled inside the whole food value chain from field to fork in order to formulate functional foods and nutraceuticals. Nonetheless, it is important to implement environmentally friendly industrial extraction procedures. Moreover, despite so many above reports, there is still a need for human and animal studies, as well as studies in the field in the case of plants, to confirm the protective effect of such phytochemicals against diseases.

Taking into account the European Union's emphasis on the development of a circular economy and reducing the carbon footprint, it is expected that the effective application of these wastes will be carried out and that regulations will be developed in accordance with needs.

Author Contributions: Conceptualization, M.O., I.K. and W.O.; resources, W.O., I.K.; Visualisation, M.O., I.K. and T.B.; writing—original draft preparation, M.O., I.K. and T.B.; writing—review and editing, M.O. All authors have read and agreed to the published version of the manuscript.

Funding: This research received no external funding.

Institutional Review Board Statement: Not applicable.

Informed Consent Statement: Not applicable.

Data Availability Statement: Not applicable.

Conflicts of Interest: The authors declare no conflict of interest.

References

1. Santana-Méridas, O.; González-Coloma, A.; Sánchez-Vioque, R. Agricultural residues as a source of bioactive natural products. *Phytochem. Rev.* **2012**, *11*, 447–466. [CrossRef]
2. FAOSTAT (Statistics Division of Food and Agriculture Organization of the United Nations). Available online: https://www.fao.org/faostat/en/#data/QCL (accessed on 28 June 2022).
3. Marić, M.; Grassino, A.N.; Zhu, Z.; Barba, F.J.; Brnčić, M.; Brnčić, S.R. An overview of the traditional and innovative approaches for pectin extraction from plant food wastes and by-products: Ultrasound-, microwaves-, and enzyme-assisted extraction. *Trends Food Sci. Technol.* **2018**, *76*, 28–37. [CrossRef]
4. Kasapidou, E.; Sossidou, E.; Mitlianga, P. Fruit and vegetable co-products as functional feed ingredients in farm animal nutrition for improved product quality. *Agriculture* **2018**, *5*, 1020–1034. [CrossRef]
5. Casas-Godoy, L.; Campos-Valdez, A.R.; Alcázar-Valle, M.; Barrera-Martínez, I. Comparison of Extraction Techniques for the Recovery of Sugars, Antioxidant and Antimicrobial Compounds from Agro-Industrial Wastes. *Sustainability* **2022**, *14*, 5956. [CrossRef]
6. Ngwasiri, P.N.; Ambindei, W.A.; Adanmengwi, V.A.; Ngwi, P.; Mah, A.T.; Ngangmou, N.T.; Fonmboh, D.J.; Ngwabie, N.M.; Ngassoum, M.B.; Aba, E.R. Review Paper on Agro-food Waste and Food by-Product Valorization into Value Added Products for Application in the Food Industry: Opportunities and Challenges for Cameroon Bioeconomy. *Asian J. Biotechnol. Bioresour. Technol.* **2022**, *8*, 32–61. [CrossRef]
7. Rodrigues, F.; Nunes, M.A.; Alves, R.C.; Oliveira, M.B.P. Applications of recovered bioactive compounds in cosmetics and other products. In *Handbook of Coffee Processing By-Products*; Academic Press: London, UK, 2017; pp. 195–220.
8. Pestana-Bauer, V.R.; Zambiazi, R.C.; Mendonça, C.R.; Beneito-Cambra, M.; Ramis-Ramos, G. γ-Oryzanol and tocopherol contents in residues of rice bran oil refining. *Food Chem.* **2012**, *134*, 1479–1483. [CrossRef] [PubMed]
9. Jiang, D.; Zhuang, D.; Fu, J.; Huang, Y.; Wen, K. Bioenergy potential from crop residues in China: Availability and distribution. *Renew. Sustain. Energy Rev.* **2012**, *16*, 1377–1382. [CrossRef]
10. Searle, S.; Malins, C. *Availability of Cellulosic Residues and Wastes in the EU 2013*; The International Council on Clean Transportation: Washington, DC, USA, 2013; p. 11.
11. Ben Taher, I.; Fickers, P.; Chniti, S.; Hassouna, M. Optimization of enzymatic hydrolysis and fermentation conditions for improved bioethanol production from potato peel residues. *Biotechnol. Prog.* **2017**, *33*, 397–406. [CrossRef] [PubMed]
12. Yanli, Y.; Peidong, Z.; Wenlong, Z.; Yongsheng, T.; Yonghong, Z.; Lisheng, W. Quantitative appraisal and potential analysis for primary biomass resources for energy utilization in China. *Renew. Sustain. Energy Rev.* **2010**, *14*, 3050–3058. [CrossRef]
13. Oleszek, M.; Tys, J.; Wiącek, D.; Król, A.; Kuna, J. The possibility of meeting greenhouse energy and CO_2 demands through utilisation of cucumber and tomato residues. *BioEnergy Res.* **2016**, *9*, 624–632. [CrossRef]
14. Gabhane, J.; William, S.P.; Gadhe, A.; Rath, R.; Vaidya, A.N.; Wate, S. Pretreatment of banana agricultural waste for bio-ethanol production: Individual and interactive effects of acid and alkali pretreatments with autoclaving, microwave heating and ultrasonication. *Waste Manag.* **2014**, *34*, 498–503. [CrossRef] [PubMed]
15. Cruz, M.G.; Bastos, R.; Pinto, M.; Ferreira, J.M.; Santos, J.F.; Wessel, D.F.; Coelho, E.; Coimbra, M.A. Waste mitigation: From an effluent of apple juice concentrate industry to a valuable ingredient for food and feed applications. *J. Clean. Prod.* **2018**, *193*, 652–660. [CrossRef]
16. Muhlack, R.A.; Potumarthi, R.; Jeffery, D.W. Sustainable wineries through waste valorisation: A review of grape marc utilisation for value-added products. *Waste Manag.* **2018**, *72*, 99–118. [CrossRef] [PubMed]

17. Rezzadori, K.; Benedetti, S.; Amante, E.R. Proposals for the residues recovery: Orange waste as raw material for new products. *Food Bioprod. Process.* **2012**, *90*, 606–614. [CrossRef]
18. Kusbiantoro, A.; Embong, R.; Aziz, A.A. Strength and microstructural properties of mortar containing soluble silica from sugarcane bagasse ash. *Key Eng. Mater.* **2018**, *765*, 269–274. [CrossRef]
19. Zheng, R.; Su, S.; Zhou, H.; Yan, H.; Ye, J.; Zhao, Z.; You, L.; Fu, X. Antioxidant/antihyperglycemic activity of phenolics from sugarcane (*Saccharum officinarum* L.) bagasse and identification by UHPLC-HR-TOFMS. *Ind. Crops Prod.* **2017**, *101*, 104–114. [CrossRef]
20. Ishak NA, I.M.; Kamarudin, S.K.; Timmiati, S.N.; Sauid, S.M.; Karim, N.A.; Basri, S. Green synthesis of platinum nanoparticles as a robust electrocatalyst for methanol oxidation reaction: Metabolite profiling and antioxidant evaluation. *J. Clean. Prod.* **2023**, *382*, 135111. [CrossRef]
21. Rocha, G.J.; Nascimento, V.M.; Goncalves, A.R.; Silva, V.F.; Martin, C. Influence of mixed sugarcane bagasse samples evaluated by elemental and physical–chemical composition. *Ind. Crops Prod.* **2015**, *64*, 52–58. [CrossRef]
22. Mohan, P.R.; Ramesh, B.; Redyy, O.V. Production and optimization of ethanol from pretreated sugarcane bagasse using *Sacchromyces bayanus* in simultaneous saccharification and fermentation. *Microbiol. J.* **2012**, *2*, 52–63. [CrossRef]
23. Xi, Y.L.; Dai, W.Y.; Xu, R.; Zhang, J.H.; Chen, K.Q.; Jiang, M.; Wei, P.; Ouyang, P.K. Ultrasonic pretreatment and acid hydrolysis of sugarcane bagasse for succinic acid production using *Actinobacillus succinogenes*. *Bioprocess Biosyst. Eng.* **2013**, *36*, 1779–1785. [CrossRef]
24. Zhao, Z.; Yan, H.; Zheng, R.; Khan, M.S.; Fu, X.; Tao, Z.; Zhang, Z. Anthocyanins characterization and antioxidant activities of sugarcane (*Saccharum officinarum* L.) rind extracts. *Ind. Crops Prod.* **2018**, *113*, 38–45. [CrossRef]
25. Nieder-Heitmann, M.; Haigh, K.F.; Görgens, J.F. Process design and economic analysis of a biorefinery co-producing itaconic acid and electricity from sugarcane bagasse and trash lignocelluloses. *Bioresour. Technol.* **2018**, *262*, 159–168. [CrossRef] [PubMed]
26. Zhao, Y.; Chen, M.; Zhao, Z.; Yu, S. The antibiotic activity and mechanisms of sugarcane (*Saccharum officinarum* L.) bagasse extract against food-borne pathogens. *Food Chem.* **2015**, *185*, 112–118. [CrossRef]
27. Al Arni, S.; Drake, A.F.; Del Borghi, M.; Converti, A. Study of aromatic compounds derived from sugarcane bagasse. Part I: Effect of pH. *Chem. Eng. Technol.* **2010**, *33*, 895–901. [CrossRef]
28. González-Bautista, E.; Santana-Morales, J.C.; Ríos-Fránquez, F.J.; Poggi-Varaldo, H.M.; Ramos-Valdivia, A.C.; Cristiani-Urbina, E.; Ponce-Noyola, T. Phenolic compounds inhibit cellulase and xylanase activities of Cellulomonas flavigena PR-22 during saccharification of sugarcane bagasse. *Fuel* **2017**, *196*, 32–35. [CrossRef]
29. Zheng, R.; Su, S.; Li, J.; Zhao, Z.; Wei, J.; Fu, X.; Liu, R.H. Recovery of phenolics from the ethanolic extract of sugarcane (*Saccharum officinarum* L.) baggase and evaluation of the antioxidant and antiproliferative activities. *Ind. Crops Prod.* **2017**, *107*, 360–369. [CrossRef]
30. Van der Pol, E.; Bakker, R.; Van Zeeland, A.; Garcia, D.S.; Punt, A.; Eggink, G. Analysis of by-product formation and sugar monomerization in sugarcane bagasse pretreated at pilot plant scale: Differences between autohydrolysis, alkaline and acid pretreatment. *Bioresour. Technol.* **2015**, *181*, 114–123. [CrossRef]
31. Lv, G.; Wu, S.; Lou, R.; Yang, Q. Analytical pyrolysis characteristics of enzymatic/mild acidolysis lignin from sugarcane bagasse. *Cellulose Chemistry and Technology* **2010**, *44*, 335–342.
32. Michelin, M.; Ximenes, E.; Polizeli, M.; Ladisch, M.R. Effect of phenolic compounds from pretreated sugarcane bagasse on cellulolytic and hemicellulolytic activities. *Bioresour. Technol.* **2016**, *199*, 275–278. [CrossRef]
33. Juttuporn, W.; Thiengkaew, P.; Rodklongtan, A.; Rodprapakorn, M.; Chitprasert, P. Ultrasound-assisted extraction of antioxidant and antibacterial phenolic compounds from steam-exploded sugarcane bagasse. *Sugar Technol.* **2018**, *20*, 599–608. [CrossRef]
34. Treedet, W.; Suntivarakorn, R. Design and operation of a low cost bio-oil fast pyrolysis from sugarcane bagasse on circulating fluidized bed reactor in a pilot plant. *Fuel Process. Technol.* **2018**, *179*, 17–31. [CrossRef]
35. Krishnan, C.; Sousa, L.C.; Jin, M.; Chang, L.; Dale, B.E.; Balan, V. Alkalibased AFEX pretreatment for the conversion of sugarcane bagasse and cane leaf residues to ethanol. *Biotechnol. Bioeng.* **2010**, *107*, 441–450. [CrossRef] [PubMed]
36. Zhu, Z.S.; Zhu, M.J.; Xu, W.X.; Liang, L. Production of bioethanol from sugarcane bagasse using NH_4OH-H_2O_2 pretreatment and simultaneous saccharification and co-fermentation. *Biotechnol. Bioprocess Eng.* **2012**, *17*, 316–325. [CrossRef]
37. Guilherme, A.A.; Dantas, P.V.; Santos, E.S.; Fernandes, F.A.; Macedo, G.R. Evaluation of composition, characterization and enzymatic hydrolysis of pretreated sugarcane bagasse. *Braz. J. Chem. Eng.* **2015**, *32*, 23–33. [CrossRef]
38. Chandel, A.K.; da Silva, S.S.; Carvalho, W.; Singh, O.V. Sugarcane bagasse and leaves: Foreseeable biomass of biofuel and bio-products. *J. Chem. Technol. Biotechnol.* **2012**, *87*, 11–20. [CrossRef]
39. Guo, J.; Zhang, J.; Wang, W.; Liu, T.; Xin, Z. Isolation and identification of bound compounds from corn bran and their antioxidant and angiotensin I-converting enzyme inhibitory activities. *Eur. Food Res. Technol.* **2015**, *241*, 37–47. [CrossRef]
40. Bujang, J.S.; Zakaria, M.H.; Ramaiya, S.D. Chemical constituents and phytochemical properties of floral maize pollen. *PLoS ONE* **2021**, *16*, e0247327. [CrossRef]
41. Dong, J.; Cai, L.; Zhu, X.; Huang, X.; Yin, T.; Fang, H.; Ding, Z. Antioxidant activities and phenolic compounds of cornhusk, corncob and stigma maydis. *J. Braz. Chem. Soc.* **2014**, *25*, 1956–1964. [CrossRef]
42. Li, Q.; Somavat, P.; Singh, V.; Chatham, L.; Gonzalez de Mejia, E. A comparative study of anthocyanin distribution in purple and blue corn coproducts from three conventional fractionation processes. *Food Chem.* **2017**, *231*, 332–339. [CrossRef]

43. Haslina, H.; Eva, M. Extract corn silk with variation of solvents on yield, total phenolics, total flavonoids and antioxidant activity. *Indones. Food Nutr. Prog.* **2017**, *14*, 21–28. [CrossRef]
44. Tian, S.; Sun, Y.; Chen, Z. Extraction of flavonoids from corn silk and biological activities in vitro. *J. Food Qual.* **2021**, *2021*, 1–9. [CrossRef]
45. Lao, F.; Giusti, M.M. Extraction of purple corn (*Zea mays* L.) cob pigments and phenolic compounds using food-friendly solvents. *J. Cereal Sci.* **2018**, *80*, 87–93. [CrossRef]
46. Chen, L.; Yang, M.; Mou, H.; Kong, Q. Ultrasound-assisted extraction and characterization of anthocyanins from purple corn bran. *J. Food Preserv.* **2017**, *42*, e13377. [CrossRef]
47. Barba, F.J.; Rajha, H.N.; Debs, E.; Abi-Khattar, A.M.; Khabbaz, S.; Dar, B.N.; Simirgiotis, M.J.; Castagnini, J.M.; Maroun, R.G.; Louka, N. Optimization of Polyphenols' Recovery from Purple Corn Cobs Assisted by Infrared Technology and Use of Extracted Anthocyanins as a Natural Colorant in Pickled Turnip. *Molecules* **2022**, *27*, 5222. [CrossRef] [PubMed]
48. Fernandez-Aulis, F.; Hernandez-Vazquez, L.; Aguilar-Osorio, G.; Arrieta-Baez, D.; Navarro-Ocana, A. Extraction and identification of anthocyanins in corn cob and corn husk from Cacahuacintle maize. *J. Food Sci.* **2019**, *84*, 954–962. [CrossRef] [PubMed]
49. Wille, J.J.; Berhow, M.A. Bioactives derived from ripe corn tassels: A possible new natural skin whitener, 4-hydroxy-1-oxindole-3-acetic acid. *Curr. Bioact. Compd.* **2011**, *7*, 126–134. [CrossRef]
50. Khamphasan, P.; Lomthaisong, K.; Harakotr, B.; Ketthaisong, D.; Scott, M.P.; Lertrat, K.; Suriharn, B. Genotypic variation in anthocyanins, phenolic compounds, and antioxidant activity in cob and husk of purple field corn. *Agronomy* **2018**, *8*, 271. [CrossRef]
51. Brobbey, A.A.; Somuah-Asante, S.; Asare-Nkansah, S.; Boateng, F.O.; Ayensu, I. Preliminary phytochemical screening and scientific validation of the antidiabetic effect of the dried husk of *Zea mays* L. (Corn, Poaceae). *Int. J. Phytopharm.* **2017**, *7*, 1–5.
52. Thapphasaraphong, S.; Rimdusit, T.; Priprem, A.; Puthongking, P. Crops of waxy purple corn: A valuable source of antioxidative phytochemicals. *Int. J. Adv. Agric. Environ. Eng.* **2016**, *3*, 73–77.
53. Simla, S.; Boontang, S.; Harakotr, B. Anthocyanin content, total phenolic content, and antiradical capacity in different ear components of purple waxy corn at two maturation stages. *Aust. J. Crop Sci.* **2016**, *10*, 675–682. [CrossRef]
54. Deineka, V.I.; Sidorov, A.N.; Deineka, L.A. Determination of purple corn husk anthocyanins. *J. Anal. Chem.* **2016**, *71*, 1145–1150. [CrossRef]
55. Suryanto, E.; Momuat, L.I.; Rotinsulu, H.; Mewengkang, D.S. Anti-photooxidant and photoprotective activities of ethanol extract and solvent fractions from corn cob (*Zea mays*). *Int. J. ChemTech Res.* **2018**, *11*, 25–37.
56. Duangpapeng, P.; Lertrat, K.; Lomthaisong, K.; Scott, M.P.; Suriharn, B. Variability in anthocyanins, phenolic compounds and antioxidant capacity in the tassels of collected waxy corn germplasm. *Agronomy* **2019**, *9*, 158. [CrossRef]
57. Duangpapeng, P.; Ketthaisong, D.; Lomthaisong, K.; Lertrat, K.; Scott, M.P.; Suriharn, B. Corn tassel: A new source of phytochemicals and antioxidant potential for value-added product development in the agro-industry. *Agronomy* **2018**, *8*, 242. [CrossRef]
58. Žilić, S.; Vančetović, J.; Janković, M.; Maksimović, V. Chemical composition, bioactive compounds, antioxidant capacity and stability of floral maize (*Zea mays* L.) pollen. *J. Funct. Foods* **2014**, *10*, 65–74. [CrossRef]
59. Sarepoua, E.; Tangwongchai, R.; Suriharn, B.; Lertrat, K. Influence of variety and harvest maturity on phytochemical content in corn silk. *Food Chem.* **2015**, *169*, 424–429. [CrossRef] [PubMed]
60. Singh, J.; Rasane, P.; Nanda, V.; Kaur, S. Bioactive compounds of corn silk and their role in management of glycaemic response. *J. Food Sci. Technol.* **2022**, 1–16. [CrossRef]
61. Ren, S.C.; Qiao, Q.Q.; Ding, X.L. Antioxidative activity of five flavones glycosides from corn silk (*Stigma maydis*). *Czech J. Food Sci.* **2013**, *31*, 148–155. [CrossRef]
62. Galanakis, C.M. Functionality of food components and emerging technologies. *Foods* **2021**, *10*, 128. [CrossRef]
63. Roh, K.B.; Kim, H.; Shin, S.; Kim, Y.S.; Lee, J.A.; Kim, M.O.; Jung, E.; Lee, J.; Park, D. Anti-inflammatory effects of *Zea mays* L. husk extracts. *BMC Complement. Altern. Med.* **2016**, *16*, 298–306. [CrossRef]
64. Boeira, C.P.; Flores, D.C.B.; Lucas, B.N.; Santos, D.; Flores, E.M.M.; Reis, F.L.; Morandini, M.L.B.; Morel, A.F.; Rosa, C.S.D. Extraction of antioxidant and antimicrobial phytochemicals from corn stigma: A promising alternative to valorization of agricultural residues. *Ciência Rural.* **2022**, *52*, e20210535. [CrossRef]
65. Wang, L.; Yu, Y.; Fang, M.; Zhan, C.; Pan, H.; Wu, Y.; Gong, Z. Antioxidant and antigenotoxic activity of bioactive extracts from corn tassel. *J. Huazhong Univ. Sci. Technol.-Med. Sci.* **2014**, *34*, 131–136. [CrossRef] [PubMed]
66. Habeebullah, S.F.; Grejsen, H.D.; Jacobsen, C. Potato peel extract as a natural antioxidant in chilled storage of minced horse mackerel (*Trachurus trachurus*): Effect on lipid and protein oxidation. *Food Chem.* **2012**, *131*, 843–851.
67. Mohdaly, A.A.; Hassanien, M.F.; Mahmoud, A.; Sarhan, M.A.; Smetanska, I. Phenolics extracted from potato, sugar beet, and sesame processing by-products. *Int. J. Food Prop.* **2013**, *16*, 1148–1168. [CrossRef]
68. Lappalainen, K.; Kärkkäinen, J.; Joensuu, P.; Lajunen, M. Modification of potato peel waste with base hydrolysis and subsequent cationization. *Carbohydr. Polym.* **2015**, *132*, 97–103. [CrossRef]
69. Chang, K. Polyphenol antioxidants from potato peels: Extraction optimization and application to stabilizing lipid oxidation in foods. In Proceedings of the National Conference on Undergraduate Research (NCUR) 2019, New York, NY, USA, 11–13 April 2019.

70. Wijngaard, H.H.; Ballay, M.; Brunton, N. The optimisation of extraction of antioxidants from potato peel by pressurised liquids. *Food Chem.* **2012**, *133*, 1123–1130. [CrossRef]
71. Frontuto, D.; Carullod, D.; Harrison, S.M.; Brunton, N.P.; Ferrari, G.; Lyng, J.G.; Patar, G. Optimization of pulsed electric fields-assisted extraction of polyphenols from potato peels using response surface methodology. *Food Bioprocess Technol.* **2019**, *12*, 1708–1720. [CrossRef]
72. Javed, A.; Ahmad, A.; Tahir, A.; Shabbir, U.; Nouman, M.; Hameed, A. Potato peel waste-its nutraceutical, industrial and biotechnological applacations. *AIMS Agric. Food* **2019**, *4*, 807–823. [CrossRef]
73. Samarin, A.M.; Poorazarang, H.; Hematyar, N.; Elhamirad, A. Phenolics in potato peels: Extraction and utilization as natural antioxidants. *World Appl. Sci. J.* **2012**, *18*, 191–195.
74. Chamorro, S.; Cueva-Mestanza, R.; de Pascual-Teresa, S. Effect of spray drying on the polyphenolic compounds present in purple sweet potato roots: Identification of new cinnamoylquinic acids. *Food Chem.* **2021**, *345*, 128679. [CrossRef]
75. Paniagua-García, A.I.; Hijosa-Valsero, M.; Garita-Cambronero, J.; Coca, M.; Díez-Antolínez, R. Development and validation of a HPLC-DAD method for simultaneous determination of main potential ABE fermentation inhibitors identified in agro-food waste hydrolysates. *Microchem. J.* **2019**, *150*, 104147. [CrossRef]
76. Sarwari, G.; Sultana, B.; Sarfraz, R.A.; Zia, M.A. Cytotoxicity, antioxidant and antimutagenic potential evaluation of peels of edible roots and tubers. *Int. Food Res. J.* **2019**, *26*, 1773–1779.
77. Wu, Z.G.; Xu, H.Y.; Ma, Q.; Cao, Y.; Ma, J.N.; Ma, C.M. Isolation, identification and quantification of unsaturated fatty acids, amides, phenolic compounds and glycoalkaloids from potato peel. *Food Chem.* **2012**, *135*, 2425–2429. [CrossRef] [PubMed]
78. Silva-Beltran, N.P.; Chaidez-Quiroz, C.; Lopez-Cuevas, O.; Ruiz-Cruz, S.; Lopez-Mata, M.A.; Del-Toro-Sanchez, C.L.; Marquez-Rios, E.; Ornelas-Paz, J. Phenolic compounds of potato peel extracts: Their antioxidant activity and protection against human enteric viruses. *J. Microbiol. Biotechnol.* **2017**, *27*, 234–241. [CrossRef]
79. Chen, C.C.; Lin, C.; Chen, M.H.; Chiang, P.Y. Stability and quality of anthocyanin in purple sweet potato extracts. *Foods* **2019**, *8*, 393. [CrossRef]
80. Ji, X.; Rivers, L.; Zielinski, Z.; Xu, M.; MacDougall, E.; Jancy, S.; Zhang, S.; Wang, Y.; Chapman, R.G.; Keddy, P.; et al. Quantitative analysis of phenolic components and glycoalkaloids from 20 potato clones and in vitro evaluation of antioxidant, cholesterol uptake, and neuroprotective activities. *Food Chem.* **2012**, *133*, 1177–1187. [CrossRef]
81. Hossain, M.B.; Aguilo-Aguayo, I.; Lyng, J.G.; Brunton, N.P.; Rai, D.K. Effect of pulsed electric field and pulsed light pre-treatment on the extraction of steroidal alkaloids from potato peels. *Innov. Food Sci. Emerg. Technol.* **2015**, *29*, 9–14. [CrossRef]
82. Rodríguez-Martínez, B.; Gullón, B.; Yáñez, R. Identification and recovery of valuable bioactive compounds from potato peels: A comprehensive review. *Antioxidants* **2021**, *10*, 1630. [CrossRef]
83. Albishi, T.; John, J.A.; Al-Khalifa, A.S.; Shahidi, F. Phenolic content and antioxidant activities of selected potato varieties and their processing by-products. *J. Funct. Foods* **2013**, *5*, 590–600. [CrossRef]
84. Kumari, B.; Tiwari, B.K.; Hossain, M.B.; Rai, D.K.; Brunton, N.P. Ultrasound-assisted extraction of polyphenols from potato peels: Profiling and kinetic modelling. *Int. J. Food Sci. Technol.* **2017**, *52*, 1432–1439. [CrossRef]
85. Friedman, M.; Kozukue, N.; Kim, H.J.; Choi, S.H.; Mizuno, M. Glycoalkaloid, phenolic, and flavonoid content and antioxidative activities of conventional nonorganic and organic potato peel powders from commercial gold, red and Russet potatoes. *J. Food Compos. Anal.* **2017**, *62*, 69–75. [CrossRef]
86. Alves-Filho, E.G.; Sousa, V.M.; Ribeiro, P.R.; Rodrigues, S.; de Brito, E.S.; Tiwari, B.K.; Fernandes, F.A. Single-stage ultrasound-assisted process to extract and convert α-solanine and α-chaconine from potato peels into β-solanine and β-chaconine. *Biomass Convers. Biorefinery* **2018**, *8*, 689–697. [CrossRef]
87. Hossain, M.B.; Tiwari, B.K.; Gangopadhyay, N.; O'Donnell, C.P.; Brunton, N.P.; Rai, D.K. Ultrasonic extraction of steroidal alkaloids from potato peel waste. *Ultrason. Sonochemistry* **2014**, *21*, 1470–1476. [CrossRef] [PubMed]
88. Rytel, E.; Czopek, A.T.; Aniolowska, M.; Hamouz, K. The influence of dehydrated potatoes processing on the glycoalkaloids content in coloured-fleshed potato. *Food Chem.* **2013**, *141*, 2495–2500. [CrossRef]
89. Singh, L.; Kaur, S.; Aggarwal, P. Techno and bio functional characterization of industrial potato waste for formulation of phytonutrients rich snack product. *Food Biosci.* **2022**, *49*, 101824. [CrossRef]
90. Hillebrand, S.; Husing, B.; Schliephake, U.; Trautz, D.; Herrmann, M.E.; Winterhalter, P. Effect of thermal processing on the content of phenols in pigmented potatoes (*Solanum tuberosum* L.). *Ernaehrungs-Umsch.* **2011**, *58*, 349–353.
91. Singh, A.; Sabally, K.; Kubow, S.; Donnelly, D.J.; Gariepy, Y.; Orsat, V.; Raghavan, G.S. Microwave-assisted extraction of phenolic antioxidants from potato peels. *Molecules* **2011**, *16*, 2218–2232. [CrossRef]
92. Maldonado, A.F.; Mudge, E.; Gänzle, M.G.; Scheber, A. Extraction and fractionation of phenolic acids and glycoalkaloids from potato peels using acidified water/ethanol-based solvents. *Food Res. Int.* **2014**, *65*, 27–34. [CrossRef]
93. Akyol, H.; Riciputi, Y.; Capanoglu, E.; Caboni, M.F.; Verardo, V. Phenolic compounds in the potato and its by-products: An overview. *Int. J. Mol. Sci.* **2016**, *17*, 835. [CrossRef]
94. Venturi, F.; Bartolini, S.; Sanmartin, C.; Orlando, M.; Taglieri, I.; Macaluso, M.; Lucchesini, M.; Trivellini, A.; Zinnai, A.; Mensuali, A. Potato peels as a source of novel green extracts suitable as antioxidant additives for fresh-cut fruits. *Appl. Sci.* **2019**, *9*, 2431. [CrossRef]
95. Gebrechristos, H.Y.; Chen, W. Utilization of potato peel as eco-friendly products: A review. *Food Sci. Nutr.* **2018**, *6*, 1352–1356. [CrossRef] [PubMed]

96. Amado, I.R.; Franco, D.; Sanchez, M.; Zapata, C.; Vazques, J.A. Optimisation of antioxidant extraction from *Solanum tuberosum* potato peel waste by surface response methodology. *Food Chem.* **2014**, *165*, 290–299. [CrossRef] [PubMed]
97. Hsieh, Y.L.; Yeh, Y.H.; Lee, Y.T.; Huang, C.Y. Dietary potato peel extract reduces the toxicity of cholesterol oxidation products in rats. *J. Funct. Foods* **2016**, *27*, 461–471. [CrossRef]
98. Yang, G.; Cheon, S.Y.; Chung, K.S.; Lee, S.J.; Hong, C.H.; Lee, K.T.; Jang, D.S.; Jeong, J.C.; Kwon, O.K.; Nam, J.H.; et al. *Solanum tuberosum* L. young epidermis extract inhibits mite antigen-induced atopic dermatitis in NC/Nga mice by regulating the Th1/Th2 balance and expression of filaggrin. *J. Med. Food* **2015**, *18*, 1013–1021. [CrossRef] [PubMed]
99. Khawla, B.J.; Sameh, M.; Imen, G.; Donyes, F.; Dhouha, G.; Raoudha, E.G.; Oumèma, N.E. Potato peel as feedstock for bioethanol production: A comparison of acidic and enzymatic hydrolysis. *Ind. Crops Prod.* **2014**, *52*, 144–149. [CrossRef]
100. Wu, D. Recycle technology for potato peel waste processing: A review. *Procedia Environ. Sci.* **2016**, *31*, 103–107. [CrossRef]
101. Liang, S.; Han, Y.; Wei, L.; McDonald, A.G. Production and characterization of bio-oil and bio-char from pyrolysis of potato peel wastes. *Biomass Convers. Biorefin.* **2015**, *5*, 237–246. [CrossRef]
102. Abdelraof, M.; Hasanin, M.S.; El-Saied, H. Ecofriendly green conversion of potato peel wastes to high productivity bacterial cellulose. *Carbohydr. Polym.* **2019**, *211*, 75–83. [CrossRef]
103. Elkahoui, S.; Levin, C.; Bartley, G.; Yokoyama, W.; Friedman, M. Dietary supplementation of potato peel powders prepared from conventional and organic russet and nonorganic gold and red potatoes reduces weight gain in mice on a high-fat diet. *J. Agric. Food Chem.* **2018**, *66*, 6064–6072. [CrossRef]
104. Chimonyo, M. A review of the utility of potato by-products as a feed resource for smallholder pig production. *Anim. Feed. Sci. Technol.* **2017**, *227*, 107–117.
105. Apel, C.; Lyng, J.G.; Papoutsis, K.; Harrison, S.M.; Brunton, N.P. Screening the effect of different extraction methods (ultrasound-assisted extraction and solid–liquid extraction) on the recovery of glycoalkaloids from potato peels: Optimization of the extraction conditions using chemometric tools. *Food Bioprod. Process.* **2019**, *119*, 277–286. [CrossRef]
106. Khan, M.T.; Shah, A.S.; Safdar, N.; Rani, S.; Bilal, H.; Hashim, M.M.; Basir, A.; Rahman ZShah, S.A. Polyphenoles extraction from the potato peel and their utilization in biscuit. *Pure Appl. Biol.* **2017**, *6*, 1269–1275. [CrossRef]
107. Ding, X.; Zhu, F.; Yang, Y.; Li, M. Purification, antitumor activity in vitro of steroidal glycoalkaloids from black nightshade (*Solanum nigrum* L.). *Food Chem.* **2013**, *141*, 1181–1186. [CrossRef] [PubMed]
108. Kenny, O.M.; McCarthy, C.M.; Brunton, N.P.; Hossain, M.B.; Rai, D.K.; Collins, S.G.; Jones, P.W.; Maguire, A.R.; O'Brien, N.M. Anti-inflammatory properties of potato glycoalkaloids in stimulated Jurkat and Raw 264.7 mouse macrophages. *Life Sci.* **2013**, *92*, 775–782. [CrossRef] [PubMed]
109. Anjum, S.; Rana, S.; Dasila, K.; Agnihotri, V.; Pandey, A.; Pande, V. Comparative nutritional and antimicrobial analysis of Himalayan black and yellow soybean and their okara. *J. Sci. Food Agric.* **2022**, *102*, 5358–5367. [CrossRef]
110. Park, J.; Choi, I.; Kim, Y. Cookies formulated from fresh okara using starch, soy flour and hydroxypropyl methylcellulose have high quality and nutritional value. *LWT-Food Sci. Technol.* **2015**, *63*, 660–666. [CrossRef]
111. Ostermann-Porcel, M.V.; Quiroga-Panelo, N.; Rinaldoni, A.N.; Campderrós, M.E. Incorporation of okara into gluten-free cookies with high quality and nutritional value. *J. Food Qual.* **2017**, *2017*, 1–8. [CrossRef]
112. Guimarães, R.M.; Silva, T.E.; Lemes, A.C.; Boldrin MC, F.; da Silva MA, P.; Silva, F.G.; Egea, M.B. Okara: A soybean by-product as an alternative to enrich vegetable paste. *LWT* **2018**, *92*, 593–599. [CrossRef]
113. Šibul, F.; Orčić, D.; Vasić, M.; Anačkov, G.; Nađpal, J.; Savić, A.; Mimica-Dukić, N. Phenolic profile, antioxidant and anti-inflammatory potential of herb and root extracts of seven selected legumes. *Ind. Crops Prod.* **2016**, *83*, 641–653. [CrossRef]
114. Liu, W.; Zhang, H.X.; Wu, Z.L.; Wang, Y.J.; Wang, L.J. Recovery of isoflavone aglycones from soy whey wastewater using foam fractionation and acidic hydrolysis. *J. Agric. Food Chem.* **2013**, *61*, 7366–7372. [CrossRef]
115. Kumar, V.; Chauhan, S.S. Daidzein Induces Intrinsic Pathway of Apoptosis along with ER α/β Ratio Alteration and ROS Production. *Asian Pac. J. Cancer Prev. APJCP* **2021**, *22*, 603. [CrossRef] [PubMed]
116. Pabich, M.; Marciniak, B.; Kontek, R. Phenolic Compound Composition and Biological Activities of Fractionated Soybean Pod Extract. *Appl. Sci.* **2021**, *11*, 10233. [CrossRef]
117. Singh, P.; Krishnaswamy, K. Sustainable zero-waste processing system for soybeans and soy by-product valorization. *Trends Food Sci. Technol.* **2022**, *128*, 331–344. [CrossRef]
118. Bragagnolo, F.S.; Funari, C.S.; Ibáñez, E.; Cifuentes, A. Metabolomics as a tool to study underused soy parts: In search of bioactive compounds. *Foods* **2021**, *10*, 1308. [CrossRef] [PubMed]
119. Hsu, W.H.; Chen, S.Y.; Lin, J.H.; Yen, G.C. Application of saponins extract from food byproducts for the removal of pesticide residues in fruits and vegetables. *Food Control* **2022**, *136*, 108877. [CrossRef]
120. Freitas, S.C.; Alves da Silva, G.; Perrone, D.; Vericimo, M.A.; dos S. Baião, D.; Pereira, P.R.; Paschoalin, V.M.F.; Del Aguila, E.M. Recovery of antimicrobials and bioaccessible isoflavones and phenolics from soybean (*Glycine max*) meal by aqueous extraction. *Molecules* **2018**, *24*, 74. [CrossRef] [PubMed]
121. Silva, F.D.O.; Perrone, D. Characterization and Stability of Bioactive Compounds from Soybean Meal. *LWT Food Sci. Technol.* **2015**, *63*, 992–1000. [CrossRef]
122. Wang, Q.; Ge, X.; Tian, X.; Zhang, Y.; Zhang, J.; Zhang, P. Soy isoflavone: The multipurpose phytochemical (Review). *Biomed. Rep.* **2013**, *1*, 697–701. [CrossRef]

123. Zhou, X.; Shen, P.; Wang, W.; Zhou, J.; Raj, R.; Du, Z.; Xu, S.; Wang, W.; Yu, B.; Zhang, J. Derivatization of Soyasapogenol A through Microbial Transformation for Potential Anti-inflammatory Food Supplements. *J. Agric. Food Chem.* **2021**, *69*, 6791–6798. [CrossRef]
124. Laranjeira, T.; Costa, A.; Faria-Silva, C.; Ribeiro, D.; de Oliveira, J.M.P.F.; Simões, S.; Ascenso, A. Sustainable valorization of tomato by-products to obtain bioactive compounds: Their potential in inflammation and cancer management. *Molecules* **2022**, *27*, 1701. [CrossRef]
125. Alsuhaibani, A.M. Chemical composition and ameliorative effect of tomato on isoproterenol-induced myocardial infarction in rats. *Asian J. Clin. Nutr.* **2018**, *10*, 1–7. [CrossRef]
126. Padalino, L.; Conte, A.; Lecce, L.; Likyova, D.; Sicari, V.; Pellicano, T.M.; Poiana, M.; Del Nobile, M.A. Functional pasta with tomato by-product as a source of antioxidant compounds and dietary fibre. *Czech J. Food Sci.* **2017**, *35*, 48–56.
127. Bakic, M.T.; Pedisic, S.; Zoric, Z.; Dragovic-Uzelac, V.; Grassino, A.N. Effect of microwave-assisted extraction on polyphenols recovery from tomato peel waste. *Acta Chim. Slov.* **2019**, *66*, 367–377. [CrossRef]
128. Gutiérrez-del-Río, I.; López-Ibáñez, S.; Magadán-Corpas, P.; Fernández-Calleja, L.; Pérez-Valero, Á.; Tuñón-Granda, M.; Miguélez, E.M.; Villar, C.J.; Lombó, F. Plant Nutraceuticals as Natural Antioxidant Agents in Food Preservation. *Antioxidants* **2021**, *10*, 1264. [CrossRef]
129. Valta, K.; Damala, P.; Panaretou, V.; Orli, E.; Moustakas, K.; Loizidou, M. Review and assessment of waste and wastewater treatment from fruits and vegetables processing industries in Greece. *Waste Biomass Valorization* **2017**, *8*, 1629–1648. [CrossRef]
130. Fritsch, C.; Staebler, A.; Happel, A.; Cubero Márquez, M.A.; Aguiló-Aguayo, I.; Abadias, M.; Gallur, M.; Cigognini, I.M.; Montanari, A.; López, M.J.; et al. Processing, valorization and application of bio-waste derived compounds from potato, tomato, olive and cereals: A Review. *Sustainability* **2017**, *9*, 1492. [CrossRef]
131. Perea-Dominguez, X.P.; Hernandez-Gastelum, L.Z.; Olivas-Olguin, H.R.; Espinosa-Alonso, L.G.; Valdez-Morales, M.; Medina-Godoy, S. Phenolic composition of tomato varieties and an industrial tomato by-product: Free, conjugated and bound phenolics and antioxidant activity. *J. Food Sci. Technol.* **2018**, *55*, 3453–3461. [CrossRef]
132. Coelho, M.; Pereira, R.; Rodrigues, A.S.; Teixeira, J.A.; Pintado, M.E. Extraction of tomato by-products' bioactive compounds using ohmic technology. *Food Bioprod. Process.* **2019**, *117*, 329–339. [CrossRef]
133. Nour, V.; Panaite, T.D.; Ropota, M.; Turcu, R.; Trandafir, I.; Corbu, A.R. Nutritional and bioactive compounds in dried tomato processing waste. *CyTA J. Food* **2018**, *16*, 222–229. [CrossRef]
134. Elbadrawy, E.; Sello, A. Evaluation of nutritional value and antioxidant activity of tomato peel extracts. *Arab. J. Chem.* **2016**, *9*, S1010–S1018. [CrossRef]
135. Ćetković, G.; Savatović, S.; Čanadović-Brunet, J.; Djilas, S.; Vulić, J.; Mandić, A.; Četojević-Simin, D. Valorisation of phenolic composition, antioxidant and cell growth activities of tomato waste. *Food Chem.* **2012**, *133*, 938–945. [CrossRef]
136. Aires, A.; Carvalho, R.; Saavedra, M.J. Reuse potential of vegetable wastes (broccoli, green bean and tomato) for the recovery of antioxidant phenolic acids and flavonoids. *Int. J. Food Sci. Technol.* **2017**, *52*, 98–107. [CrossRef]
137. Navarro-González, I.; García-Valverde, V.; García-Alonso, M.; Periago, M.J. Chemical profile, functional and antioxidant properties of tomato peel fiber. *Food Res. Int.* **2011**, *44*, 1528–1535. [CrossRef]
138. Kalogeropoulos, N.; Chiou, A.; Pyriochou, V.; Peristeraki, A.; Karathanos, V.T. Bioactive phytochemicals in industrial tomatoes and their processing by-products. *LWT-Food Sci. Technol.* **2012**, *49*, 213–216. [CrossRef]
139. Di Donato, P.; Taurisano, V.; Tommonaro, G.; Pasquale, V.; Jimenez, J.M.; de Pascual, T.S.; Poli, A.; Nicolaus, B. Biological properties of polyphenols extracts from agro industry's wastes. *Waste Biomass Valorization* **2018**, *9*, 1567–1578. [CrossRef]
140. García-Valverde, V.; Navarro-González, I.; García Alonso, J.; Periago, M. Antioxidant bioactive compounds in selected industrial processing and fresh consumption tomato cultivars. *Food Bioprocess Technol.* **2013**, *6*, 391–402. [CrossRef]
141. Szabo, K.; Diaconeasa, Z.; Catoi, A.F.; Vodnar, D.C. Screening of ten tomato varieties processing waste for bioactive components and their related antioxidant and antimicrobial activities. *Antioxidants* **2019**, *8*, 292. [CrossRef]
142. Valdez-Morales, M.; Espinosa-Alonso, L.G.; Espinoza-Torres, L.C.; Delgado-Vargas, F.; Medina-Godoy, S. Phenolic content and antioxidant and antimutagenic activities in tomato peel, seeds and by-products. *J. Agric. Food Chem.* **2014**, *62*, 5281–5289. [CrossRef]
143. Kumar, M.; Tomar, M.; Bhuyan, D.J.; Punia, S.; Grasso, S.; Sa, A.G.A.; Carciofi, B.A.M.; Arrutia, F.; Changan, S.; Singh, S.; et al. Tomato (*Solanum lycopersicum* L.) seed: A review on bioactives and biomedical activities. *Biomed. Pharmacother.* **2021**, *142*, 112018. [CrossRef]
144. Concha-Meyer, A.; Palomo, I.; Plaza, A.; Gadioli Tarone, A.; Junior MR, M.; Sáyago-Ayerdi, S.G.; Fuentes, E. Platelet anti-aggregant activity and bioactive compounds of ultrasound-assisted extracts from whole and seedless tomato pomace. *Foods* **2020**, *9*, 1564. [CrossRef]
145. Fărcaș, A.C.; Socaci, S.A.; Michiu, D.; Biriș, S.; Tofană, M. Tomato waste as a source of biologically active compounds. *Bull. UASVM Food Sci. Technol.* **2019**, *76*, 85–88. [CrossRef] [PubMed]
146. Markovic, K.; Krbavcic, I.P.; Krpan, M.; Bicanic, D.; Vahcic, N. The lycopene content in pulp and peel of five fresh tomato cultivars. *Acta Aliment.* **2010**, *39*, 90–98. [CrossRef]
147. Stoica, R.M.; Tomulescu, C.; Căṣărică, A.; Soare, M.G. Tomato by-products as a source of natural antioxidants for pharmaceutical and food industries—A mini-review. *Sci. Bull. Ser. F Biotechnol.* **2018**, *22*, 200–204.

148. Górecka, D.; Wawrzyniak, A.; Jędrusek-Golińska, A.; Dziedzic, K.; Hamułka, J.; Kowalczewski, P.Ł.; Walkowiak, J. Lycopene in tomatoes and tomato products. *Open Chem.* **2020**, *18*, 752–756. [CrossRef]
149. Campestrini, L.H.; Melo, P.S.; Peres, L.E.; Calhelha, R.C.; Ferreira, I.C.; Alencar, S.M. A new variety of purple tomato as a rich source of bioactive carotenoids and its potential health benefits. *Heliyon* **2019**, *5*, e02831. [CrossRef] [PubMed]
150. Grassino, A.N.; Djakovic, S.; Bosiljkov, T.; Halambek, J.; Zorić, Z.; Dragović-Uzelac, V.; Petrović, M.; Brnčić, S.R. Valorisation of tomato peel waste as a sustainable source for pectin, polyphenols and fatty acids recovery using sequential extraction. *Waste Biomass Valorization* **2019**, *11*, 4593–4611. [CrossRef]
151. Grassino, A.N.; Pedistić, S.; Dragović-Uzelac, V.; Karlović, S.; Ježek, D.; Bosiljkov, T. Insight into high-hydrostatic pressure extraction of polyphenols from tomato peel waste. *Plant Foods Hum. Nutr.* **2020**, *75*, 427–433. [CrossRef]
152. Lucera, A.; Costa, C.; Marinelli, V.; Saccotelli, M.A.; Del Nobile, M.A.; Conte, A. Fruit and vegetable by-products to fortify spreadable cheese. *Antioxidants* **2018**, *7*, 61. [CrossRef]
153. Lim, W.; Li, J. Co-expression of onion chalcone isomerase in Del/Ros1-expressing tomato enhances anthocyanin and flavonol production. *Plant Cell Tissue Organ Cult.* **2017**, *128*, 113–124. [CrossRef]
154. Zuorro, A.; Lavecchia, R.; Medici, F.; Piga, L. Enzyme-assisted production of tomato seed oil enriched with lycopene from tomato pomace. *Food Bioprocess Technol.* **2013**, *6*, 3499–3509. [CrossRef]
155. Eller, F.J.; Moser, J.K.; Kenar, J.A.; Taylor, S.L. Extraction and analysis of tomato seed oil. *J. Am. Oil Chem. Soc.* **2010**, *87*, 755–762. [CrossRef]
156. Pellicanò, T.M.; Sicari, V.; Loizzo, M.R.; Leporini, M.; Falco, T.; Poiana, M. Optimizing the supercritical fluid extraction process of bioactive compounds from processed tomato skin by-products. *Food Sci. Technol.* **2019**, *40*, 692–697. [CrossRef]
157. Marti, R.; Rosello, S.; Cebolla-Cornejo, J. Tomato as a source of carotenoids and polyphenols targeted to cancer prevention. *Cancers* **2016**, *8*, 58. [CrossRef] [PubMed]
158. Savatović, S.; Cetkovic, G.; Canadanovic-Brunet, J.; Djilas, S. Tomato waste: A potential source of hydrophilic antioxidants. *Int. J. Food Sci. Nutr.* **2012**, *63*, 129–137. [CrossRef] [PubMed]
159. Nour, V.; Ionica, M.E.; Trandafir, I. Bread enriched in lycopene and other bioactive compounds by addition of dry tomato waste. *J. Food Sci. Technol.* **2015**, *52*, 8260–8267. [CrossRef]
160. Abid, Y.; Azabou, S.; Jridi, M.; Khemakhem, I.; Bouaziz, M.; Attia, H. Storage stability of traditional Tunisian butter enriched with antioxidant extract from tomato processing by-products. *Food Chem.* **2017**, *15*, 476–482. [CrossRef]
161. Trombino, S.; Cassano, R.; Procopio, D.; Di Gioia, M.L.; Barone, E. Valorization of tomato waste as a source of carotenoids. *Molecules* **2021**, *26*, 5062. [CrossRef]
162. Ho, K.K.; Ferruzzi, M.G.; Liceaga, A.M.; San Martin-Gonzales, M.F. Microwave-assisted extraction of lycopene in tomato peels: Effect of extraction conditions on all-trans and cis-isomer yields. *LWT-Food Sci. Technol.* **2015**, *62*, 160–168. [CrossRef]
163. Horuz, T.I.; Belibagli, K.B. Encapsulation of tomato peel extract into nanofibers and its application in model food. *Food Process. Preserv.* **2019**, *43*, e14090. [CrossRef]
164. Hernández-Carranza, P.; Ávila-Sosa, R.; Guerrero-Beltrán, J.A.; Navarro-Cruz, A.R.; Corona-Jiménez, E.; Ochoa-Velasco, C.E. Optimization of antioxidant compounds extraction from fruit by-products: Apple pomace, orange and banana peel. *J. Food Process. Preserv.* **2016**, *40*, 103–115. [CrossRef]
165. Afsharnezhad, M.; Shahangian, S.S.; Panahi, E.; Sariri, R. Evaluation of the antioxidant activity of extracts from some fruit peels. *Casp. J. Environ. Sci.* **2017**, *15*, 213–222.
166. Kabir, M.R.; Hasan, M.M.; Islam, M.R.; Haque, A.R.; Hasan, S.K. Formulation of yogurt with banana peel extracts to enhance storability and bioactive properties. *J. Food Process. Preserv.* **2021**, *45*, e15191. [CrossRef]
167. Chaudhry, F.; Ahmad, M.L.; Hayat, Z.; Ranjha MM, A.N.; Chaudhry, K.; Elboughdiri, N.; Asmari, M.; Uddin, J. Extraction and Evaluation of the Antimicrobial Activity of Polyphenols from Banana Peels Employing Different Extraction Techniques. *Separations* **2022**, *9*, 165. [CrossRef]
168. Rebello LP, G.; Ramos, A.M.; Pertuzatti, P.B.; Barcia, M.T.; Castillo-Muñoz, N.; Hermosín-Gutiérrez, I. Flour of banana (Musa AAA) peel as a source of antioxidant phenolic compounds. *Food Res. Int.* **2014**, *55*, 397–403. [CrossRef]
169. Behiry, S.I.; Okla, M.K.; Alamri, S.A.; El-Hefny, M.; Salem, M.Z.; Alaraidh, I.A.; Ali, H.M.; Al-Ghtani, S.M.; Monroy, J.C.; Salem, A.Z. Antifungal and antibacterial activities of Musa paradisiaca L. peel extract: HPLC analysis of phenolic and flavonoid contents. *Processes* **2019**, *7*, 215. [CrossRef]
170. Kandasamy, S.; Ramu, S.; Aradhya, S.M. In vitro functional properties of crude extracts and isolated compounds from banana pseudostem and rhizome. *J. Sci. Food Agric.* **2016**, *96*, 1347–1355. [CrossRef] [PubMed]
171. Avram, I.; Gatea, F.; Vamanu, E. Functional Compounds from Banana Peel Used to Decrease Oxidative Stress Effects. *Processes* **2022**, *10*, 248. [CrossRef]
172. Nofianti, T.; Ahmad, M.; Irda, F. Comparison of antihyperglycemic activity of different parts of klutuk banana (*Musa balbisiana* colla). *Int. J. Appl. Pharm.* **2021**, *13*, 57–61. [CrossRef]
173. Vu, H.T.; Scarlett, C.J.; Vuong, Q.V. Encapsulation of phenolic-rich extract from banana (*Musa cavendish*) peel. *J. Food Sci. Technol.* **2020**, *57*, 2089–2098. [CrossRef]
174. Buendía-Otero, M.J.; Jiménez-Corzo, D.J.; Caamaño De Ávila, Z.I.; Restrepo, J.B. Chromatographic analysis of phytochemicals in the peel of *Musa paradisiaca* to synthesize silver nanoparticles. *Rev. Fac. De Ing. Univ. De Antioq.* **2022**, *103*, 130–137. [CrossRef]

175. Padam, B.S.; Tin, H.S.; Chye, F.Y.; Abdullah, M.I. Banana by-products: An under-utilized renewable food biomass with great potential. *J. Food Sci. Technol.* **2014**, *51*, 3527–3545. [CrossRef] [PubMed]
176. Vani, R.; Bhandari, A.; Jain, Y.A. Inhibition Effects Of Banana And Orange Peel Extract On The Corrosion Of Bright Steel In Acidic Media. In *IOP Conference Series: Materials Science and Engineering*; IOP Publishing: Bristol, UK, 2021; Volume 1065, p. 012029. [CrossRef]
177. CSO (Central Statistical Office in Poland). Production of Agricultural and Horticultural Crops in 2021. 2022. Available online: https://stat.gov.pl/en/topics/agriculture-forestry/agricultural-and-horticultural-crops/production-of-agricultural-and-horticultural-crops-in-2021,2,6.html (accessed on 29 June 2022).
178. Fernandes, P.A.; Ferreira, S.S.; Bastos, R.; Ferreira, I.; Cruz, M.T.; Pinto, A.; Coelho, E.; Passos, C.P.; Coimbra, M.A.; Cardoso, S.M.; et al. Apple pomace extract as a sustainable food ingredient. *Antioxidants* **2019**, *8*, 189. [CrossRef] [PubMed]
179. Uyttebroek, M.; Vandezande, P.; Van Dael, M.; Vloemans, S.; Noten, B.; Bongers, B.; Porto-Carrero, M.; Unamunzaga, M.M.; Bulut, M.; Lemmens, B. Concentration of phenolic compounds from apple pomace extracts by nanofiltration at lab and pilot scale with a techno-economic assessment. *J. Food Process Eng.* **2018**, *41*, e12629. [CrossRef]
180. Barreira, J.C.; Arraibi, A.A.; Ferreira, I.C. Bioactive and functional compounds in apple pomace from juice and cider manufacturing: Potential use in dermal formulations. *Trends Food Sci. Technol.* **2019**, *90*, 76–87. [CrossRef]
181. Waldbauer, K.; McKinnon, R.; Kopp, B. Apple pomace as potential source of natural active compounds. *Planta Med.* **2017**, *83*, 994–1010. [CrossRef]
182. Li, W.; Yang, R.; Ying, D.; Yu, J.; Sanguansri, L.; Augustin, M.A. Analysis of polyphenols in apple pomace: A comparative study of different extraction and hydrolysis procedures. *Ind. Crops Prod.* **2020**, *147*, 112250. [CrossRef]
183. Gorjanović, S.; Micić, D.; Pastor, F.; Tosti, T.; Kalušević, A.; Ristić, S.; Zlatanović, S. Evaluation of apple pomace flour obtained industrially by dehydration as a source of biomolecules with antioxidant, antidiabetic and antiobesity effects. *Antioxidants* **2020**, *9*, 413. [CrossRef]
184. Perussello, C.A.; Zhang, Z.; Marzocchella, A.; Tiwari, B.K. Valorization of apple pomace by extraction of valuable compounds. *Compr. Rev. Food Sci. Food Saf.* **2017**, *16*, 776–796. [CrossRef]
185. Oleszek, M.; Pecio, Ł.; Kozachok, S.; Lachowska-Filipiuk, Ż.; Oszust, K.; Frąc, M. Phytochemicals of apple pomace as prospect bio-fungicide agents against mycotoxigenic fungal species—In vitro experiments. *Toxins* **2019**, *11*, 361. [CrossRef]
186. Ramirez-Ambrosi, M.; Abad-Garcia, B.; Viloria-Bernal, M.; Garmon-Lobato, S.; Berrueta, L.A.; Gallo, B. A new ultrahigh performance liquid chromatography with diode array detection coupled to electrospray ionization and quadrupole time-of-flight mass spectrometry analytical strategy for fast analysis and improved characterization of phenolic compounds in apple products. *J. Chromatogr. A* **2013**, *1316*, 78–91.
187. Mohammed, E.T.; Mustafa, Y.F. Coumarins from Red Delicious apple seeds: Extraction, phytochemical analysis, and evaluation as antimicrobial agents. *Syst. Rev. Pharm.* **2020**, *11*, 64–70.
188. Khalil, R.R.; Mustafa, Y.F. Phytochemical, antioxidant and antitumor studies of coumarins extracted from Granny Smith apple seeds by different methods. *Syst. Rev. Pharm.* **2020**, *11*, 57–63.
189. Pingret, D.; Fabiano-Tixier, A.S.; Le Bourvellec, C.; Renard, C.M.; Chemat, F. Lab and pilot-scale ultrasound-assisted water extraction of polyphenols from apple pomace. *J. Food Eng.* **2012**, *111*, 73–81. [CrossRef]
190. Woźniak, Ł.; Szakiel, A.; Pączkowski, C.; Marszałek, K.; Skąpska, S.; Kowalska, H.; Jędrzejczak, R. Extraction of triterpenic acids and phytosterols from apple pomace with supercritical carbon dioxide: Impact of process parameters, modelling of kinetics, and scaling-up study. *Molecules* **2018**, *23*, 2790. [CrossRef]
191. Delgado-Pelayo, R.; Gallardo-Guerrero, L.; Hornero-Méndez, D. Chlorophyll and carotenoid pigments in the peel and flesh of commercial apple fruit varieties. *Food Res. Int.* **2014**, *65*, 272–281. [CrossRef]
192. Walia, M.; Rawat, K.; Bhushan, S.; Padwad, Y.S.; Singh, B. Fatty acid composition, physicochemical properties, antioxidant and cytotoxic activity of apple seed oil obtained from apple pomace. *J. Sci. Food Agric.* **2014**, *94*, 929–934. [CrossRef]
193. Skinner, R.C.; Gigliotti, J.C.; Ku, K.M.; Tou, J.C. A comprehensive analysis of the composition, health benefits, and safety of apple pomace. *Nutr. Rev.* **2018**, *76*, 893–909. [CrossRef]
194. Gołębiewska, E.; Kalinowska, M.; Yildiz, G. Sustainable Use of Apple Pomace (AP) in Different Industrial Sectors. *Materials* **2022**, *15*, 1788. [CrossRef]
195. Rana, S.; Kumar, S.; Rana, A.; Padwad, Y.; Bhushan, S. Biological activity of phenolics enriched extracts from industrial apple pomace. *Ind. Crops Prod.* **2021**, *160*, 113158. [CrossRef]
196. Cargnin, S.T.; Gnoatto, S.B. Ursolic acid from apple pomace and traditional plants: A valuable triterpenoid with functional properties. *Food Chem.* **2017**, *220*, 477–489. [CrossRef]
197. Silva, G.N.; Maria, N.R.; Schuck, D.C.; Cruz, L.N.; de Moraes, M.S.; Nakabashi, M.; Graebin, C.; Gosmann, G.; Garcia, C.R.S.; Gnoatto, S.C. Two series of new semisynthetic triterpene derivatives: Differences in anti-malarial activity, cytotoxicity and mechanism of action. *Malar. J.* **2013**, *12*, 1–7. [CrossRef] [PubMed]
198. Arraibi, A.A.; Liberal, Â.; Dias, M.I.; Alves, M.J.; Ferreira, I.C.; Barros, L.; Barreira, J.C. Chemical and bioactive characterization of Spanish and Belgian apple pomace for its potential use as a novel dermocosmetic formulation. *Foods* **2021**, *10*, 1949. [CrossRef] [PubMed]
199. Zhang, T.; Wei, X.; Miao, Z.; Hassan, H.; Song, Y.; Fan, M. Screening for antioxidant and antibacterial activities of phenolics from Golden Delicious apple pomace. *Chem. Cent. J.* **2016**, *10*, 1–9. [CrossRef] [PubMed]

200. Haghighi, M.; Rezaei, K. Designing an all-apple-pomace-based functional dessert formulation. *Br. Food J.* **2013**, *115*, 409–424. [CrossRef]
201. Liu, B.; Liu, J.; Zhang, C.; Liu, J.; Jiao, Z. Enzymatic preparation and antioxidant activity of the phloridzin oxidation product. *J. Food Biochem.* **2018**, *42*, e12475. [CrossRef]
202. Vera, R.; Figueredo, F.; Díaz-Gómez, A.; Molinari, A. Evaluation of Fuji apple peel extract as a corrosion inhibitor for carbon steel in a saline medium. *Int. J. Electrochem. Sci.* **2018**, *13*, 4139–4159. [CrossRef]
203. Kruczek, M.; Gumul, D.; Kačániová, M.; Ivanišhová, E.; Mareček, J.; Gambuś, H. Industrial Apple Pomace By-Products As A Potential Source Of Pro-Health Compounds In Functional Food. *J. Microbiol. Biotechnol. Food Sci.* **2017**, *7*, 22–26. [CrossRef]
204. Rabetafika, H.N.; Bchir, B.; Blecker, C.; Richel, A. Fractionation of apple by-products as source of new ingredients: Current situation and perspectives. *Trends Food Sci. Technol.* **2014**, *40*, 99–114. [CrossRef]
205. Luo, H.; Li, L.; Tang, J.; Zhang, F.; Zhao, F.; Sun, D.; Zheng, F.; Wang, X. Amygdalin inhibits HSC-T6 cell proliferation and fibrosis through the regulation of TGF-β/CTGF. *Mol. Cell. Toxicol.* **2016**, *12*, 265–271. [CrossRef]
206. Song, Z.; Xu, X. Advanced research on anti-tumor effects of amygdalin. *J. Cancer Res. Ther.* **2014**, *10*, 3–7.
207. Teixeira, A.; Baenas, N.; Dominguez-Perles, R.; Barros, A.; Rosa, E.; Moreno, D.A.; Garcia-Viguera, C. Natural bioactive compounds from winery by-products as health promoters: A review. *Int. J. Mol. Sci.* **2014**, *15*, 15638–15678. [CrossRef] [PubMed]
208. Pintać, D.; Majkić, T.; Torović, L.; Orčić, D.; Beara, I.; Simin, N.; Mimica–Dukić, N.; Lesjak, M. Solvent selection for efficient extraction of bioactive compounds from grape pomace. *Ind. Crops Prod.* **2018**, *111*, 379–390. [CrossRef]
209. Eyiz, V.; Tontul, I.; Turker, S. Optimization of green extraction of phytochemicals from red grape pomace by homogenizer assisted extraction. *J. Food Meas. Charact.* **2020**, *14*, 39–47. [CrossRef]
210. Farías-Campomanes, A.M.; Rostagno, M.A.; Meireles MA, A. Production of polyphenol extracts from grape bagasse using supercritical fluids: Yield, extract composition and economic evaluation. *J. Supercrit. Fluids* **2013**, *77*, 70–78. [CrossRef]
211. Wang, X.; Tong, H.; Chen, F.; Gangemi, J.D. Chemical characterization and antioxidant evaluation of muscadine grape pomace extract. *Food Chem.* **2010**, *123*, 1156–1162. [CrossRef]
212. Daniel, T.; Ben-Shachar, M.; Drori, E.; Hamad, S.; Permyakova, A.; Ben-Cnaan, E.; Tam, J.; Kerem, Z.; Rosenzweig, T. Grape pomace reduces the severity of non-alcoholic hepatic steatosis and the development of steatohepatitis by improving insulin sensitivity and reducing ectopic fat deposition in mice. *J. Nutr. Biochem.* **2021**, *98*, 108867. [CrossRef] [PubMed]
213. Wittenauer, J.; Mäckle, S.; Sußmann, D.; Schweiggert-Weisz, U.; Carle, R. Inhibitory effects of polyphenols from grape pomace extract on collagenase and elastase activity. *Fitoterapia* **2015**, *101*, 179–187. [CrossRef]
214. Jara-Palacios, M.J.; Hernanz, D.; Cifuentes-Gomez, T.; Escudero-Gilete, M.L.; Heredia, F.J.; Spencer, J.P. Assessment of white grape pomace from winemaking as source of bioactive compounds, and its antiproliferative activity. *Food Chem.* **2015**, *183*, 78–82. [CrossRef]
215. Gonçalves, G.A.; Soares, A.A.; Correa, R.C.; Barros, L.; Haminiuk, C.W.; Peralta, R.M.; Ferreira, I.C.F.R.; Bracht, A. Merlot grape pomace hydroalcoholic extract improves the oxidative and inflammatory states of rats with adjuvant-induced arthritis. *J. Funct. Foods* **2017**, *33*, 408–418. [CrossRef]
216. Jara-Palacios, M.J.; Rodríguez-Pulido, F.J.; Hernanz, D.; Escudero-Gilete, M.L.; Heredia, F.J. Determination of phenolic substances of seeds, skins and stems from white grape marc by near-infrared hyperspectral imaging. *Aust. J. Grape Wine Res.* **2016**, *22*, 11–15. [CrossRef]
217. Balea, Ş.S.; Pârvu, A.E.; Pârvu, M.; Vlase, L.; Dehelean, C.A.; Pop, T.I. Antioxidant, Anti-Inflammatory and Antiproliferative Effects of the Vitis vinifera L. var. Fetească Neagră and Pinot Noir Pomace Extracts. *Front. Pharmacol.* **2020**, *11*, 990. [CrossRef] [PubMed]
218. Drosou, C.; Kyriakopoulou, K.; Bimpilas, A.; Tsimogiannis, D.; Krokida, M. A comparative study on different extraction techniques to recover red grape pomace polyphenols from vinification byproducts. *Ind. Crops Prod.* **2015**, *75*, 141–149. [CrossRef]
219. Negro, C.; Aprile, A.; Luvisi, A.; De Bellis, L.; Miceli, A. Antioxidant activity and polyphenols characterization of four monovarietal grape pomaces from Salento (Apulia, Italy). *Antioxidants* **2021**, *10*, 1406. [CrossRef] [PubMed]
220. Iora, S.R.; Maciel, G.M.; Zielinski, A.A.; da Silva, M.V.; Pontes PV, D.A.; Haminiuk, C.W.; Granato, D. Evaluation of the bioactive compounds and the antioxidant capacity of grape pomace. *Int. J. Food Sci. Technol.* **2015**, *50*, 62–69. [CrossRef]
221. Silva DS, M.E.; Grisi CV, B.; da Silva, S.P.; Madruga, M.S.; da Silva, F.A.P. The technological potential of agro-industrial residue from grape pulping (*Vitis* spp.) for application in meat products: A review. *Food Biosci.* **2022**, *49*, 101877. [CrossRef]
222. Gerardi, G.; Cavia-Saiz, M.; Muniz, P. From winery by-product to healthy product: Bioavailability, redox signaling and oxidative stress modulation by wine pomace product. *Crit. Rev. Food Sci. Nutr.* **2021**, *62*, 1–23. [CrossRef] [PubMed]
223. Anastasiadi, M.; Pratsinis, H.; Kletsas, D.; Skaltsounis, A.L.; Haroutounian, S.A. Grape stem extracts: Polyphenolic content and assessment of their *in vitro* antioxidant properties. *LWT-Food Sci. Technol.* **2012**, *48*, 316–322. [CrossRef]
224. Aliakbarian, B.; Fathi, A.; Perego, P.; Dehghani, F. Extraction of antioxidants from winery wastes using subcritical water. *J. Supercrit. Fluids* **2012**, *65*, 18–24. [CrossRef]
225. Álvarez, E.; Rodiño-Janeiro, B.K.; Jerez, M.; Ucieda-Somoza, R.; Núñez, M.J.; González-Juanatey, J.R. Procyanidins from grape pomace are suitable inhibitors of human endothelial NADPH oxidase. *J. Cell. Biochem.* **2012**, *113*, 1386–1396. [CrossRef]
226. Mendoza, L.; Yañez, K.; Vivanco, M.; Melo, R.; Cotoras, M. Characterization of extracts from winery by-products with antifungal activity against *Botrytis cinerea*. *Ind. Crops Prod.* **2013**, *43*, 360–364. [CrossRef]

227. Aizpurua-Olaizola, O.; Navarro, P.; Vallejo, A.; Olivares, M.; Etxebarria, N.; Usobiaga, A. Microencapsulation and storage stability of polyphenols from Vitis vinifera grape wastes. *Food Chem.* **2016**, *190*, 614–621. [CrossRef] [PubMed]
228. Alibade, A.; Kaltsa, O.; Bozinou, E.; Athanasiadis, V.; Palaiogiannis, D.; Lalas, S.; Makris, D.P. Stability of microemulsions containing red grape pomace extract obtained with a glycerol/sodium benzoate deep eutectic solvent. *OCL* **2022**, *29*, 28. [CrossRef]
229. Soares SC, S.; de Lima, G.C.; Laurentiz, A.C.; Féboli, A.; Dos Anjos, L.A.; de Paula Carlis, M.S.; da Silva Filardi, R.; de Laurentiz RD, S. In vitro anthelmintic activity of grape pomace extract against gastrointestinal nematodes of naturally infected sheep. *Int. J. Vet. Sci. Med.* **2018**, *6*, 243–247. [CrossRef] [PubMed]
230. Silvan, J.M.; Gutiérrez-Docio, A.; Moreno-Fernandez, S.; Alarcón-Cavero, T.; Prodanov, M.; Martinez-Rodriguez, A.J. Procyanidin-rich extract from grape seeds as a putative tool against Helicobacter pylori. *Foods* **2020**, *9*, 1370. [CrossRef]
231. Quiñones, M.; Guerrero, L.; Suarez, M.; Pons, Z.; Aleixandre, A.; Arola, L.; Muguerza, B. Low-molecular procyanidin rich grape seed extract exerts antihypertensive effect in males spontaneously hypertensive rats. *Food Res. Int.* **2013**, *51*, 587–595. [CrossRef]
232. Tournour, H.H.; Segundo, M.A.; Magalhães, L.M.; Barreiros, L.; Queiroz, J.; Cunha, L.M. Valorization of grape pomace: Extraction of bioactive phenolics with antioxidant properties. *Ind. Crops Prod.* **2015**, *74*, 397–406. [CrossRef]
233. Della Vedova, L.; Ferrario, G.; Gado, F.; Altomare, A.; Carini, M.; Morazzoni, P.; Aldini, G.; Baron, G. Liquid Chromatography–High-Resolution Mass Spectrometry (LC-HRMS) Profiling of Commercial Enocianina and Evaluation of Their Antioxidant and Anti-Inflammatory Activity. *Antioxidants* **2022**, *11*, 1187. [CrossRef]
234. Hübner, A.A.; Sarruf, F.D.; Oliveira, C.A.; Neto, A.V.; Fischer, D.C.; Kato, E.T.; Lourenço, F.R.; Baby, A.R.; Bacchi, E.M. Safety and photoprotective efficacy of a sunscreen system based on grape pomace (*Vitis vinifera* L.) phenolics from winemaking. *Pharmaceutics* **2020**, *12*, 1148. [CrossRef]
235. Gavrilaș, S.; Calinovici, I.; Chiș, S.; Ursachi, C.Ș.; Raț, M.; Munteanu, F.D. White Grape Pomace Valorization for Remediating Purposes. *Appl. Sci.* **2022**, *12*, 1997. [CrossRef]
236. Olt, V.; Báez, J.; Jorcin, S.; López, T.; Fernández, A.; Medrano, A. Development of a potential functional yogurt using bioactive compounds obtained from the by-product of the production of Tannat red wine. *Biol. Life Sci. Forum* **2021**, *6*, 93.
237. Asmat-Campos, D.; Bravo Huivin, E.; Avalos-Vera, V. Valorization of agro-industrial waste in a circular economy environment: Grape pomace as a source of bioactive compounds for its application in nanotechnology. In Proceedings of the 19th LACCEI International Multi-Conference for Engineering, Education, and Technology: "Prospective and Trends in Technology and Skills for Sustainable Social Development" "Leveraging Emerging Technologies to Construct the Future", Buenos Aires, Argentina, 21–23 July 2021. [CrossRef]
238. Andrés, A.I.; Petrón, M.J.; Adámez, J.D.; López, M.; Timón, M.L. Food by-products as potential antioxidant and antimicrobial additives in chill stored raw lamb patties. *Meat Sci.* **2017**, *129*, 62–70. [CrossRef] [PubMed]
239. Biniari, K.; Xenaki, M.; Daskalakis, I.; Rusjan, D.; Bouza, D.; Stavrakaki, M. Polyphenolic compounds and antioxidants of skin and berry grapes of Greek Vitis vinifera cultivars in relation to climate conditions. *Food Chem.* **2020**, *307*, 125518. [CrossRef] [PubMed]
240. Bordiga, M.; Travaglia, F.; Locatelli, M. Valorisation of grape pomace: An approach that is increasingly reaching its maturity–a review. *Int. J. Food Sci. Technol.* **2019**, *54*, 933–942. [CrossRef]
241. Chen, Y.; Wen, J.; Deng, Z.; Pan, X.; Xie, X.; Peng, C. Effective utilization of food wastes: Bioactivity of grape seed extraction and its application in food industry. *J. Funct. Foods* **2020**, *73*, 104113. [CrossRef]
242. Crupi, P.; Dipalmo, T.; Clodoveo, M.L.; Toci, A.T.; Coletta, A. Seedless table grape residues as a source of polyphenols: Comparison and optimization of non-conventional extraction techniques. *Eur. Food Res. Technol.* **2018**, *244*, 1091–1100. [CrossRef]
243. Mainente, F.; Menin, A.; Alberton, A.; Zoccatelli, G.; Rizzi, C. Evaluation of the sensory and physical properties of meat and fish derivatives containing grape pomace powders. *Int. J. Food Sci. Technol.* **2019**, *54*, 952–958. [CrossRef]
244. Gárcia-Lomillo, J.; González-SanJosé, M. Applications of wine pomace in the food industry: Approaches and functions. *Compr. Rev. Food Sci. Food Saf.* **2017**, *16*, 3–22. [CrossRef] [PubMed]
245. Liu, N.; Li, X.; Zhao, P.; Zhang, X.; Qiao, O.; Huang, L.; Gao, W. A review of chemical constituents and health-promoting effects of citrus peels. *Food Chem.* **2021**, *365*, 130585. [CrossRef]
246. Yaqoob, M.; Aggarwal, P.; Rasool, N.; Baba, W.N.; Ahluwalia, P.; Abdelrahman, R. Enhanced functional properties and shelf stability of cookies by fortification of kinnow derived phytochemicals and residues. *J. Food Meas. Charact.* **2021**, *15*, 2369–2376. [CrossRef]
247. Karetha, K.; Gadhvi, K.; Vyas, S. Peelings of citrus fruits as a precious resource of phytochemical and vital bioactive medicines during Covid: 19 periods. *Int. J. Bot. Stud.* **2020**, *5*, 342–344.
248. Benayad, O.; Bouhrim, M.; Tiji, S.; Kharchoufa, L.; Addi, M.; Drouet, S.; Hano, C.; Lorenzo, J.M.; Bendaha, H.; Bnouham, M.; et al. Phytochemical profile, α-glucosidase, and α-amylase inhibition potential and toxicity evaluation of extracts from *Citrus aurantium* (L) peel, a valuable by-product from Northeastern Morocco. *Biomolecules* **2021**, *11*, 1555. [CrossRef] [PubMed]
249. Barbosa, P.D.P.M.; Ruviaro, A.R.; Macedo, G.A. Comparison of different Brazilian citrus by-products as source of natural antioxidants. *Food Sci. Biotechnol.* **2018**, *27*, 1301–1309. [CrossRef] [PubMed]
250. Liew, S.S.; Ho, W.Y.; Yeap, S.K.; Sharifudin SA, B. Phytochemical composition and in vitro antioxidant activities of Citrus sinensis peel extracts. *PeerJ* **2018**, *6*, e5331. [CrossRef] [PubMed]
251. Jorge, N.; Silva AC, D.; Aranha, C.P. Antioxidant activity of oils extracted from orange (*Citrus sinensis*) seeds. *An. Da Acad. Bras. De Ciên.* **2016**, *88*, 951–958. [CrossRef]

252. Olfa, T.; Gargouri, M.; Akrouti, A.; Brits, M.; Gargouri, M.; Ben Ameur, R.; Pieters, L.; Foubert, K.; Magné, C.; Soussi, A.; et al. A comparative study of phytochemical investigation and antioxidative activities of six citrus peel species. *Flavour Fragr. J.* **2021**, *36*, 564–575. [CrossRef]
253. Lee, G.J.; Lee, S.Y.; Kang, N.G.; Jin, M.H. A multi-faceted comparison of phytochemicals in seven citrus peels and improvement of chemical composition and antioxidant activity by steaming. *LWT* **2022**, *160*, 113297. [CrossRef]
254. Šafranko, S.; Ćorković, I.; Jerković, I.; Jakovljević, M.; Aladić, K.; Šubarić, D.; Jokić, S. Green extraction techniques for obtaining bioactive compounds from mandarin peel (Citrus unshiu var. Kuno): Phytochemical analysis and process optimization. *Foods* **2021**, *10*, 1043. [CrossRef]
255. Huang, Q.; Liu, J.; Hu, C.; Wang, N.; Zhang, L.; Mo, X.; Li, G.; Liao, H.; Huang, H.; Ji, S.; et al. Integrative analyses of transcriptome and carotenoids profiling revealed molecular insight into variations in fruits color of Citrus Reticulata Blanco induced by transplantation. *Genomics* **2022**, *114*, 110291. [CrossRef]
256. Saini, A.; Panesar, P.S.; Bera, M.B. Valuation of Citrus reticulata (kinnow) peel for the extraction of lutein using ultrasonication technique. *Biomass Convers. Biorefinery* **2021**, *11*, 2157–2165. [CrossRef]
257. Lopresto, C.G.; Petrillo, F.; Casazza, A.A.; Aliakbarian, B.; Perego, P.; Calabrò, A. A non-conventional method to extract D-limonene from waste lemon peels and comparison with traditional Soxhlet extraction. *Sep. Purif. Technol.* **2014**, *137*, 13–20. [CrossRef]
258. Okino Delgado, C.H.; Fleuri, L.F. Orange and mango by-products: Agro-industrial waste as source of bioactive compounds and botanical versus commercial description—A review. *Food Rev. Int.* **2016**, *32*, 1–14. [CrossRef]
259. Yang, X.; Kang, S.M.; Jeon, B.T.; Kim, Y.D.; Ha, J.H.; Kim, Y.T.; Jeon, Y.J. Isolation and identification of an antioxidant flavonoid compound from citrus-processing by-product. *J. Sci. Food Agric.* **2011**, *91*, 1925–1927. [CrossRef] [PubMed]
260. Fava, F.; Zanaroli, G.; Vannini, L.; Guerzoni, E.; Bordoni, A.; Viaggi, D.; Robertson, J.; Waldron, K.; Bald, C.; Esturo, A.; et al. New advances in the integrated management of food processing by-products in Europe: Sustainable exploitation of fruit and cereal processing by-products with the production of new food products (NAMASTE EU). *New Biotechnol.* **2013**, *30*, 647–655. [CrossRef] [PubMed]
261. Lv, K.; Zhang, L.; Zhao, H.; Ho, C.T.; Li, S. Recent study on the anticancer activity of nobiletin and its metabolites. *J. Food Bioact.* **2021**, *14*. [CrossRef]
262. Gao, Z.; Wang, Z.Y.; Guo, Y.; Chu, C.; Zheng, G.D.; Liu, E.H.; Li, F. Enrichment of polymethoxyflavones from Citrus reticulata 'Chachi' peels and their hypolipidemic effect. *J. Chromatogr. B* **2019**, *1124*, 226–232. [CrossRef]
263. Zeng, S.-L.; Li, S.-Z.; Xiao, P.-T.; Cai, Y.-Y.; Chu, C.; Chen, B.-Z.; Li, P.; Li, J.; Liu, E.H. Citrus polymethoxyflavones attenuate metabolic syndrome by regulating gut microbiome and amino acid metabolism. *Sci. Adv.* **2020**, *6*, eaax6208. [CrossRef]
264. Chiechio, S.; Zammataro, M.; Barresi, M.; Amenta, M.; Ballistreri, G.; Fabroni, S.; Rapisarda, P. A standardized extract prepared from red orange and lemon wastes blocks high-fat diet-induced hyperglycemia and hyperlipidemia in mice. *Molecules* **2021**, *26*, 4291. [CrossRef]
265. Barbosa PD, P.M.; Ruviaro, A.R.; Martins, I.M.; Macedo, J.A.; LaPointe, G.; Macedo, G.A. Enzyme-assisted extraction of flavanones from citrus pomace: Obtention of natural compounds with anti-virulence and anti-adhesive effect against Salmonella enterica subsp. enterica serovar Typhimurium. *Food Control* **2021**, *120*, 107525. [CrossRef]
266. Lamine, M.; Gargouri, M.; Rahali, F.Z.; Mliki, A. Recovering and characterizing phenolic compounds from citrus by-product: A way towards agriculture of subsistence and sustainable bioeconomy. *Waste Biomass Valorization* **2021**, *12*, 4721–4731. [CrossRef]
267. Gunwantrao, B.B.; Bhausaheb, S.K.; Ramrao, B.S.; Subhash, K.S. Antimicrobial activity and phytochemical analysis of orange (Citrus aurantium L.) and pineapple (Ananas comosus (L.) Merr.) peel extract. *Ann. Phytomed.* **2016**, *5*, 156–160. [CrossRef]
268. Khan, N.H.; Qian, C.J.; Perveen, N. Phytochemical screening, antimicrobial and antioxidant activity determination of citrus maxima peel. *Pharm. Pharmacol. Int. J.* **2018**, *6*, 279–285.
269. Khan, J.; Sakib, S.A.; Mahmud, S.; Khan, Z.; Islam, M.N.; Sakib, M.A.; Emran, T.B.; Simal-Gandara, J. Identification of potential phytochemicals from Citrus limon against main protease of SARS-CoV-2: Molecular docking, molecular dynamic simulations and quantum computations. *J. Biomol. Struct. Dyn.* **2021**, *40*, 1–12. [CrossRef] [PubMed]
270. Achimón, F.; Leal, L.E.; Pizzolitto, R.P.; Brito, V.D.; Alarcón, R.; Omarini, A.B.; Zygadlo, J.A. Insecticidal and antifungal effects of lemon, orange, and grapefruit peel essential oils from Argentina. *Agriscientia* **2022**, *39*, 71–82.
271. Liu, Y.; Benohoud, M.; Yamdeu JH, G.; Gong, Y.Y.; Orfila, C. Green extraction of polyphenols from citrus peel by-products and their antifungal activity against Aspergillus flavus. *Food Chem. X* **2021**, *12*, 100144. [CrossRef] [PubMed]
272. Jiang, H.; Chen, H.; Jin, C.; Mo, J.; Wang, H. Nobiletin flavone inhibits the growth and metastasis of human pancreatic cancer cells via induction of autophagy, G0/G1 cell cycle arrest, and inhibition of NF-kB signalling pathway. *J. Buon* **2020**, *25*, 1070–1075.
273. Ozkan, A.D.; Kaleli, S.; Onen, H.I.; Sarihan, M.; Eskiler, G.G.; Yigin, A.K.; Akdogan, M. Anti-inflammatory effects of nobiletin on TLR4/TRIF/IRF3 and TLR9/IRF7 signaling pathways in prostate cancer cells. *Immunopharmacol. Immunotoxicol.* **2020**, *42*, 93–100. [CrossRef] [PubMed]
274. Hanafy, S.M.; El-Shafea, A.; Mohamed, Y.; Saleh, W.D.; Fathy, H.M. Chemical profiling, in vitro antimicrobial and antioxidant activities of pomegranate, orange and banana peel-extracts against pathogenic microorganisms. *J. Genet. Eng. Biotechnol.* **2021**, *19*, 1–10. [CrossRef] [PubMed]
275. Abbattista, R.; Ventura, G.; Calvano, C.D.; Cataldi, T.R.; Losito, I. Bioactive compounds in waste by-products from olive oil production: Applications and structural characterization by mass spectrometry techniques. *Foods* **2021**, *10*, 1236. [CrossRef]

276. Martakos, I.; Katsianou, P.; Koulis, G.; Efstratiou, E.; Nastou, E.; Nikas, S.; Dasenaki, M.; Pentogennis, M.; Thomaidis, N. Development of Analytical Strategies for the Determination of Olive Fruit Bioactive Compounds Using UPLC-HRMS and HPLC-DAD. Chemical Characterization of Kolovi Lesvos Variety as a Case Study. *Molecules* 2021, *26*, 7182. [CrossRef]
277. Dermeche, S.; Nadour, M.; Larroche, C.; Moulti-Mati, F.; Michaud, P. Olive mill wastes: Biochemical characterizations and valorization strategies. *Process Biochem.* 2013, *48*, 1532–1552. [CrossRef]
278. Darvishzadeh, P.; Orsat, V. Microwave-assisted extraction of antioxidant compounds from Russian olive leaves and flowers: Optimization, HPLC characterization and comparison with other methods. *J. Appl. Res. Med. Aromat. Plants* 2022, *27*, 100368. [CrossRef]
279. Russo, E.; Spallarossa, A.; Comite, A.; Pagliero, M.; Guida, P.; Belotti, V.; Caviglia, D.; Schito, A.M. Valorization and Potential Antimicrobial Use of Olive Mill Wastewater (OMW) from Italian Olive Oil Production. *Antioxidants* 2022, *11*, 903. [CrossRef] [PubMed]
280. D'Antuono, I.; Kontogianni, V.G.; Kotsiou, K.; Linsalata, V.; Logrieco, A.F.; Tasioula-Margari, M.; Cardinali, A. Polyphenolic characterization of Olive Mill Waste Waters, coming from Italian and Greek olive cultivars, after membrane technology. *Food Res. Int.* 2014, *65*, 301–310. [CrossRef]
281. Alu'datt, M.H.; Alli, I.; Ereifej, K.; Alhamad, M.; Al-Tawaha, A.R.; Rababah, T. Optimisation, characterisation and quantification of phenolic compounds in olive cake. *Food Chem.* 2010, *123*, 117–122. [CrossRef]
282. Zhao, H.; Avena-Bustillos, R.J.; Wang, S.C. Extraction, Purification and In Vitro Antioxidant Activity Evaluation of Phenolic Compounds in California Olive Pomace. *Foods* 2022, *11*, 174. [CrossRef]
283. Benincasa, C.; Pellegrino, M.; Romano, E.; Claps, S.; Fallara, C.; Perri, E. Qualitative and Quantitative Analysis of Phenolic Compounds in Spray-Dried Olive Mill Wastewater. *Front. Nutr.* 2022, *8*, 782693. [CrossRef]
284. Ladhari, A.; Zarrelli, A.; Ghannem, M.; Ben Mimoun, M. Olive wastes as a high-potential by-product: Variability of their phenolic profiles, antioxidant and phytotoxic properties. *Waste Biomass Valorization* 2021, *12*, 3657–3669. [CrossRef]
285. Poerschmann, J.; Weiner, B.; Baskyr, I. Organic compounds in olive mill wastewater and in solutions resulting from hydrothermal carbonization of the wastewater. *Chemosphere* 2013, *92*, 1472–1482. [CrossRef]
286. Uribe, E.; Pasten, A.; Lemus-Mondaca, R.; Vega-Gálvez, A.; Quispe-Fuentes, I.; Ortiz, J.; Di Scala, K. Comparison of Chemical Composition, Bioactive Compounds and Antioxidant Activity of Three Olive-Waste Cakes. *J. Food Biochem.* 2015, *39*, 189–198. [CrossRef]
287. Akli, H.; Grigorakis, S.; Kellil, A.; Loupassaki, S.; Makris, D.P.; Calokerinos, A.; Mati, A.; Lydakis-Simantiris, N. Extraction of Polyphenols from Olive Leaves Employing Deep Eutectic Solvents: The Application of Chemometrics to a Quantitative Study on Antioxidant Compounds. *Appl. Sci.* 2022, *12*, 831. [CrossRef]
288. Taamalli, A.; Arraez-Roman, D.; Barrajon-Catalan, E.; Ruiz-Torres, V.; Perez-Sanchez, A.; Herrero, M.; Ibanñez, E.; Micol, V.; Zarrouk, M.; Segura-Carretero, A.; et al. Use of advanced techniques for the extraction of phenolic compounds from Tunisian olive leaves: Phenolic composition and cytotoxicity against human breast cancer cells. *Food Chem. Toxicol.* 2012, *50*, 1817–1825. [CrossRef] [PubMed]
289. Servian-Rivas, L.D.; Pachón, E.R.; Rodríguez, M.; González-Miquel, M.; González, E.J.; Díaz, I. Techno-economic and environmental impact assessment of an olive tree pruning waste multiproduct biorefinery. *Food Bioprod. Process.* 2022, *134*, 95–108. [CrossRef]
290. Yeniçeri, M.; Filik, A.G.; Filik, G. The Effect of Some Selected Fruit Wastes for Poultry Feed on Growth Performance of Broilers. *Palandöken J. Anim. Sci. Technol. Econ.* 2022, *1*, 33–41.
291. Kreatsouli, K.; Fousteri, Z.; Zampakas, K.; Kerasioti, E.; Veskoukis, A.S.; Mantas, C.; Gkoutsidis, P.; Ladas, D.; Petrotos, K.; Kouretas, D.; et al. A Polyphenolic Extract from Olive Mill Wastewaters Encapsulated in Whey Protein and Maltodextrin Exerts Antioxidant Activity in Endothelial Cells. *Antioxidants* 2019, *8*, 280. [CrossRef] [PubMed]
292. Lafka, T.I.; Lazou, A.E.; Sinanoglou, V.J.; Lazos, E.S. Phenolic and antioxidant potential of olive oil mill wastes. *Food Chem.* 2011, *125*, 92–98. [CrossRef]
293. Visioli, F.; Romani, A.; Mulinacci, N.; Zarini, S.; Conte, D.; Vincieri, F.F.; Galli, G. Antioxidant and other biological activities of olive mill waste waters. *J. Agric. Food Chem.* 1999, *47*, 3397–3401. [CrossRef]
294. Di Mauro, M.D.; Fava, G.; Spampinato, M.; Aleo, D.; Melilli, B.; Saita, M.G.; Centonze, G.; Maggiore, R.; D'Antona, N. Polyphenolic Fraction from Olive Mill Wastewater: Scale-Up and in Vitro Studies for Ophthalmic Nutraceutical Applications. *Antioxidants* 2019, *8*, 462. [CrossRef]
295. Robles-Almazan, M.; Pulido-Moran, M.; Moreno-Fernandez, J.; Ramirez-Tortosa, C.; Rodriguez-Garcia, C.; Quiles, J.L.; Ramirez-Tortosa, M.C. Hydroxytyrosol: Bioavailability, toxicity, and clinical applications. *Food Res. Int.* 2018, *105*, 654–667. [CrossRef]
296. Bernini, R.; Merendino, N.; Romani, A.; Velotti, F. Naturally occurring hydroxytyrosol: Synthesis and anticancer potential. *Curr. Med. Chem.* 2013, *20*, 655–670. [CrossRef]
297. Benincasa, C.; La Torre, C.; Plastina, P.; Fazio, A.; Perri, E.; Caroleo, M.C.; Gallelli, L.; Cannataro, R.; Cione, E. Hydroxytyrosyl Oleate: Improved Extraction Procedure from Olive Oil and By-Products, and In Vitro Antioxidant and Skin Regenerative Properties. *Antioxydants* 2019, *8*, 233. [CrossRef]
298. Obied, H.K.; Allen, M.S.; Bedgood, D.R. Bioscreening of Australian olive mill waste extracts: Biophenol content, antioxidant, antimicrobial and molluscicidal activities. *Food Chem. Toxicol.* 2007, *45*, 1238–1248. [CrossRef] [PubMed]

299. Yangui, T.; Sayadi, S.; Gargoubi, A.; Dhouib, A. Fungicidal effect of hydroxytyrosol rich preparations from olive mill wastewater against Verticillium dahliae. *Crop Prot.* **2010**, *29*, 1208–1213. [CrossRef]
300. Abdel-Razek, A.G.; Badr, A.; Shehata, G. Characterization of Olive Oil By-products: Antioxidant Activity, Its Ability to Reduce Aflatoxigenic Fungi Hazard and Its Aflatoxins. *Annu. Res. Rev. Biol.* **2017**, *14*, 1–14. [CrossRef]
301. Abi-Khattar, A.M.; Rajha, N.; Abdel-Massih, M.; Maroun, G.; Louka, N.; Debs, E. Intensification of Polyphenol Extraction from Olive Leaves Using Ired-Irrad, an Environmentally-Friendly Innovative Technology. *Antioxidants* **2019**, *8*, 227. [CrossRef]
302. Bavaro, S.L.; D'Antuono, I.; Cozzi, G.; Haidukowski, M.; Cardinali, A.; Logrieco, A.F. Inhibition of aflatoxin B_1 production by verbascoside and other olive polyphenols. *World Mycotoxin J.* **2016**, *9*, 545–553. [CrossRef]
303. Schaffer, S.; Müller, W.E.; Eckert, G.P. Cytoprotective effects of olive mill waste water extract and its main constituent hydroxytyrosol in PC12 cells. *Pharmacol. Res.* **2010**, *62*, 322–327. [CrossRef]
304. Palos-Hernández, A.; Fernández MY, G.; Burrieza, J.E.; Pérez-Iglesias, J.L.; González-Paramás, A.M. Obtaining green extracts rich in phenolic compounds from underexploited food by-products using natural deep eutectic solvents. Opportunities and challenges. *Sustain. Chem. Pharm.* **2022**, *29*, 100773. [CrossRef]

Disclaimer/Publisher's Note: The statements, opinions and data contained in all publications are solely those of the individual author(s) and contributor(s) and not of MDPI and/or the editor(s). MDPI and/or the editor(s) disclaim responsibility for any injury to people or property resulting from any ideas, methods, instructions or products referred to in the content.

Article

Chemical Composition Profiling and Antifungal Activity of Saffron Petal Extract

Nadia Naim [1,2], Marie-Laure Fauconnier [3], Nabil Ennahli [1], Abdessalem Tahiri [4], Mohammed Baala [4], Ilham Madani [2], Said Ennahli [1,*] and Rachid Lahlali [4,*]

1. Department of Arboriculture-Viticulture, Ecole Nationale d'Agriculture de Meknès, Km10, Rte Haj Kaddour, BP S/40, Meknès 50001, Morocco
2. Faculty of Sciences, Moulay Ismail University, Meknes 50001, Morocco
3. Gembloux AgroBiotech, University of Liege, 5030 Gembloux, Belgium
4. Phytopathology Unit, Department of Plant Protection, Ecole Nationale d'Agriculture de Meknès, Km10, Rte Haj Kaddour, BP S/40, Menkes 50001, Morocco
* Correspondence: sennahli@enameknes.ac.ma (S.E.); rlahlali@enameknes.ac.ma (R.L.)

Abstract: Numerous fungal plant pathogens can infect fresh fruits and vegetables during transit and storage conditions. The resulting infections were mainly controlled by synthetic fungicides, but their application has many drawbacks associated with the threatened environment and human health. Therefore, the use of natural plants with antimicrobial potential could be a promising alternative to overcome the side effects of fungicides. In this regard, this study aimed at evaluating the antifungal activity potential of saffron petal extract (SPE) against three mains important fungal pathogens: *Rhizopus stolonifer*, *Penicillium digitatum* and *Botritys cinerea*, which cause rot decay on the tomato, orange and apple fruits, respectively. In addition, the organic composition of SPE was characterized by attenuated total reflection Fourier transform infrared (ATR-FT-IR) spectroscopy and its biochemical, and gas chromatography-mass spectrometry (GC-MS) analyses were carried out. The obtained results highlighted an increased inhibition rate of the mycelial growth and spore germination of the three pathogenic fungi with increasing SPE concentrations. The mycelial growth and spore germination were completely inhibited at 10% of the SPE for *Rhizopus stolonifer* and *Penicillium digitatum* and at 5% for *B. cinerea*. Interestingly, the in vivo test showed the complete suppression of *Rhizopus* rot by the SPE at 10%, and a significant reduction of the severity of grey mold disease (37.19%) and green mold, when applied at 5 and 10%, respectively. The FT-IR spectra showed characteristic peaks and a variety of functional groups, which confirmed that SPE contains phenolic and flavonoid components. In addition, The average value of the total phenolic content, flavonoid content and half-maximal inhibitory concentration (IC_{50}) were 3.09 ± 0.012 mg GAE/g DW, 0.92 ± 0.004 mg QE/g DW and 235.15 ± 2.12 µg/mL, respectively. A volatile analysis showed that the most dominant component in the saffron petal is 2(5H)-Furanone (92.10%). Taken together, it was concluded that SPE could be used as an alternative to antioxidant and antifungal compounds for the control of postharvest diseases in fruits.

Keywords: saffron petal extracts; antifungal effect; postharvest diseases; biochemical analysis; GC-MS; FT-IR

1. Introduction

Saffron (*Crocus sativus* L.) is one of the most valuable medicinal plants worldwide. The flowers of the saffron are a combination of six petals, three stamens, and three red stigmas [1]. The dried red stigma of the saffron flowers is one of the most expensive spices in the world [2,3]. It is widely used as a spice and as a coloring and flavoring agent in the preparation of various foods, cosmetics preparation and disease treatments. The saffron is also well known for its pharmacological benefits, such as antioxidant [4], anti-inflammatory [5], antihypertensive and hypolipidemic [6], antidepressant [7] and antitumor activities [8]. Recently, a new study demonstrated its anti-inflammatory and antiviral potential against severe COVID-19 symptoms [9].

In saffron production, great amounts of floral bio-residues are generated (92.6 g per 100 g of flowers). For every kilogram of the produced spice, about 63 kg of floral bio-residues are generated (about 53 kg of petals, 9 kg of stamens, 1 kg of styles, 1500 kg of leaves,100 kg of spathes and 100 kg of corms [10]). The saffron petal, as a by-product, is available for free and produced in large amounts, compared to the saffron stigma; but in general, they are not used as a food component and are thrown away after harvesting [11] or used to feed domestic animals [12] (Moshiri et al., 2006). Diverse compounds are identified in saffron petals, such as the phenolic content and antioxidant activity [13]. Flavonols, such as kaempferol, quercetin, isorhamnetin, and anthocyanins, such as delphinidin, petunidin and malvidin, are isolated from the saffron petals [14].

Several properties of the saffron floral bio-residues have been demonstrated, such as antityrosinase [15], antidepressant [12], antinociceptive and anti-inflammatory activities [16], antifungal and cytotoxic against tumor cell lines [17], arterial pressure reducer [18] and antibacterial [19]. Therefore, saffron petals might be considered as an appropriate source for different purposes. Regarding the toxicity of saffron petals, the toxicity of the stigma is greater than the petals (the IC_{50} values of the saffron stigma and petals, in mice, were 1.6 and 6 g/kg, respectively) [20].

Fruits and vegetables are metabolically active and subjected to senescence changes that need to be controlled, to maintain their long-term quality and shelf life [21]. Generally, the postharvest decay of fruit and vegetables is caused by several plant pathogens, in particular fungi and bacteria, resulting in severe losses during packing and storing [22]. The most important fungal pathogens the cause postharvest diseases in fruits belong to the *Alternaria*, *Aspergillus*, *Botrytis*, *Fusarium*, *Geotrichum*, *Gloeosporium*, *Mucor*, *Monilinia*, *Penicillium*, and *Rhizopus* genera. These pathogens are mainly controlled using synthetic fungicides, which have several drawbacks, such as high costs, risks associated with handling, residue persistence on food, and therefore a high risk for human health and the environment [23]. As a result, consumers tend to look for residue-free products, thereby, farmers are shifting towards natural alternatives, to protect their fruit during the storing period.

Plants produce several secondary metabolites that have a biocidal action against postharvest pathogens [24]. These compounds are associated with the plant immune system and can play an important role as fungal inhibitors [25]. Numerous studies have highlighted the antimicrobial properties of natural plant extracts, basically due to their richness, with different classes of phenolic compounds [26]. In this regard, Kaveh [27] reported that the phytochemical composition of saffron petals and stigma was flavonoids, anthocyanins, alkaloids, carbohydrate glycosides, tannins, terpenes, steroids and saponins, which are useful in extending the shelf life of fresh-cut fruits, such as the watermelon [27]. Therefore, this study aims to evaluate the antifungal activity of saffron petal extracts (SPEs) in controlling postharvest diseases in fruit caused by *Rhizopus stolonifer*, *Penicillium digitatum* and *Botrytis cinerea*. In addition, the ATR-FTIR, GS-MS and biochemical analysis were performed to decipher the organic and chemical profiling of SPE.

2. Results

2.1. Antifungal Activity of the Saffron Petal Extract (SPE) on the Mycelial Growth

The effect of the SPE on the mycelial growth of *R. stolonifer* was revealed to be significant ($p < 0.05$) (Figure 1). The four SPE concentrations significantly reduced the mycelial growth with inhibition rates ranging from 37.62 to 100%. A complete inhibition was obtained with 10% of the SPE, which was comparable to that obtained with the fungicidal difenoconazole (1 ppm). Additionally, the IC_{50} value was determined using the linear regression equation (y = 8.007x + 19.23; R^2 = 0.99). The estimated IC_{50} was 3.84%.

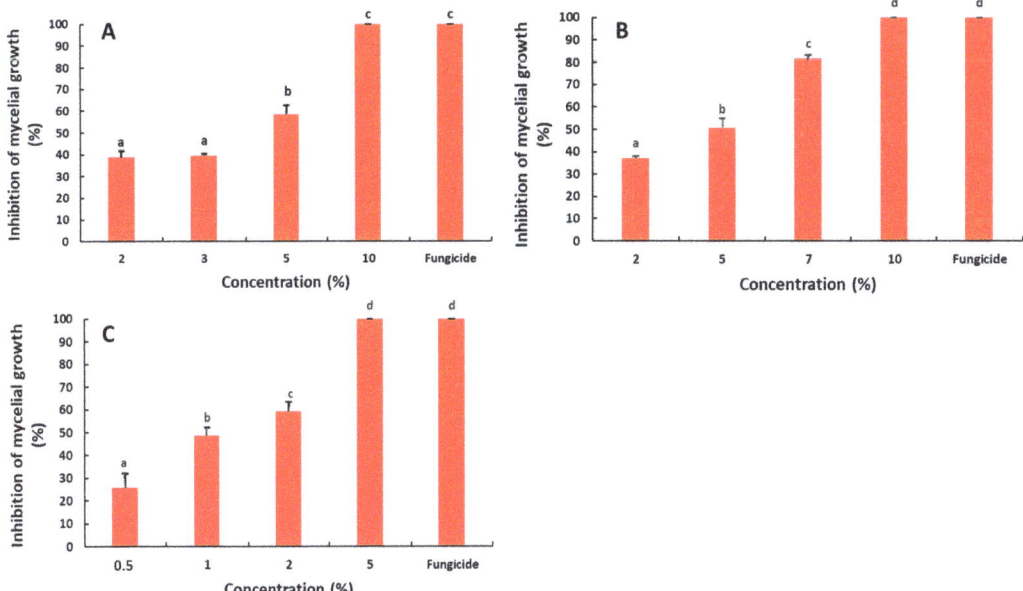

Figure 1. Effect of the saffron petal extract on the mycelial growth of postharvest fungal pathogens *R. stolonifera* (**A**), *P. digitatum* (**B**) and *B. cinerea* (**C**). The different letters (a–d) represent the statistically significant differences between the concentrations, according to Duncan's test ($p < 0.05$).

The impact of the SPE on the mycelial growth of *P. digitatum* was evaluated (Figure 1). All tested concentrations showed a significant reduction of the mycelial growth. The inhibition rate increased with the increasing SPE concentration with the percentage ranging from 37.06 to 100%. The complete inhibition was obtained with the highest concentration of the SPE (10%). This result was comparable to that obtained with the fungicidal difenoconazole (1 ppm). Furthermore, the IC_{50} value was 3.91%, according to the linear regression curve ($y = 8.312x + 17.46$, $R^2 = 0.95$).

Regarding the effect of the SPE on the mycelial growth of *B. cinerea*, the results evidenced the same trend (Figure 1). The effect was significant with inhibition rates ranging from 25.96 to 100%. The highest inhibition rate (100%) was observed at 5% of the SPE and it was statistically comparable to that of the fungicidal difenoconazole (1 ppm). Moreover, the IC_{50} value was 1.56%, according to the linear regression equation ($y = 15.04x + 26.45$, $R^2 = 0.96$).

2.2. Antifungal Activity of the Saffron Petal Extract (SPE) on the Spore Germination

The possible effect of the SPE on the spore germination of postharvest fungal pathogens was also evaluated (Figure 2). The effect was revealed as significant ($p < 0.05$). The inhibition rates of the spore germination of *R. stolonifer* ranged from 46.04 to 100%, with the highest rate observed at 10% of the SPE. The IC_{50} was 2.06%, according to the linear regression equation ($y = 6.481x + 36.63$; $R^2 = 0.98$).

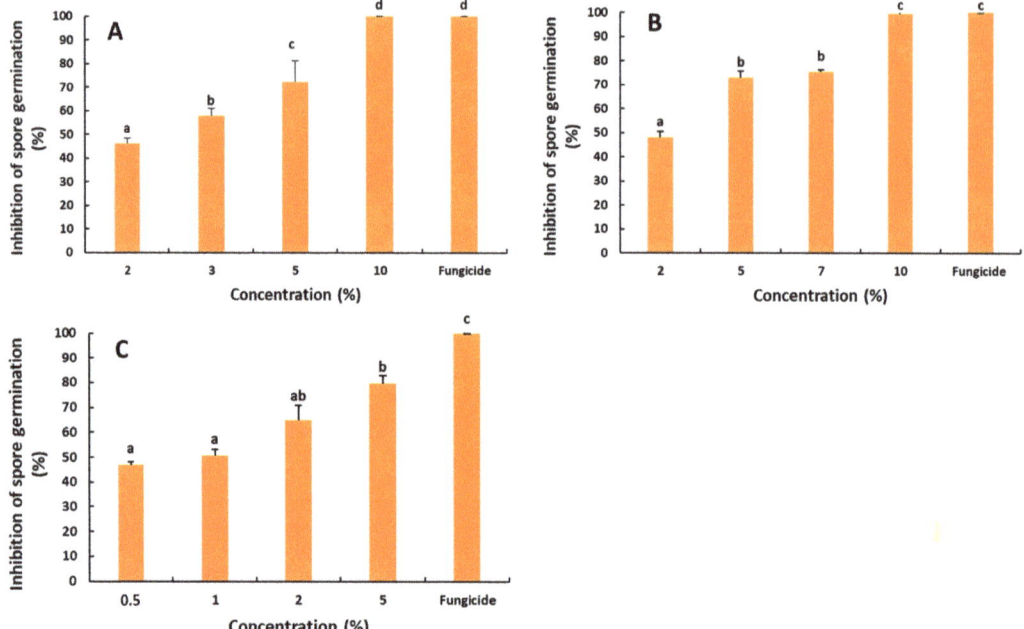

Figure 2. Effect of the saffron petal extract on the spore germination of postharvest fungal pathogens. *R. stolonifera* (**A**), *P. digitatum* (**B**) and *B. cinerea* (**C**). The different letters (a–d) represent the statistically significant differences between the concentrations, according to Duncan's test ($p < 0.05$).

Concerning the impact of the SPE on the spore germination of *P. digitatum*, the results presented in Figure 2 denote a significant difference in the inhibition rates of the spore germination, with respect to the SPE concentrations ($p < 0.05$). The inhibition rates ranged from 48.09 to 99.47%. The spore germination was completely inhibited at the concentration of 10% SPE after 24 h of incubation. A similar result was obtained with the fungicidal difenoconazole. Furthermore, the IC_{50} was 2.07%, according to the linear regression equation (y = 6.11x + 37.28; R^2 = 0.96).

Likewise, the effect of the SPE on the spore germination of *B. cinerea* was significant (Figure 2). The highest inhibition rate (79.70%) was obtained with 5% of the SPE and the fungicidal difenoconazole (100%). The IC_{50} was 0.66, based on the linear regression curve (y = 7.20x + 45.24; R^2 = 0.96).

2.3. Effect of the Saffron Petal Extract on the Rot Decay Development

To confirm the effectiveness of the SPE in controlling the rot decay in fruit, trials were conducted and the disease severity was determined for each fungi (Figure 3). The results showed that the SPE at 2, 3 and 5% reduced the severity of *R. stolonifer* to 63.75, 62.66 and 57.96%. While, at 10% of the SPE, the disease was completely controlled (0% severity). This result was similar to that obtained with difenoconazole (1 ppm).

For green mold on the orange, the obtained results underlined a slight reduction in the disease severity, when compared with the untreated control. The highest reduction rate was registered at 10% of the SPE with 66.55%. This result was lower than that obtained with the fungicidal difenoconazole, which completely inhibited the disease development.

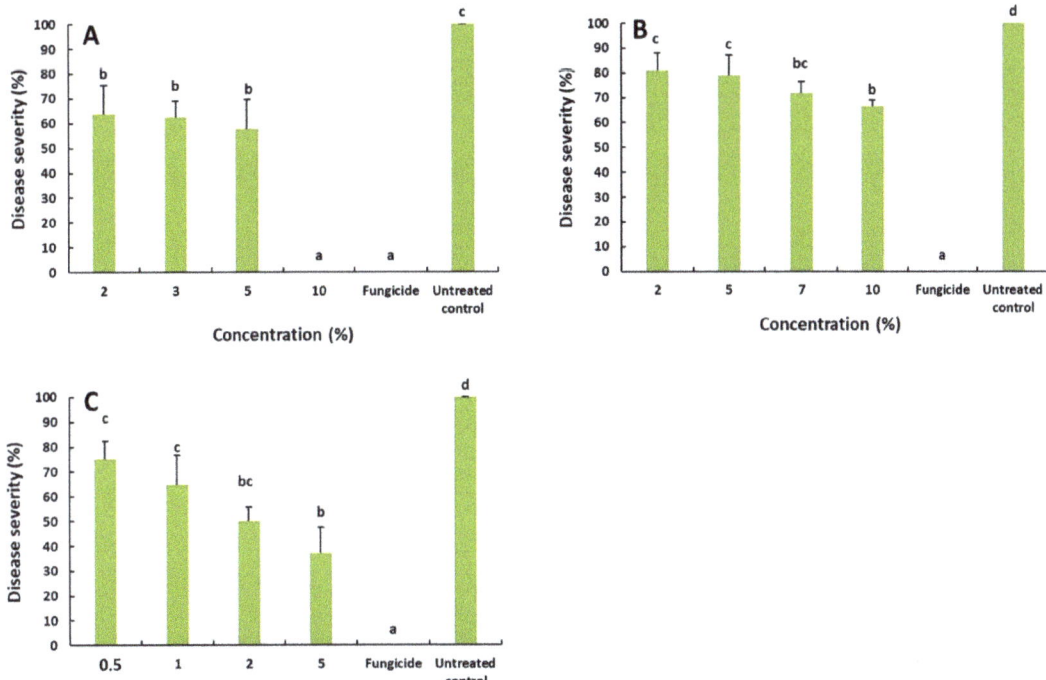

Figure 3. Effect of the saffron petal extract on the development of rot decay caused by *R. stolonifer* (**A**) on the tomato, *P. digitatum* (**B**) on the orange and *B. cinerea* (**C**) on the apple fruit. The different letters (a–d) represent the statistically significant differences between concentrations, according to Duncan's test ($p < 0.05$).

The disease severity, due to *B. cinerea* on the apple, was significantly reduced with reduction rates varying from 75.12 to 37.19%. The highest reduction rate was obtained with 5% of the SPE.

2.4. Chemical Composition

2.4.1. FTIR Analysis of the Organic Composition

The ATR-FTIR spectrum was used to identify the functional groups of the active components of the SPE. The obtained ATR-FTIR spectrum of the SPE sample is shown in Figure 4. The results showed distinct peaks characteristic of the functional groups. These functional groups were identified for the saffron petals, based on the literature [28–31]. The absorption band at 3300 cm^{-1} corresponds to the stretching vibration of the O-H hydroxyl group (water or phenol and alcohol). The characteristic absorption bands at 2922 and 2850 cm^{-1} were attributed to the asymmetrical and symmetrical C-H stretch vibrations of methylene [32]. The band at 1733 cm^{-1} is due to the stretching of the carbonyl and ester groups. The band at 1607 cm^{-1} is assigned to the –C=C group and conjugated C=O group. Other characteristic vibrations of the saffron petals, attributed to the monoterpenes, are located at 1408 and 1370 cm^{-1}. In addition, the spectrum showed the strong band at 1016 cm^{-1}, associated with the presence of the carbohydrates group. The intensity of the bands, in ascending order, was 0.05 (3300 cm^{-1}), 0.043 (1016 cm^{-1}), 0.042 (2918 cm^{-1}), 0.035 (2850 cm^{-1}), 0.023 (1607 and 1370 cm^{-1}), 0.22 (1409 cm^{-1}), 0.021 (1640 cm^{-1}) and 0.018 (1733 cm^{-1}). The band at 3300 cm^{-1} was mainly associated with the effect of the antioxidant and antifungal, while other bands were related to the lipid acyl chains, carbonyl ester group, phenolic, aromatic groups and the presence of cell wall components (Table 1).

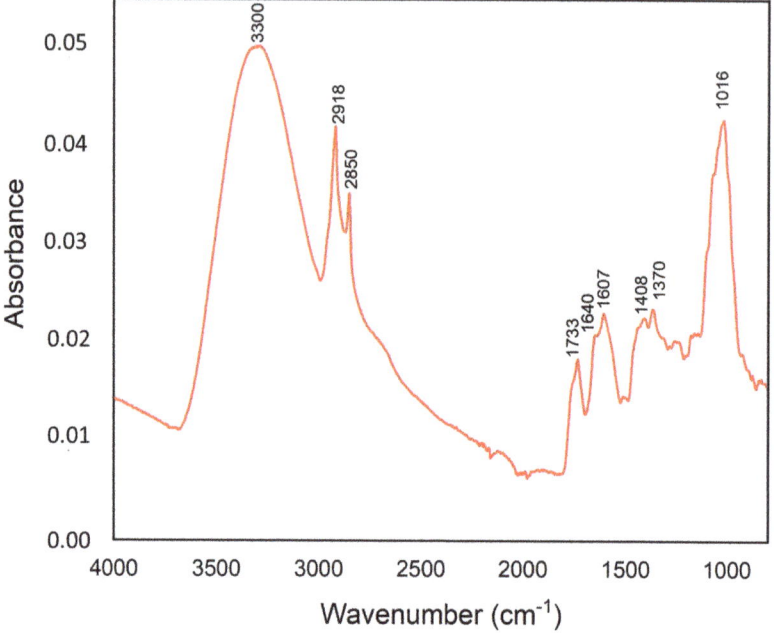

Figure 4. Averaged ATR-FTIR spectrum of the saffron petal powder in the mid-infrared region (4000–800 cm^{-1}). This IR spectrum is an average of three replicates, each one corresponding to the accumulation of 128 scans.

Table 1. Assignment (tentative) of the infrared bands observed in the saffron petal powder, based on the literature [31,32].

Wavenumber (cm^{-1})	Group	Characteristics
3300	O-H str. of the hydroxyl group	Hydroxyl of the phenolic compounds
2918	C-H str. (asym) of CH2	Aliphatic C-H from the lipid acyl chains
2850	C-H str. (sym) of CH2 from	Aliphatic C-H from the lipid acyl chains
1733	C-O stretching vibration	Carbonyl ester group (lipid)
1640	C=O and C=C stretching vibratons of cis-alkene	Carboxylic groups, hemicellulose or amide groups in proteins
1607	–C=C group of alkenes and conjugated C=O group	Aromatic group, phenolic ring, pectin ester group
1408	C-H stretching	Aromatic group
1370	CH$_2$ scissors vibration	Xyloglucan, cellulose
1016	C-O stretchings	Pectins

2.4.2. Total Phenolic, Flavonoid Contents and the DPPH Radical Scavenging Activity

The total phenolic, flavonoid contents and the DPPH radical scavenging activity in the saffron petal extract was quantified (Table 2). The average value of the total phenolic and flavonoid contents and the half-maximal inhibitory concentration (IC$_{50}$) were 3.09 ± 0.012 mg GAE/g DW, 0.92 ± 0.004 mg QE/g DW and 235.15 ± 2.12 µg/mL, respectively.

Table 2. Average levels of the total phenolic content, total flavonoid content and the DPPH radical scavenging activity.

	Total Phenolic (mg GAE/g DW)	TFC (mg QE/g DW)	DPPH (IC$_{50}$) (µg/mL)
SPE	3.09 ± 0.012	0.92 ± 0.004	235.15 ± 2.12

Values are the means of three independent replicates.

2.4.3. Volatile Composition: GC-MS

In order to identify the volatile compounds in the SPE, GC-MS chromatography was performed. The obtained results are listed in Table 3 and show that the most dominant component in the volatile fraction is 2(5H)-Furanone (92.10%). The safranal (3.56%) and limonene (1.48%) were also identified at low levels. In addition, other compounds were also found in trace amounts (Table 3).

Table 3. List of identified volatile compounds in the saffron petal by GC-MS.

Compound	Cas Number	RI Lit	RI Calculated	% Peak Area
2(5H)-Furanone	497-23-4	951	920	92.10
Limonene	138-86-3	1029.5	1033	1.48
Phenylethyl alcohol	60-12-8	1114.9	1120	0.70
3,5,5-trimethyl-3-cyclohexen-1-one	471-01-2	1429	1128	0.52
2,6,6-trimethyl-2-cyclohexene-1,4-dione	1125-21-9	1142	1150	0.51
Safranal	116-26-7	1201	1204	3.56
Carvone	99-49-0	1242	1227	0.53
Thymol	89-83-8	1290.1	1293	0.61

RI lit: The RI theoretical value was found in Pherobase in the same column.

3. Discussion

The control of postharvest pathogens of fruits and vegetables is mainly achieved by applying fungicides in pre/postharvest periods, which might have several disadvantages, such as the persistence of residues on fruits, which is a high risk for human health and the environment, the high cost and the appearance of fungicide resistant strains in the pathogen population [23]. In this study, the effect of the saffron petal extract was investigated for the control of postharvest diseases in fruits as a potential alternative strategy to replace the use of chemicals. It was known that plants are capable of producing a range variety of secondary metabolites that have antifungal activities against major postharvest pathogens [24]. These compounds are associated with the immune plant system and can play a major role as fungal inhibitors [25]. The saffron petal is the main by-product of *Crocus sativus*, that is produced in large quantities and is known for its several properties, particularly its antimicrobial potential, which could be a good alternative for controlling postharvest fungal infections. Furthermore, the antifungal effect of the saffron petal extract was evaluated against three most important fungal pathogens causing postharvest damage to the tomato, orange and apple.

To the best of our knowledge, there is currently no report on the ability of the saffron petal extract to suppress postharvest diseases. The promising findings from this study showed a great inhibitory effect of the petals of the saffron, suggested that the saffron petal extract might have metabolites with a higher antifungal activity against *R. stolonifer* on the tomato and a moderate significant reduction of grey mold on the apple and a slight inhibition of green mold on the orange. These findings evidenced that the saffron petal extract has antifungal [17] and antimicrobial effects [27]. In this regard, our in vitro trials showed that the mycelial growth and spore germination of *R. stolonifer* and *P. digitatum* were completely inhibited at 10% of the petal extract. Interestingly, the growth of *B. cinerea* was inhibited at 5% of the SPE. Previous studies demonstrated the ability of plant extracts to reduce postharvest fungal diseases [24]. Jasso de Rodríguez et al. [33] reported that the mycelial growth of *R. stolonifer* was completely stopped at 3 g/L of the *Flourensia* spp extract. A similar result was obtained in another study in which the complete inhibition of the spore germination of *P. digitatum* and *B. cinerea* was observed when the pomegranate peel aqueous extract was used at a concentration of 12 g/L after 20 h of incubation [34]. Furthermore, Gholamnezhad [35] highlighted the in vitro efficacy of seven plant extracts (neem, fennel, lavender, thyme, pennyroyal, salvia and asafetida) to reduce the mycelial growth of *B. cinerea* [35]. Interestingly, our results showed that the inhibition rate of the mycelial growth and spore germination increased with the increasing SPE concentrations, regardless of the fungal species. These results were confirmed by the in vivo trials in which the disease severity was reduced with the increasing SPE concentration. López-Anchondo et al. [36] found that the antifungal effect is proportional to the increase in the concentration of the extract and the *Prosopis glandulosa* extract had an antifungal index of 55% for *R. stolonifer*. Interestingly, the SPE at 10%, completely suppressed the disease in artificially injured and inoculated fruit by *R. stolonifer* (0% severity) and result was similar to the fungicidal difenoconazole (1 µg/mL). The SPE had no phytotoxic effect on the tissues of the tomato fruit. This finding is very interesting, compared to other studies conducted using other plant extracts. Lopez-Anchondo et al., 2020 found that the application of the *P. glandulosa* extract displayed less efficiency in controlling the *Rhizopus* species [36]. Moreover, our results demonstrated that applying the SPE at 5%, significantly reduce the disease severity of grey mold (37.19%) on the apple, compared to the untreated control in which the disease severity reached 100%. In a similar study, Gholamnezhad [35] found that the *Azadirachta indica* methanolic and aqueous extracts, applied at 25%, significantly reduced the disease on the wounded area by 52 and 89%, respectively, compared to the control [35]. Surprisingly, a slight reduction of the disease severity, due *P. digitatum*, was obtained at 10% of the SPE.

In order to understand the mechanisms by which the SPE control postharvest fungal pathogens, a series of chemical analyses were undertaken in this study. Among them, the FT-IR spectroscopy, which is an effective tool to detect different chemical components in food products [37,38]. The obtained results revealed that the SPE has potent antifungal properties, which may be attributed to the presence of many chemical components, including phenols-alcohols (O-H), aromatic group and monoterpene composites (C-H), which can be the main chemical compounds that affect the biological activity of saffron petals. This result was confirmed by the phytochemical quality of the SPE, which highlighted the implication of the phenolic and flavonoid components contained in the SPE in its microbial activity. The phenolic contents are highlighted as very powerful antimicrobial agents that exert a direct effect by neutralizing the microbial systems and damaging the hyphae [39]. Anthocyanins are responsible for the attractive color of the saffron petals, among which delphinidin, petunidin and malvidin glycosides represent 30% of the total content of the phenolic compounds in the petals [1]. Likewise, De Leon-Zapata et al. [40] reported that the fungal inhibition is correlated to the concentration of the bioactive compounds of the tarbush leaf extract, and especially to the gallic acid and flavonoids [38]. They found that, in vitro, the highest inhibition mycelial growth of *R. stolonifer* was 67.40% at 4 g/L.

Flavonoids are important constituents of plants because of the scavenging ability conferred by their hydroxyl groups. The flavonoids may contribute directly to anti-oxidative and antimicrobial actions [41]. Indeed, Termentzi and Kokkalou [42] found that the saffron petal is a good potential source of quercetin, kaempferol and naringenin, which are relatively highly resistant flavonols to thermal degradation [42]. In addition, saffron petals have been shown to have a higher antioxidant activity and their beneficial effects, derived from phenolic compounds, are usually attributed to their antioxidant activity [43,44]. These results are consistent with several previous studies [13,18,45]. In addition, several volatile compounds were found in the SPE, of which furanone is the most predominant. Interestingly, a previous study evidenced the biological activity of furanone against some germs [46]. Similarly, several studies reported that a large number of halogenated furanones and related synthetic analogues, were later discovered to inhibit the biofilm formation in a variety of pathogens [47–49]. Therefore, the richness of the SPE with furanone might explain its higher antifungal activity in this study. Ultimately, compounds of natural origin with an antifungal activity are present in several plants [50]. The plant activity is determined by the plant genotype and depends on their chemical composition, which is influenced by several factors, including environmental conditions and geographical location [51]. The mechanisms of action by which plant extracts suppress the growth of postharvest fungal pathogens, are multiple and include the disturbances in the cell membrane function, the disruption of the energy activity and damage of the cytoplasmic membrane [52]. In addition, a previous study conducted by Ma et al. [53] also focused on the control of *B. cinerea* by using honokiol, a poly-phenolic compound obtained from *Magnolia officinalis*. It was found that honokiol significantly inhibited the mycelial growth and reduced the virulence of *B. cinerea*. It was demonstrated also that honokiol altered the mitochondrial membrane potential with the accumulation of the reactive oxygen species. Moreover, some key genes involved in the fungal pathogenicity have their expression down-regulated. In a recent study, Mastino et al. [54] underlined that the phenolic compounds represent a rich source of protectants and biocides, which can be used as alternative strategies for the control of postharvest diseases in fruits [54]. Rubio-Moraga et al. [55] pointed out that saponins and phenolic compounds could be responsible for the fungicidal activity detected in internal parts of the corms, against five fungi [55]. According to Zhang et al. [56], The effectiveness of the antifungal activity of the plant extracts is correlated with the extraction process, particularly the interaction between the solvent and the raw material, which allows its dissolution and separation from the solid matrix, depending on the solvent/solid ratio, particle size, temperature and the timing of the extraction [56]. Furthermore, the use of innovative processing techniques, such as microwave-assisted extraction, ultrasound-assisted extraction and ohmic heating assisted extraction, was proved to have a substantial effect on the antifungal activity of the jackfruit extract against fungal pathogens *Colletotrichum gloeosporioides* and *Penicillium italicum* [57]. Thereby, natural molecules generated by the plant present many advantages for the consumer because it protects against toxic substances produced, either by postharvest fungal pathogens or biocontrol antagonists, and therefore they present an additive food for human health [58].

4. Materials and Methods

4.1. Collection and Preparation of the Saffron Petal Aqueous Extract

The dry saffron petals were collected in November 2021 after pruning the harvest from a saffron farm in Serghina/Boulmane. The petals are placed in an oven at 37 °C to drive out the humidity. The saffron petals were crushed using an automated grinder and then stored until use. For the in vitro test, different concentrations (0.5, 1, 2, 3, 5, 7, and 10%) of the appropriate amount of the powder were added to 100 mL of distilled water, to achieve the desired concentration. The suspensions obtained were brought to a boil, filtered and mixed with potato dextrose agar (PDA). Then, they were autoclaved for 20 min at 121 °C, before being distributed into 9 cm diameter Petri dishes [52–54].

4.2. Fungal Pathogens

The fungal pathogens used to assess the efficacy of the aqueous extract of the saffron petals were *P. digitatum, B. cinerea* and *R. stolonifer*, which were provided by the laboratory of the Department of Plant Protection and Environment, Phytopathology Unit, Ecole Nationale d'Agriculture, Meknes, Morocco. Prior to the testing, the sub-fungal isolates were subcultured on a potato dextrose agar medium (PDA). The spore suspension was obtained by scraping the fungus and mixing it with 20 mL of sterile distilled water (SDW). The resulting liquid was filtered through a sterile filter, to remove the hyphal fragments and medium debris after centrifugation.

4.3. Fruit Preparation

Navel oranges (Lane late), Golden delicious apples and tomatoes were used to study the in vivo effects of the saffron petal extract on green rot caused by *P. digitatum*, and gray rot caused by *B. cinerea* and *Rhizopus* rot, respectively. All fruits were bought from the local market in the town of Meknes. They were washed, disinfected with 2% (v/v) sodium hypochlorite, rinsed three times in sterile distilled water and then air dried for 1 h at room temperature under a laminar flow cabinet. Once dried, two artificial wounds (4 mm in diameter and 3 mm in depth) were performed on both equatorial sides of each fruit with a sterile cork-borer [59].

4.4. Antifungal Activity of the Saffron Petal Extract (SPE) on the Mycelial Growth

The agar dilution method was used to determine the ability of the saffron petal extract to inhibit the mycelial growth of *P. digitatum*, *B. cinerea* and *R. stolonifer*. The saffron petal extract was tested at different concentrations: 0.5, 1, 2, and 5% for *B. cinerea*, 2, 5, 7 and 10% for *P. digitatum*, and 2, 3, 5 and 10%, and for *R. stolonifer*. Each Petri plate was aseptically inoculated with each pathogen, using a 5 mm mycelium taken from a 7-day-old colony. The Petri dishes were sealed with parafilm and incubated at 25 °C for 5 days. The pathogens cultured in PDA without the extract, served as a control. Each treatment was repeated three times and the antifungal activity that was expressed as the inhibition rate was compared to the control and was calculated after 5 days of incubation, according to the following formula:

Mycelial growth inhibition rate (MGI) = [(colony diameter on control treatment − colony diameter on SPE treatment)/colony diameter on control treatment] × 100

4.5. Effect of the Saffron Petal Extract on the Spore Germination

The method used to study the effect of the saffron petal extract on the spore germination of each fungus consisted of mixing the spore suspension (1×10^4 spores/mL) with each aqueous extract concentration at an equal volume (1 v/1 v) as following: 0.5, 1, 2, and 5% for *B. cinerea*, 2, 5, 10, and 12% for *P. digitatum*, and 2, 3, 5, and 10% for *R. stolonifer*. The control consisted of using the same amount of spore suspension without the plant extract. The mixtures were incubated at 24 °C in sterile micro-centrifuge tubes. The spore germination was examined under a light microscope after 24 h. At least 100 spores were observed for each replicate at 40× magnification. The inhibition rate of the spore germination was determined, according to the following formula:

$$GI\ (\%) = [(Gc - Gt)/Gc] \times 100$$

where, Gc and Gt represent the mean number of the germinated spores in the control and treated tubes, respectively.

4.6. Effect of the Saffron Petal Extract on the Rot Decay Development

The in vivo test consisted of treating the disinfected and wounded fruits with 50 µL of the plant extract at different concentrations. Following 2 h of incubation at room temperature, under a laminar flow cabinet, each wound was inoculated with 20 µL of the spore suspension concentrated at 1×10^4 spores/mL. The fruits treated with sterile distilled water (SDW) and difenoconazole fungicide (15 µL/10 mL) were served as controls. The treated fruits were weighed and placed in plastic bags and incubated in darkness at 24 °C with 95% relative humidity (RH). Two experiments were performed over time with three replicates for each concentration. Then, 7 days later, the disease severity (%) was calculated for all treatments (plant extract, water control and fungicide control), according to the following formula:

Disease Severity (%) = [(average lesion diameter of treatment/average lesion diameter of control)] × 100

4.7. Chemical Composition Analysis of the Saffron Petal
4.7.1. FTIR Analysis

A ground and homogenized saffron petal sample was scanned in the wavelength range of 4000–400 cm^{-1} with a spectral resolution of 4 cm^{-1} using the FTIR spectrometer (PerkinElmer, Waltham, MA, USA) and the characteristic peaks and their functional groups were detected. The FTIR peak values were recorded. The analysis was repeated three times and the averaged spectrum was used.

4.7.2. Determination of the Total Phenolic and Flavonoid Contents and the DPPH Radical Scavenging Activity

The total phenolic and flavonoid contents were determined for the SPE concentration 10 mg/mL. The extraction was based on a method previously described by Ghanbari et al. [60] using methanolic solutions of the extract.

The total phenolic content (TPC) of the saffron petal extract was determined by a colorimetric method, based on the procedure described by Ghanbari et al. [60]. Briefly, 0.5 mL of extract was added to 2.5 mL of Folin–Ciocalteu (FC) reagent (1:10) and incubated for 5 min at room temperature. Then, 2 mL of 7.5% sodium carbonate solution was added. Once shaken, the mixture was incubated in a hot water bath at 45 °C for 15 min. Finally, the absorbance was recorded at 765 nm. The results were expressed as mg of the gallic acid equivalent (GAE/g sample dry weight (DW)).

The total flavonoid content was measured by the aluminium chloride method using quercetin as a standard and described by Ghanbari et al. [60]: 0.3 mL of 5% $NaNO_2$ solution was added to 0.5 mL of the methanolic extract. The mixture was incubated in the dark at room temperature for 6 min. Thereafter, 0.6 mL of 10% $AlCl_3$ was added and incubated for 5 min. Finally, 3 mL of NaOH 1M was added, and the final volume was adjusted to 10 mL with distilled water. The absorbance was read at 510 nm after 15 min incubation. The total flavonoid content values were expressed as mg of the quercetin equivalent (QE) per g DW.

The methanolic DPPH solution 0.5 mM (1.5 mL) was added to 0.75 mL of prepared 50, 100 and 300 µg/mL extract concentrations [60,61]. Then, 20 min later, the absorbance was determined at 517 nm with 80% methanol as blank. The same concentrations of ascorbic acid were used as a positive control. The percentage of the inhibition was determined, according to the following formula: Inhibition rate (%) = ((A control − A sample)/A control) × 100, where A sample is the absorbance value of the sample and A control is the absorbance of the control. Following the calculation of the percentage of the inhibition, a linear regression model was established, based on the concentration and percentage of the inhibition.

4.7.3. GC-MS Analysis

The volatile components analysis of the saffron was carried out using gas chromatography-mass spectrometry (GC-MS) equipped with an Agilent 7890A system (A.01.01, Wilmington, DE, USA) and a mass selective detector 5975 Network MSD and coupled to a MPS automatic sampling system, as described previously by Naim et al. [62]. The chromatographic separation was performed on a HP-5MS capillary column (30 m × 0.25 mm, film thickness 0.17 mm), and the following temperature program was used: 60 °C held for 3 min, then increased to 210 °C at a rate of 4 °C/min, then held at 210 °C for 15 min, then increased to 300 °C at a rate of 10 °C/min, and finally held at 300 °C for 15 min. Helium was used as the carrier gas at a constant flow of 1 mL/min. For the quantification, the results are presented as a percentage of the peak area, considering a response factor of the fiber. Mass Hunter Version B.06.00 (Agilent Technologies) was used for the data acquisition and processing. The identification of the components was based on the comparison of the obtained mass spectrum with those from the commercial databases (NIST17 and Wiley) and by comparison with the retention index (RI) of each peak from the literature (Pherobase). The experimental retention index (RI) of the compounds were calculated following the injection of a mixture of n-alkanes C8-C20 (Sigma Aldrich, Darmstadt, Germany).

4.8. Statistical Analysis

The statistical analysis was performed using SPSS V25 software (version 25, IBM SPSS Statistics 20, New York, NY, USA) and the datasets were expressed as the mean ± standard deviation. Duncan's multiple analysis was used for the means separation at a significance level of $p \leq 0.05$. The linear regression equation of the mycelial growth and the spore germination inhibition rates versus the logarithm of the SPE concentrations were performed to calculate the half-maximal effective concentration (IC_{50}).

5. Conclusions

In this study, the chemical composition analysis of the saffron petal extract was carried out and its antifungal activity was investigated. In light of these findings, it was concluded that the SPE could be used to reduce postharvest fruit infections caused by fungal pathogens, such as *R. stolonifer, B. cinerea* and *P. digitatum*. The antifungal activity of the SPE might be explained by its antioxidant power and its richness in phenolic and flavonoid contents. In addition, the use of the SPE does not present any risks to both the user and consumer. Therefore, this study has shed light on new opportunities of using the SPE to control postharvest fruit infections and could be used as an alternative to chemical products. However, further investigations are needed to assess the effectiveness of the SPE to control fungal plant diseases in large-scale trials.

Author Contributions: Conceptualization, N.N., S.E. and R.L.; methodology, N.N. and R.L.; software, N.N.; validation, A.T., S.E. and R.L.; formal analysis, S.E. and R.L.; investigation, N.N.; resources, A.T. and R.L.; data curation, N.N., N.E., M.B. and M.-L.F.; writing—original draft preparation, N.N.; writing—review and editing, R.L., S.E. and M.-L.F.; supervision, S.E., I.M. and R.L.; project administration, S.E.; funding acquisition, S.E. All authors have read and agreed to the published version of the manuscript.

Funding: This research did not receive an external funding.

Institutional Review Board Statement: Not applicable.

Informed Consent Statement: Not applicable.

Data Availability Statement: Data will be made available upon request.

Acknowledgments: This research was financially supported by the Phytopathology Unit, Department of Plant Protection and the Department of Arboriculture-Viticulture of the Ecole Nationale d'Agriculture de Meknès.

Conflicts of Interest: The authors declare no conflict of interest.

References

1. Serrano-Diaz, J.; Sanchez, A.M.; Martinez-Tome, M.; Winterhalter, P.; Alonso, G.L. Flavonoid Determination in the Quality Control of *Floral Bioresidues* from (*Crocus Sativus*, L.). *J. Agric. Food Chem.* **2014**, *62*, 3125–3133. [CrossRef] [PubMed]
2. Cardone, L.; Castronuovo, D.; Perniola, M.; Cicco, N.; Candido, V. Saffron (*Crocus sativus*, L.), the King of Spices: An Overview. *Sci. Hortic.* **2020**, *272*, 109560. [CrossRef]
3. Kafi, M.; Kamili, A.N.; Husaini, A.M.; Ozturk, M.; Altay, V. An Expensive Spice Saffron (*Crocus sativus*, L.): A Case Study from Kashmir, Iran, and Turkey. In *Global Perspectives on Underutilized Crops*; Springer: Berlin, Germany, 2018; pp. 109–149.
4. Armellini, R.; Peinado, I.; Pittia, P.; Scampicchio, M.; Heredia, A.; Andres, A. Effect of Saffron (*Crocus sativus*, L.) Enrichment on Antioxidant and Sensorial Properties of Wheat Flour Pasta. *Food Chem.* **2018**, *254*, 55–63. [CrossRef] [PubMed]
5. Ashktorab, H.; Soleimani, A.; Singh, G.; Amin, A.; Tabtabaei, S.; Latella, G.; Stein, U.; Akhondzadeh, S.; Solanki, N.; Gondré-Lewis, M.C.; et al. Saffron: The Golden Spice with Therapeutic Properties on Digestive Diseases. *Nutrients* **2019**, *11*, 943. [CrossRef] [PubMed]
6. Ghaffari, S.; Roshanravan, N. Saffron: An Updated Review on Biological Properties with Special Focus on Cardiovascular Effects. *Biomed. Pharmacother.* **2019**, *109*, 21–27. [CrossRef] [PubMed]
7. Lopresti, A.L.; Drummond, P.D. Efficacy of Curcumin, and a Saffron/Curcumin Combination for the Treatment of Major Depression: A Randomised, Double-Blind, Placebo-Controlled Study. *J. Affect. Disord.* **2017**, *207*, 188–196. [CrossRef]
8. Moradzadeh, M.; Kalani, M.R.; Avan, A. The Antileukemic Effects of Saffron (*Crocus sativus* L.) and Its Related Molecular Targets: A Mini Review. *J. Cell. Biochem.* **2019**, *120*, 4732–4738. [CrossRef]
9. Mentis, A.F.A.; Dalamaga, M.; Lu, C.; Polissiou, M.G. Saffron for "Toning down" COVID-19-Related Cytokine Storm: Hype or Hope? A Mini-Review of Current Evidence. *Metab. Open* **2021**, *11*, 100111. [CrossRef]
10. Serrano-Díaz, J.; Sánchez, A.M.; Maggi, L.; Martínez-Tomé, M.; García-Diz, L.; Murcia, M.A.; Alonso, G.L. Increasing the Applications of Crocus Sativus Flowers as Natural Antioxidants. *J. Food Sci.* **2012**, *77*, C1162–C1168. [CrossRef]
11. Nasab, B.F. Evaluation of Antibacterial Activities of Hydroalcoholic Extract of Saffron Petals on Some Bacterial Pathogens. *J. Med. Bacteriol.* **2019**, *8*, 8–20.
12. Moshiri, E.; Basti, A.A.; Noorbala, A.A.; Jamshidi, A.H.; Abbasi, S.H.; Akhondzadeh, S. *Crocus sativus* L. (Petal) in the Treatment of Mild-to-Moderate Depression: A Double-Blind, Randomized and Placebo-Controlled Trial. *Phytomedicine* **2006**, *13*, 607–611. [CrossRef]

13. Sánchez-Vioque, R.; Rodríguez-Conde, M.F.; Reina-Ureña, J.V.; Escolano-Tercero, M.A.; Herraiz-Peñalver, D.; Santana-Méridas, O. In Vitro Antioxidant and Metal Chelating Properties of Corm, Tepal and Leaf from Saffron (*Crocus sativus*, L.). *Ind. Crops Prod.* **2012**, *39*, 149–153. [CrossRef]
14. Goupy, P.; Vian, M.A.; Chemat, F.; Caris-Veyrat, C. Identification and Quantification of Flavonols, Anthocyanins and Lutein Diesters in Tepals of Crocus Sativus by Ultra Performance Liquid Chromatography Coupled to Diode Array and Ion Trap Mass Spectrometry Detections. *Ind. Crops Prod.* **2013**, *44*, 496–510. [CrossRef]
15. Li, C.Y.; Lee, E.J.; Wu, T.S. Antityrosinase Principles and Constituents of the Petals of *Crocus Ativus*. *J. Nat. Prod.* **2004**, *67*, 437–440. [CrossRef]
16. Hosseinzadeh, H.; Younesi, H.M. Antinociceptive and Anti-Inflammatory Effects of *Crocus sativus* L. Stigma and Petal Extracts in Mice. *BMC Pharmacol.* **2002**, *2*, 1–8.
17. Zheng, C.J.; Li, L.; Ma, W.H.; Han, T.; Qin, L.P. Chemical Constituents and Bioactivities of the Liposoluble Fraction from Different Medicinal Parts of *Crocus sativus*. *Pharm. Biol.* **2011**, *49*, 756–763. [CrossRef]
18. Tuberoso, C.I.G.; Rosa, A.; Montoro, P.; Fenu, M.A.; Pizza, C. Antioxidant Activity, Cytotoxic Activity and Metabolic Profiling of Juices Obtained from Saffron (*Crocus sativus* L.) Floral by-Products. *Food Chem.* **2016**, *199*, 18–27. [CrossRef]
19. Ahmadi Shadmehri, A.; Namvar, F.; Miri, H.; Yaghmaei, P.; Nakhaei Moghaddam, M. Cytotoxicity, Antioxidant and Antibacterial Activities of Crocus Sativus Petal Extract. *J. Res. Appl. Basic Med. Sci.* **2019**, *5*, 69–76.
20. Karimi, G.H.; Taiebi, N.; Hosseinzadeh, A.; Shirzad, F. Evaluation of Subacute Toxicity of Aqueous Extract of *Crocus sativus* L. Stigma and Petal in Rats. *Sci. Inf. Database* **2004**, *3*, 29–35.
21. Mahajan, P.V.; Caleb, O.J.; Singh, Z.; Watkins, C.B.; Geyer, M. Postharvest Treatments of Fresh Produce. *Philos. Trans. R. Soc. A Math. Phys. Eng. Sci.* **2014**, *372*, 20130309. [CrossRef]
22. Ruffo Roberto, S.; Youssef, K.; Hashim, A.F.; Ippolito, A. Nanomaterials as Alternative Control Means against Postharvest Diseases in Fruit Crops. *Nanomaterials* **2019**, *9*, 1752. [CrossRef] [PubMed]
23. Hosseini, S.; Amini, J.; Saba, M.K.; Karimi, K.; Pertot, I. Preharvest and Postharvest Application of Garlic and Rosemary Essential Oils for Controlling Anthracnose and Quality Assessment of Strawberry Fruit During Cold Storage. *Front. Microbiol.* **2020**, *11*, 1–15. [CrossRef] [PubMed]
24. El Khetabi, A.; Lahlali, R.; Ezrari, S.; Radouane, N.; Lyousfi, N.; Banani, H.; Askarne, L.; Tahiri, A.; El Ghadraoui, L.; Belmalha, S.; et al. Role of Plant Extracts and Essential Oils in Fighting against Postharvest Fruit Pathogens and Extending Fruit Shelf Life: A Review. *Trends Food Sci. Technol.* **2022**, *120*, 402–417. [CrossRef]
25. Palou, L.; Ali, A.; Fallik, E.; Romanazzi, G. GRAS, Plant and Animal-Derived Compounds as Alternatives to Conventional Fungicides for the >control of Postharvest Diseases of Fresh Horticultural Produce. *Postharvest Biol. Technol.* **2016**, *122*, 41–52. [CrossRef]
26. Álvarez-Martínez, F.J.; Barrajón-Catalán, E.; Encinar, J.A.; Rodríguez-Díaz, J.C.; Micol, V. Antimicrobial Capacity of Plant Polyphenols against Gram-Positive Bacteria: A Comprehensive Review. *Curr. Med. Chem.* **2020**, *27*, 2576–2606. [CrossRef]
27. Kaveh, H. Effect of Saffron Petal Extract on Retention Quality of Fresh-Cut Watermelon Cubes. *Saffron Agron. Technol. Eff.* **2016**, *4*, 301–311. [CrossRef]
28. Wilson, R.H.; Smith, A.C.; Kacuráková, M.; Saunders, P.K.; Wellner, N.; Waldron, K.W. The Mechanical Properties and Molecular Dynamics of Plant Cell Wall Polysaccharides Studied by Fourier-Transform Infrared Spectroscopy. *Plant Physiol.* **2000**, *124*, 397–406. [CrossRef]
29. Lahlali, R.; Song, T.; Chu, M.; Karunakaran, C.; Yu, F.; Wei, Y.; Peng, G. Synchrotron-Based Spectroscopy and Imaging Reveal Changes in the Cell-Wall Composition of Barley Leaves in Defence Responses to *Blumeria Graminis* f. Sp. *Tritici*. *Can. J. Plant Pathol.* **2019**, *41*, 457–467. [CrossRef]
30. Naumann, A.; Heine, G.; Rauber, R. Efficient Discrimination of Oat and Pea Roots by Cluster Analysis of Fourier Transform Infrared (FTIR) Spectra. *Field Crops Res.* **2010**, *119*, 78–84. [CrossRef]
31. Lee, F.Y.; Htar, T.T.; Akowuah, G.A. ATR-FTIR and Spectrometric Methods for the Assay of Crocin in Commercial Saffron Spices (*Crocus savitus* L.). *Int. J. Food Prop.* **2015**, *18*, 1773–1783. [CrossRef]
32. Kumar, S.; Lahlali, R.; Liu, X.; Karunakaran, C. Infrared Spectroscopy Combined with Imaging: A New Developing Analytical Tool in Health and Plant Science. *Appl. Spectrosc. Rev.* **2016**, *51*, 466–483. [CrossRef]
33. Jasso de Rodríguez, D.; Salas-Méndez, E.D.J.; Rodríguez-García, R.; Hernández-Castillo, F.D.; Díaz-Jiménez, M.L.V.; Sáenz-Galindo, A.; González-Morales, S.; Flores-López, M.L.; Villarreal-Quintanilla, J.A.; Peña-Ramos, F.M.; et al. Antifungal Activity in Vitro of Ethanol and Aqueous Extracts of Leaves and Branches of *Flourensia* Spp. against Postharvest Fungi. *Ind. Crops Prod.* **2017**, *107*, 499–508. [CrossRef]
34. Nicosia, M.G.L.D.; Pangallo, S.; Raphael, G.; Romeo, F.V.; Strano, M.C.; Rapisarda, P.; Droby, S.; Schena, L. Control of Postharvest Fungal Rots on Citrus Fruit and Sweet Cherries Using a Pomegranate Peel Extract. *Postharvest Biol. Technol.* **2016**, *114*, 54–61. [CrossRef]
35. Gholamnezhad, J. Effect of Plant Extracts on Activity of Some Defense Enzymes of Apple Fruit in Interaction with Botrytis Cinerea. *J. Integr. Agric.* **2019**, *18*, 115–123. [CrossRef]
36. López-Anchondo, A.N.; de la López-Cruz, D.; Gutiérrez-Reyes, E.; Castañeda-Ramírez, J.C.; de la Fuente-Salcido, N.M. Antifungal Activity In Vitro and In Vivo of Mesquite Extract (*Prosopis Glandulosa*) Against Phytopathogenic Fungi. *Indian J. Microbiol.* **2021**, *61*, 85–90. [CrossRef]

37. Snyder, A.B.; Sweeney, C.F.; Rodriguez-Saona, L.E.; Giusti, M.M. Rapid Authentication of Concord Juice Concentration in a Grape Juice Blend Using Fourier-Transform Infrared Spectroscopy and Chemometric Analysis. *Food Chem.* **2014**, *147*, 295–301. [CrossRef]
38. Balabin, R.M.; Smirnov, S.V. Melamine Detection by Mid-and near-Infrared (MIR/NIR) Spectroscopy: A Quick and Sensitive Method for Dairy Products Analysis Including Liquid Milk, Infant Formula, and Milk Powder. *Talanta* **2011**, *85*, 562–568. [CrossRef]
39. Alsaggaf, M.S.; Moussa, S.H.; Tayel, A.A. Application of Fungal Chitosan Incorporated with Pomegranate Peel Extract as Edible Coating for Microbiological, Chemical and Sensorial Quality Enhancement of Nile *Tilapia* Fillets. *Int. J. Biol. Macromol.* **2017**, *99*, 499–505. [CrossRef]
40. De León-Zapata, M.A.; Pastrana-Castro, L.; Rua-Rodríguez, M.L.; Alvarez-Pérez, O.B.; Rodríguez-Herrera, R.; Aguilar, C.N. Experimental Protocol for the Recovery and Evaluation of Bioactive Compounds of Tarbush against Postharvest Fruit Fungi. *Food Chem.* **2016**, *198*, 62–67. [CrossRef]
41. Sun, L.; Zhang, J.; Lu, X.; Zhang, L.; Zhang, Y. Evaluation to the Antioxidant Activity of Total Flavonoids Extract from Persimmon (*Diospyros kaki* L.) Leaves. *Food Chem. Toxicol.* **2011**, *49*, 2689–2696. [CrossRef]
42. Termentzi, A.; Kokkalou, E. LC-DAD-MS (ESI+) Analysis and Antioxidant Capacity of Crocus Sativus Petal Extracts. *Planta Med.* **2008**, *74*, 573–581. [CrossRef] [PubMed]
43. Heim, K.E.; Tagliaferro, A.R.; Bobilya, D.J. Flavonoid Antioxidants: Chemistry, Metabolism and Structure-Activity Relationships. *J. Nutr. Biochem.* **2002**, *13*, 572–584. [CrossRef] [PubMed]
44. Fazeli-Nasab, B.; Rahnama, M.; Mazarei, A. Correlation between Antioxidant Activity and Antibacterial Activity of Nine Medicinal Plant Extracts. *J. Maz. Univ. Med. Sci.* **2017**, *27*, 63–78.
45. Goli, S.A.H.; Mokhtari, F.; Rahimmalek, M. Phenolic Compounds and Antioxidant Activity from Saffron (*Crocus sativus*, L.) Petal. *J. Agric. Sci.* **2012**, *4*, 175.
46. Gómez, A.C.; Lyons, T.; Mamat, U.; Yero, D.; Bravo, M.; Daura, X.; Elshafee, O.; Brunke, S.; Gahan, C.G.M.; O'Driscoll, M. Synthesis and Evaluation of Novel Furanones as Biofilm Inhibitors in Opportunistic Human Pathogens. *Eur. J. Med. Chem.* **2022**, *242*, 114678. [CrossRef] [PubMed]
47. Hentzer, M.; Givskov, M. Pharmacological Inhibition of Quorum Sensing for the Treatment of Chronic Bacterial Infections. *J. Clin. Investig.* **2003**, *112*, 1300–1307. [CrossRef]
48. Lönn-Stensrud, J.; Landin, M.A.; Benneche, T.; Petersen, F.C.; Scheie, A.A. Furanones, Potential Agents for Preventing Staphylococcus Epidermidis Biofilm Infections? *J. Antimicrob. Chemother.* **2009**, *63*, 309–316. [CrossRef]
49. Han, Y.; Hou, S.; Simon, K.A.; Ren, D.; Luk, Y.Y. Identifying the Important Structural Elements of Brominated Furanones for Inhibiting Biofilm Formation by Escherichia Coli. *Bioorg. Med. Chem. Lett.* **2008**, *18*, 1006–1010. [CrossRef]
50. Redondo-Blanco, S.; Fernandez, J.; Lopez-Ibanez, S.; Miguelez, E.M.; Villar, C.J.; Lombo, F. Plant Phytochemicals in Food Preservation: Antifungal Bioactivity: A Review. *J. Food Prot.* **2020**, *83*, 163–171. [CrossRef]
51. Nandhavathy, G.; Dharini, V.; Babu, P.A.; Nambiar, R.B.; Selvam, S.P.; Sadiku, E.R.; Kumar, M.M. Determination of Antifungal Activities of Essential Oils Incorporated-Pomegranate Peel Fibers Reinforced-Polyvinyl Alcohol Biocomposite Film against Mango Postharvest Pathogens. *Mater. Today Proc.* **2021**, *38*, 923–927. [CrossRef]
52. Xin, Z.; OuYang, Q.; Wan, C.; Che, J.; Li, L.; Chen, J.; Tao, N. Isolation of Antofine from Cynanchum Atratum BUNGE (*Asclepiadaceae*) and Its Antifungal Activity against Penicillium Digitatum. *Postharvest Biol. Technol.* **2019**, *157*, 110961. [CrossRef]
53. Ma, D.; Cui, X.; Zhang, Z.; Li, B.; Xu, Y.; Tian, S.; Chen, T. Honokiol Suppresses Mycelial Growth and Reduces Virulence of Botrytis Cinerea by Inducing Autophagic Activities and Apoptosis. *Food Microbiol.* **2020**, *88*, 103411. [CrossRef]
54. Mastino, P.M.; Marchetti, M.; Costa, J.; Juliano, C.; Usai, M. Analytical Profiling of Phenolic Compounds in Extracts of Three Cistus Species from Sardinia and Their Potential Antimicrobial and Antioxidant Activity. *Chem. Biodivers.* **2021**, *18*, e2100053. [CrossRef]
55. Rubio-Moraga, Á.; Gómez-Gómez, L.; Trapero, A.; Castro-Díaz, N.; Ahrazem, O. Saffron Corm as a Natural Source of Fungicides: The Role of Saponins in the Underground. *Ind. Crops Prod.* **2013**, *49*, 915–921. [CrossRef]
56. Zhang, H.; Mahunu, G.K.; Castoria, R.; Yang, Q.; Apaliya, M.T. Recent Developments in the Enhancement of Some Postharvest Biocontrol Agents with Unconventional Chemicals Compounds. *Trends Food Sci. Technol.* **2018**, *78*, 180–187. [CrossRef]
57. Vázquez-González, Y.; Ragazzo-Sánchez, J.A.; Calderón-Santoyo, M. Characterization and Antifungal Activity of Jackfruit (*Artocarpus heterophyllus* Lam.) Leaf Extract Obtained Using Conventional and Emerging Technologies. *Food Chem.* **2020**, *330*, 127211. [CrossRef]
58. Gurău, F.; Baldoni, S.; Prattichizzo, F.; Espinosa, E.; Amenta, F.; Procopio, A.D.; Albertini, M.C.; Bonafè, M.; Olivieri, F. Anti-Senescence Compounds: A Potential Nutraceutical Approach to Healthy Aging. *Ageing Res. Rev.* **2018**, *46*, 14–31. [CrossRef]
59. El Khetabi, A.; Lahlali, R.; Askarne, L.; Ezrari, S.; El Ghadaroui, L.; Tahiri, A.; Hrustić, J.; Amiri, S. Efficacy Assessment of Pomegranate Peel Aqueous Extract for Brown Rot (*Monilinia spp.*) Disease Control. *Physiol. Mol. Plant Pathol.* **2020**, *110*, 101482. [CrossRef]
60. Ghanbari, J.; Khajoei-Nejad, G.; van Ruth, S.M.; Aghighi, S. The Possibility for Improvement of Flowering, Corm Properties, Bioactive Compounds, and Antioxidant Activity in Saffron (*Crocus Sativus* L.) by Different Nutritional Regimes. *Ind. Crops Prod.* **2019**, *135*, 301–310. [CrossRef]

61. Parejo, I.; Viladomat, F.; Bastida, J.; Rosas-Romero, A.; Saavedra, G.; Murcia, M.A.; Jiménez, A.M.; Codina, C. Investigation of Bolivian Plant Extracts for Their Radical Scavenging Activity and Antioxidant Activity. *Life Sci.* **2003**, *73*, 1667–1681. [CrossRef]
62. Naim, N.; Ennahli, N.; Hanine, H.; Lahlali, R.; Tahiri, A.; Fauconnier, M.L.; Madani, I.; Ennahli, S. ATR-FTIR Spectroscopy Combined with DNA Barcoding and GC-MS to Assess the Quality and Purity of Saffron (*Crocus sativus*, L.). *Vib. Spectrosc.* **2022**, *123*, 103446. [CrossRef]

The Role of *Allium subhirsutum* L. in the Attenuation of Dermal Wounds by Modulating Oxidative Stress and Inflammation in *Wistar* Albino Rats

Mongi Saoudi [1,*,†], Riadh Badraoui [2,3,*,†], Ahlem Chira [1], Mohd Saeed [2], Nouha Bouali [2], Salem Elkahoui [2], Jahoor M. Alam [2], Choumous Kallel [4] and Abdelfattah El Feki [1]

[1] Animal Ecophysiology Laboratory, Sciences Faculty of Sfax, University of Sfax, Sfax 3054, Tunisia; chiraahlem@gmail.com (A.C.); abdelfattahelfeki@fss.rnu.tn (A.E.F.)
[2] Laboratory of General Biology, Department of Biology, University of Ha'il, Ha'il 81451, Saudi Arabia; mo.saeed@uoh.edu.sa (M.S.); nouha_bmail@yahoo.fr (N.B.); s.elkahoui@uoh.edu.sa (S.E.); j.alam@uoh.edu.sa (J.M.A.)
[3] Section of Histology and Cytology, Medicine Faculty of Tunis, University of Tunis El Manar, La Rabta, Tunis 1007, Tunisia
[4] Hematology Laboratory, Hospital Habib Bourguiba, Sfax 3029, Tunisia; kallelC@yahoo.fr
* Correspondence: mongifss@yahoo.fr (M.S.); riadh.badraoui@fmt.utm.tn (R.B.); Tel.: +216-99740205 (M.S.)
† These authors contributed equally to this work.

Abstract: In our study, *Allium subhirsutum* L. (AS) was investigated to assess its phenolic profile and bioactive molecules including flavonoids and organosulfur compounds. The antioxidant potential of AS and wound healing activity were addressed using skin wound healing and oxidative stress and inflammation marker estimation in rat models. Phytochemical and antiradical activities of AS extract (ASE) and oil (ASO) were studied. The rats were randomly assigned to four groups: group I served as a control and was treated with simple ointment base, group II was treated with ASE ointment, group III was treated with ASO ointment and group IV (reference group; Ref) was treated with a reference drug "Cytolcentella® cream". Phytochemical screening showed that total phenols (215 ± 3.5 mg GAE/g) and flavonoids (172.4 ± 3.1 mg QE/g) were higher in the ASO than the ASE group. The results of the antioxidant properties showed that ASO exhibited the highest DPPH free radical scavenging potential (IC50 = 0.136 ± 0.07 mg/mL), FRAP test (IC50 = 0.013 ± 0.006 mg/mL), ABTS test (IC50 = 0.52 ± 0.03 mg/mL) and total antioxidant capacity (IC50 = 0.34 ± 0.06 mg/mL). In the wound healing study, topical application of ASO performed the fastest wound-repairing process estimated by a chromatic study, percentage wound closure, fibrinogen level and oxidative damage status, as compared to ASE, the Cytolcentella reference drug and the untreated rats. The use of AS extract and oil were also associated with the attenuation of oxidative stress damage in the wound-healing treated rats. Overall, the results provided that AS, particularly ASO, has a potential medicinal value to act as effective skin wound healing agent.

Keywords: *Allium subhirsutum* L.; wound-healing activity; antioxidant potential; inflammatory marker; oxidative stress

1. Introduction

Wound healing is a complicated and dynamic physiological process in response to tissue impairment [1]. It is a fundamental connective tissue response [2] to tissue impairment through three phases, including hemostasis and inflammation, proliferation and remodeling [3]. Cutaneous wound healing involves several mediators, such as fibroblasts, endothelial cells, blood cells, interactions with extracellular phases and granulation tissue remodeling phases [4,5]. Furthermore, reactive oxygen species (ROS) are produced in response to cutaneous injury, and act as cellular messengers to stimulate several physiological processes, such as cytokine action, cell motility and angiogenesis [4]. However, cutaneous injury affects the healing process by the overproduction of ROS and the perturbation of various enzymatic and non-enzymatic antioxidant defenses [6], particularly during the inflammatory phase [7]. Long-term instability and high concentration of ROS may cause cellular injury by damaging both proteins and membrane lipids, the perturbation of antioxidant enzymes and the breakdown of the nucleic acids, particularly DNA [8,9]. Higher concentrations of intracellular ROS might eventually lead to angiogenesis pathological damage, promoting inflammation [10,11], which makes blood flow and nutritional requirements unable to meet the needs of wound healing [12].

Many antioxidants in medicinal plant extracts are used to eliminate the negative effects of ROS-associated pathologies and/or injuries including wound healing [11,13,14]. Over the years, medicinal plants have been used to develop a variety of formulations that combat injuries such as wounds, burns and cuts [15]. Several ethno-medicinal plants have been used for medicinal applications thanks to their wide biological activities and medicinal applications due to counteracting oxidative stress potential, lesser costs and high safety margins [16–18]. Plant extracts are known to exhibit many pharmacological properties (anti-hyperlipidemic, anti-proliferative, and immunomodulatory, etc.) through the multitude amounts of natural polyphenolic antioxidants [17–19].

Garlic species are used as dietary supplements and an important ingredient for cooking in many parts of the world and their application in medicinal remedy has also increased its popularity [11,17,20]. Garlic species are known to have diverse biological activities, particularly due to their antioxidant properties. *Allium subhirsutum* L. is an aromatic plant known since antiquity. It was investigated in terms of its potential antioxidant components such as flavonoids and polyphenols [10,11,21]. Previous studies reported that it is a potential source of anticancer and antioxidant molecules [16]. It is a very rich source of valuable compounds, such as polyphenols, vitamins, flavonoids, carotenoids and carbohydrates [17]. Experimental studies showed that garlic phenolic compounds and flavonoids may promote epithelialization and stimulate new tissue growth, fluid handling and moist wound healing [22]. As regards to its pharmacological properties, garlic has been revealed to display antidiabetic, hepatoprotective, antimicrobial, renoprotective, immunomodulatory and anti-inflammatory properties [23].

Furthermore, garlic is also rich in different bioactive compounds like allicin, glutathione diallyl sulfides [24] and important minerals (selenium, manganese and zinc) which encourage its consumption. Pre-treatment with garlic significantly reduced levels of ROS, lipid peroxidation and DNA damage, and thus enhanced the antioxidant system [11,25]. Recent studies [26] revealed that the application of bioactive molecules with antioxidant activities improved wound healing and protected against oxidative damage. Wound care medicinal plants in the form of ointment could ameliorate wound healing and tissue repair with minimal side effects [27]. Previous studies reported that infections in the locations of injured skin are the main reasons for mortality in hospitalized patients with extensive burns [28]. For that reason, the application of plant medicinal preparations as local ointment with considerable antimicrobial effects can significantly reduce the risk of burn wound infections and alleviate the period of treatment [29]. Garlic has been reported to accelerate wound contraction rate, validated by a significant improvement and an increase in the rate of wound closure and a reduction in the time taken by the granulation tissue and inflammatory marker levels to fall [30].

With these considerations, the current study aimed to evaluate wound healing activity of AS extract and oil, using a skin wound healing rat model via the estimation of oxidative stress and anti-inflammatory parameters. This research on the antioxidants and in vivo biological activities of AS can improve its commercial value and help to develop new nutritional and health products.

2. Results & Discussion

2.1. Phytochemical Analysis

In the current study, the phytochemical analysis of *Allium subhirsutum* L. extract and oil showed their richness in phenolic and flavonoid compounds. Furthermore, higher contents of polyphenols and flavonoids confirmed the presence of these biomolecules in ASO.

Total polyphenols, flavonoids and tannins of *Allium subhirsutum* L. extract and oil were calculated according to the calibration curves and the phytochemical amounts are shown in Table 1. Phytochemical screening showed that total polyphenol (215 ± 3.5 mg GAE/g) and flavonoid (172.4 ± 3.1 mg QE/g) amounts are higher in the ASO than the ASE. However, the total tannin level was higher (387.5 ± 17.2 mg QE/g) in the ASE than ASO, in which it was not detected. Total polyphenols, flavonoids and tannins of *Allium subhirsutum* L. extract and oil were calculated according to the calibration curves (see Supplementary Figure S1). The richness in phenolic and flavonoid compounds have been highlighted in *Allium subhirsutum* by previous studies, including those realized by our team [11,17]. Nevertheless, the variations in such compounds might be related to the region of the plant collection.

Table 1. Amounts of total phenolic components, flavonoids, tannins and IC50 for the DPPH scavenging activity, ferric reducing antioxidant power (FRAP), ABTS antioxidant activity and total antioxidant capacities (TAC) of *Allium subhirsutum* L. extract and oil. Ascorbic acid was used as standard.

Samples and Parameters	Total Polyphenols [a] (mg GAE/g) [b]	Flavonoids [a] (mg EQ/g) [c]	Tannins [a] (mg EQ/g)	DPPH [a] IC50 (mg/mL)	FRAP [a] IC50 (mg/mL)	ABTS [a] IC50 (mg/mL)	Total Antioxidant Capacity [a] (mg VitC/g) [d]
A. subhirsutum L. extract	63.8 ± 2.36	41.7 ± 3.4	387.5 ± 17.2	0.20 ± 0.004	0.05 ± 0.004	0.54 ± 0.04	0.45 ± 0.09
A. subhirsutum L. oil	215 ± 3.5	172.4 ± 3.1	ND	0.136 ± 0.07	0.013 ± 0.006	0.52 ± 0.03	0.34 ± 0.06
Ascorbic acid	—	—	—	0.118 ± 0.006	0.08 ± 0.004	0.09 ± 0.09	0.124 ± 0.002

[a]: Data represent the mean ± SEM of three experiments; [b]: mg of gallic acid equivalent/g of dry plant extract; [c]: mg of quercetin equivalent/g of dry plant extract; [d]: mg Vitamin C equivalent/g of dry plant extract; ND: not detected; —: not tested.

2.2. Antioxidant Potential Analysis

The antioxidant properties of the extract and oil of *Allium subhirsutum* L. were assessed via several approaches: scavenging activity on DPPH free radicals, reducing power, total antioxidant activity assay by ABTS and total antioxidant capacity. The results are summarized in Table 1. The antioxidant activities of the studied *Allium subhirsutum* L. extract and oil were compared with vitamin C as a standard antioxidant. The *Allium subhirsutum* L. oil exhibited the highest DPPH free radical scavenging potential (IC50 = 0.136 ± 0.07 mg/mL), FRAP test (IC50 = 0.013 ± 0.006 mg/mL), ABTS test (IC50 = 0.52 ± 0.03 mg/mL) and total antioxidant capacity (IC50 = 0.34 ± 0.06 mg/mL), as compared to *Allium subhirsutum* L. extract. The results revealed an important difference of the DPPH, FRAP, ABTS and total antioxidant capacity tests between the standard vitamin C and the different extracts. Furthermore, the *Allium subhirsutum* L. extract and oil showed potential antioxidant activities as compared to vitamin C; thus, it is able to scavenge superoxide and peroxyl radicals.

Antioxidant activities as estimated by DPPH free radicals, reducing power, total antioxidant activity assay and total antioxidant capacities in ASO explain the ROS scavenging capacity, but it was less than the standard vitamin C. The antioxidant status of ASO is related to the major active components such as organosulfur molecules and their derivatives. Many garlic supplements such as garlic oil macerate, garlic oil, dehydrated garlic powder and aged garlic extract are currently commercially available [31].

2.3. Wound Closure

2.3.1. Chromatic Study

Considering the medicinal application of *Allium subhirsutum* L. and the in vitro antioxidant activity, the plant was further evaluated for skin lesion potential, particularly burns and wounds. Several garlic species have been evaluated in different animal models and were reported to display cutaneous wound healing [32].

The wound healing activity was checked by a chromatic assessment based on the progressive variations of both wound color and surface during the experimental study. The different phases of cicatrization of all studied groups are shown in Figure 1.

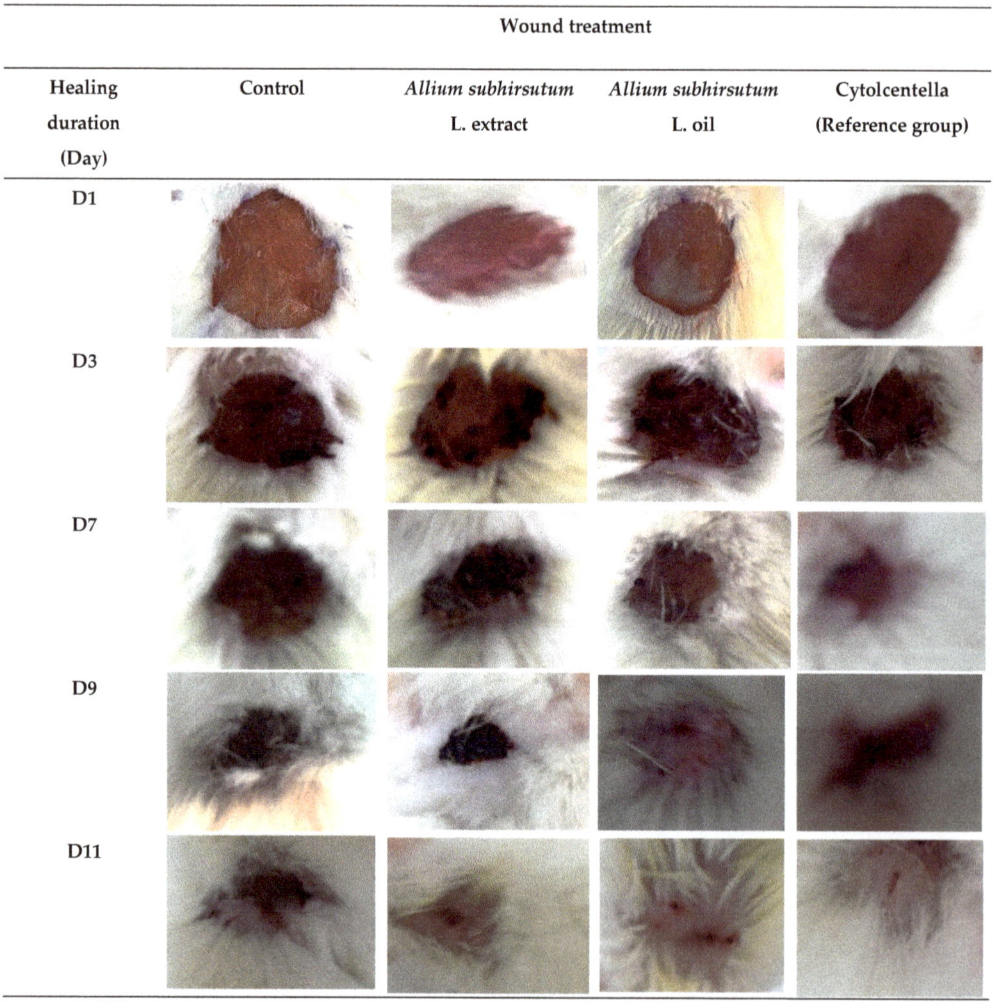

Healing duration (Day)		Wound treatment		
	Control	*Allium subhirsutum* L. extract	*Allium subhirsutum* L. oil	Cytolcentella (Reference group)
D1				
D3				
D7				
D9				
D11				

Figure 1. Photographic illustrations of wound healing process in the different experimental groups on 1, 3, 7, 9 and 11 days post-wounding.

The selected days (1, 3, 7, 9 and 11) correspond to the wound induction day, the epithelialization progress and the inflammatory evolution. The wounds' photographic representations denoted a similar surface and colored wound areas in the first three days for the different studied groups of rats. The photographs of the wound revealed a bright red color during the first day that turned dark red on the third day, which proves blood clot formation. By the seventh day of wound healing, a large inflammatory bulb in the control group was noted, while the wound surfaces of *Allium subhirsutum* L. extract and oil-treated and Cytolcentella-treated rats were smaller. From the ninth day, in the rats treated with ASO and Cytolcentella (Ref group), the crusts began to fall off revealing a red granulated tissue, which characterized completed epithelialization around the 11th day. The process was exhibited at the eleventh day to the complete wound closure in the ASO and Cytolcentella reference drug groups. However, the *Allium subhirsutum* L. extract and control group wounds showed residual scabs and healed slower. The closure was uncompleted in the control and *Allium subhirsutum* L. extract-treated groups.

The wound photographic representations of the treated groups ASO and Cytolcentella reference drug showed better and more advanced epithelial regeneration when compared to the control group (group I). This faster wound closure of *Allium subhirsutum* L. oil, as compared to the ointment by Cytolcentella reference drug, could presumably be due to the richness of *Allium subhirsutum* L., particularly polyphenols and flavonoids, and with several other bioactive compounds (sulfur-rich compounds), as demonstrated by Badraoui et al. [17] Previous findings [11,17,33] revealed that polyphenols play a key role in the proliferation of epithelial cells and the regulation of angiogenesis.

2.3.2. Effect of *Allium Subhirsutum* L. Extract and Oil on Percentage Wound Closure

The changes in the percentage of wound closure in control, *Allium subhirsutum* L. extract and oil, and the reference drug "Cytolcentella" groups were followed on some selected days (Figure 2).

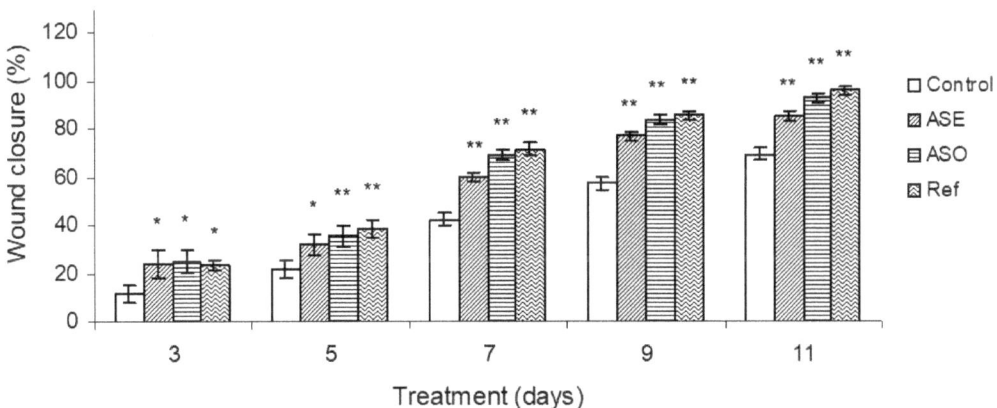

Figure 2. Effects of *Allium subhirsutum* L. extract (ASE), *Allium subhirsutum* L. oil and the reference drug "Cytolcentella®" on the percentage of wound closure in control and treated rats. Data represent the mean ± SEM for six rats. Statistically significant variations are compared as follows: ASE, ASO and Ref treated groups compared to control group. * and ** indicate significant differences when $p < 0.05$ and $p < 0.01$, respectively.

The *Allium subhirsutum* L. extract and oil group displayed a marked wound-healing potential as compared to the untreated group and the Cytolcentella reference drug group. However, the *Allium subhirsutum* L. extract showed a lower wound-healing process as compared to the *Allium subhirsutum* L. oil and Cytolcentella reference drug groups. On days 9 and 10, a rapid reduction in wound area of the *Allium subhirsutum* L. oil group was observed ($p < 0.01$), which was comparable to the Cytolcentella reference drug group.

The reference group showed the strongest wound contraction rate throughout healing days and complete healing of the wound (100%) was observed on the 11th day, while the *Allium subhirsutum* L. extract and oil group showed 81.25% and 87% healing on same day, respectively. It was also noticed that no comparable wound area evolution was observed between the ASO, ASE and Cytolcentella groups on the first 3 days.

Additionally, the morphometric assessment exhibited an increased wound contraction rate of the wounds following ASO and the Cytolcentella reference drug treatment as compared to the untreated group. Previous research using an aqueous extract of garlic (*Allium sativum*) showed a higher percentage of burn wound contraction in rats treated with 0.4% garlic topical cream (88.1%) than those treated with cream base (70.3%) [28]. This rapid wound closure may be attributed to an increase in fibroblast activity, which is crucial for normal wound contraction.

2.3.3. Effect on Inflammatory Marker

The inflammatory marker of different groups was analyzed to determine the level of fibrinogen (Figure 3), which is known as an inflammatory protein. An increased level of this protein revealed a condition of inflammation. Fibrinogen content was found to be significantly alleviated in *Allium subhirsutum* L. oil ($p < 0.001$) and the Cytolcentella reference drug ($p < 0.01$) groups, followed by *Allium subhirsutum* L. extract ($p < 0.01$) as compared to control group.

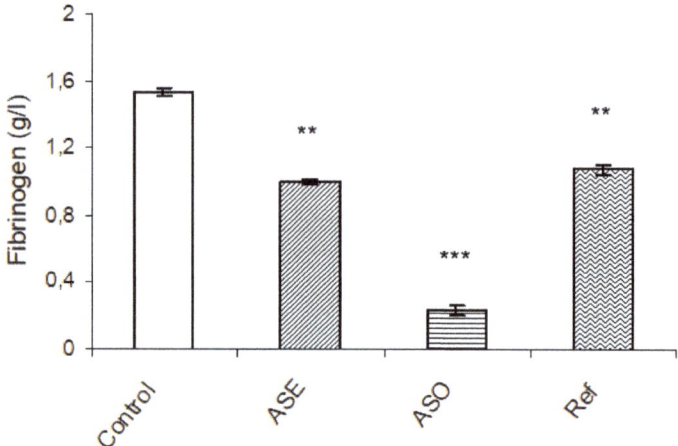

Figure 3. Effects of *Allium subhirsutum* L. extract (ASE), *Allium subhirsutum* L. oil and the reference drug "Cytolcentella®" on fibrinogen level. Data represent the mean ± SEM for six rats. Statistically significant variations are compared as follows: ASE, ASO and Ref treated groups compared to control group: ** and *** indicate significant differences when $p < 0.01$ and $p < 0.001$, respectively.

The results confirmed reduced levels of the inflammatory marker (fibrinogen content) on topical treatments with ASO and ASE as compared to the control group and the reference drug Cytolcentella group. The present study corroborates previous findings [11,34], which notified that phenolic compounds have the potency to attenuate the inflammatory markers as well as pro-inflammatory cytokines, which accelerate the mechanism of collagenation and maturation of granulation tissue.

2.4. Oxidative Stress Profile

Recent findings have shown that oxidative stress can cause cell damage [9,35–37] and delay wound healing [38]. The formation of free radicals and a low capacity to scavenge ROS are causative of skin lesions. After an overproduction of ROS, an increase in oxidative stress markers, as estimated by lipid peroxidation and protein oxidation molecules resulted in the healing process delay. The attenuation of excessive ROS generation significantly accelerates the healing process. The cells respond by developing a defense mechanism that consists of producing antioxidant enzymes, including superoxide dismutase (SOD), catalase (CAT) and glutathione peroxidase (GPx).

2.4.1. Oxidative Stress Markers of Granulation Tissue

The levels of wound tissues TBARS, CD, AOPP and CP are shown in Table 2. Results indicated that untreated control rats possessed the highest oxidative stress markers, proving the presence of an oxidative stress state in these rats. However, the application of either *Allium subhirsutum* L. extract and oil or the reference drug Cytolcentella significantly decreased the levels of TBARS, CD, AOPP and CP in the wound tissues as compared to control.

Table 2. Effects of *Allium subhirsutum* L. extract (ASE), *Allium subhirsutum* L. oil and the reference drug "Cytolcentella®" on oxidative stress markers of granulation tissue by estimation of TBARS, CD, AOPPA and CP levels.

Treatment & Parameters	TBARS (nmol MDA/mg Protein)	CD (µmol/mg Protein)	AOPP (µmol/mg Protein)	CP (µmol/mg Protein)
Control	1.38 ± 0.138	0.69 ± 0.04	0.25 ± 0.01	61.37 ± 0.37
ASE	1.08 ± 0.09 *	0.58 ± 0.13 *	0.23 ± 0.003	50.73 ± 1.28 **
ASO	0.91 ± 0.37 *	0.48 ± 0.11 **	0.21 ± 0.003 *	47.63 ± 1.09 **
Ref	0.82 ± 0.014 **	0.45 ± 0.01 ***	0.20 ± 0.006 **	41.80 ± 1.14 ***

The oxidative stress marker parameters: TBARS: Thiobarbituric acid-reactive substances; CD: conjugated dienes; AOPP: advanced oxidation of protein products; CP: carbonyl protein. Data represent the mean ± SEM for six rats. Statistically significant variations are compared as follows: ASE, ASO and Ref treated groups compared to control group. *, ** and *** indicate significant differences when $p < 0.05$, $p < 0.01$ and $p < 0.001$, respectively.

In our experiment, the treatment with ASO and ASE significantly decreased wound tissue levels TBARS, CD, AOPP and CP as compared to control rats. These results are in accordance with previous results [11–14,17,39], which reported that plants, specifically hairy garlic, possessed high antioxidant and free radical-scavenging effects. It may be attributed to the presence of active biomolecules in *Allium subhirsutum* L. oil which ultimately cause an antioxidant activity and wound repairing. The availability of bioactive molecules such polyphenols and flavonoids, and the ROS-scavenging ability of *Allium subhirsutum* L. helped in lowering the ROS levels, thus accelerating the wound closure.

2.4.2. Enzymatic Antioxidant Profile of Granulation Tissue

Several studies have shown that enzymatic antioxidant profiles such as SOD, CAT and GPx scavenge free radicals and prevent oxidative damage.

Antioxidant enzyme profiles (SOD, CAT and GPx) of control and treated rats are summarized in Table 3. The tissue antioxidant enzymatic activities of the control group were the lowest. The pre-treatment with *Allium subhirsutum* L. and the reference drug Cytolcentella showed a significant increase in the enzymatic activities as compared to the control group.

Table 3. Effects of *Allium subhirsutum* L. extract (ASE), *Allium subhirsutum* L. oil and the reference drug "Cytolcentella®" on enzymatic antioxidant profile of granulation tissue by estimation of SOD, CAT and GPx activities.

Treatment & Parameters	SOD (Units/mg Protein)	CAT (μmol H_2O_2/mg Protein)	GPx (μmol GSH/min/mg Protein)
Control	18.47 ± 0.29	50.50 ± 1.18	0.009 ± 0.0006
ASE	21.24 ± 2.71 *	53.07 ± 0.54 *	0.014 ± 0.0081 **
ASO	22.30 ± 3.81 *	57.50 ± 1.85 **	0.028 ± 0.012 ***
Ref	23.61 ± 0.99 **	69.61 ± 1.40 ***	0.037 ± 0.0003 ***

The enzymatic antioxidant profile: SOD: superoxide dismutase; CAT: catalase; GPx: glutathione peroxidase. Data represent the mean ± SEM for six rats in each group. Statistically significant variations are compared as follows: ASE, ASO and Ref treated groups compared to control group: *, ** and *** indicate significant differences when $p < 0.05$, $p < 0.01$ and $p < 0.001$, respectively.

In the current study, we observed an increase in SOD, CAT and GPx activities in the wound area in rats treated with ASO, ASE and the reference drug as compared to control rats. These results revealed that topical application of *Allium subhirsutum* L. oil and extract protected against cellular damage by the stimulation and/or the expression of the antioxidant enzymes. Our findings are in accordance with the data authored by Khan et al. [23], in which they reported that *Allium sativum* oil protected against oxidative damage in fish exposed to silver nanoparticles (Ag-NPs), and with Zammel et al. [11], where *Allium subhirsutum* was found to protect against carrageenan-induced paw edema, inflammation and oxidative damage in rats.

2.4.3. Correlation Matrix between Phytochemicals of *Allium subhirsutum* L., Oxidative Stress, Fibrinogen and Wound Reduction

Table 4 presented the correlation matrix between the antioxidant equivalent markers (polyphenols, flavonoids, tannins), the oxidative/antioxidative status, the fibrinogen level and the percentage of wound reduction (on the 11th day of treatment). As shown in Table 4, this correlation matrix revealed that AOPP oxidative stress marker, SOD and CAT enzymatic antioxidant activities were positively correlated with the antioxidant equivalent marker in *Allium subhirsutum* extract and oil (polyphenols, flavonoids and tannins), indicating its involvement in the attenuation of oxidative stress damage, as previously confirmed by several other reports [11,40].

Allium subhirsutum oil protected against oxidative damage as demonstrated by the SOD and GPx activities which were positively correlated with the polyphenols and flavonoids contents of ASO. A similar positive correlation was previously observed in *Lonicera caerulea* L. polyphenols that alleviated oxidative stress-induced intestinal environment imbalance and lipopolysaccharide-induced liver injury in high-fat diet-fed rats [41].

Table 4. Correlation matrix between phytochemicals, oxidative stress markers, fibrinogen and wound reduction.

		TBARS		CD		AOPP		CP		SOD		CAT		GPx		Fibrinogen		Wound Reduction	
	Parameters & Groups	ASE	ASO	ASE	ASO	ASE	ASO	ASE	ASO	ASE	ASO	ASE	ASO	ASE	ASO	ASE	ASO	ASE	ASO
Extract of AS	Polyphenols	−0.940	−0.140	0.824	0.037	0.544	−0.323	−0.762	−0.762	0.144	0.999 *	−0.762	0.144	−0.961	0.999 *	0.16	−0.55	−0.28	−0.87
	Flavonoids	0.630	0.981	−0.806	0.932	0.615	1.000 *	−0.362	−0.362	−0.982	−0.296	−0.362	−0.982	0.053	−0.296	−0.98	−0.60	−0.82	0.76
	Tannins	−0.174	0.787	−0.079	0.884	0.999 *	0.658	−0.942	−0.942	−0.785	0.528	−0.942	−0.785	−0.720	0.528	−0.78	−0.99 *	−0.97	0.00
Oil of AS	Polyphenols	−0.859	0.049	0.702	0.225	0.693	−0.138	−0.871	−0.871	−0.045	0.988	−0.871	−0.045	−0.996	0.988	−0.03	−0.70	−0.45	−0.76
	Flavonoids	−0.940	−0.140	0.824	0.037	0.544	−0.323	−0.762	−0.762	0.144	0.999 *	−0.762	0.144	−0.961	0.999 *	0.16	−0.55	−0.28	−0.87

Data represent the values obtained by Pearson correlation analysis. * indicate significant differences when $p < 0.05$.

3. Materials and Methods

3.1. Plant Material and Extraction

Fresh plant *Allium subhirsutum* L. cloves was procured from a local market in the Sfax region, Tunisia in October 2020. The plant specimen was washed under running water and skins of the samples were removed. For the extract preparation, *Allium subhirsutum* L. cloves were extracted and stirred with methanol at 30 °C for one night. Then, a whatmann filter paper was used to remove the particles. The residue was once more extracted, filtered, concentrated and stored until further use. The oil extraction was determined using the application of pressure as described by the method of Arisanu and Rus [42]. By this method, oil is enhanced by increased mechanical pressure on the oil-bearing material.

3.2. Phytochemical Analysis

3.2.1. Total Phenolic Content

The total phenolic content of the *Allium subhirsutum* L. extract and oil was measured using a modified colorimetric Folin–Ciocalteu method [43]. The total phenolic content was expressed as mg of gallic acid equivalents (GAE) per gram of dry weight.

3.2.2. Total Flavonoid Content

The total flavonoid content was determined by a colorimetric assay using the aluminum trichloride method according to Chang et al. [44]. Flavonoid content was expressed as mg of quercetin equivalent (QE)/gram of extract.

3.2.3. Total Tannins Content

The total tannins content of *Allium subhirsutum* L. extract and oil were determined as described by Broadhurst et al. [45] 50 µL of the extract was mixed with vanillin/methanol (3 mL, 4%). After stirring, 1.5 mL concentrated HCl was added. After 15 min, the absorbance was measured at 500 nm and the total tannins content was expressed as mg quercetin equivalent (QE)/gram of extract.

3.3. Antioxidant Potential Analysis

3.3.1. DPPH Free Radical Scavenging Assay

The DPPH• (2,2-diphenyl-1-picrylhydrazyl) free radical scavenging activities of *Allium subhirsutum* L. extract and oil were determined using the stable radical 1.1-diphenyl-2-picrylhydrazyl (DPPH), as previously reported by Kirby and Schmidt [46]. A total of 1 mL of different extract concentrations (0.06–1.0 mg $\times$ mL^{-1}) in methanol was mixed with 1 mL of DPPH radical solution in methanol 4% (*w/v*).

The absorbance of the samples and control solutions were measured at 517 nm against a blank. The antiradical activity was expressed as IC50 (µg/mL). The inhibition was calculated as follows:

$$\text{Free radical DPPH inhibition (\%)} = 100 \times (A_{control} - A_{sample})/A_{control}$$

where $A_{control}$ is the absorbance of the control reaction (without the test compound) and A_{sample} is the absorbance of the test compound. Ascorbic acid was used as a control.

3.3.2. Ferric Reducing Antioxidant Power

The reducing power was assessed using the method described by Oyaizu [47]. *Allium subhirsutum* L. extract and oil (0.06–1.0 mg $\times$ mL^{-1}) was mixed with 1 mL of sodium phosphate buffer (200 mM, pH 6.6) and 1 mL of potassium ferricyanide (1%, $K_3Fe(CN)_6$). After incubation at 50 °C for 20 min, 1 mL of trichloroacetic acid (10%) was added. The mixture was then centrifuged for 10 min at 650$\times$ *g*. An amount of 1.5 mL of the supernatant was mixed with 0.1 mL of ferric chloride (0.1%, $FeCl_3$) and 1.5 mL of deionized water. The absorbance was read at 700 nm and compared to a blank. The IC50 value (mg $\times$ mL^{-1}) was determined and compared to the ascorbic acid activity, which was used as standard.

3.3.3. Total Antioxidant Activity Assay by Radical Cation (ABTS+)

The Trolox equivalent antioxidant capacity (TEAC) determines the reduction in 2,2′-azino-bis(3-ethylbenzothiazoline-6-sulphonic acid, as previously reported by Re et al. [48] The antioxidant activity was expressed as mg TE/g extract and the IC50 was determined.

3.3.4. Total Antioxidant Capacities (TAC)

TAC of the plant substances (extract and oil) were assessed by the phosphomolybdenum method as described by Prieto et al. [49] Briefly, 0.1 mL of methanolic sample solution was mixed with 1 mL of the reagent solution (0.6 M, 28 mM and 4 mM of sulfuric acid, sodium phosphate and ammonium molybdate, respectively) and incubated in a boiling water bath for 90 min at 95 °C. After cooling at room temperature, the absorbance was determined at 695 nm and compared to a bank.

3.4. Wound Healing Assay

Due to its anti-inflammatory and antioxidant potentials, *Allium subhirsutum* L. extract and oil were tested for their wound healing in rats.

3.4.1. Animals

A total of 24 male albino *Wistar* rats weighing between 230–270 g were used for this study. The rats were purchased from the Faculty of Sciences of Gabes, Tunisia. The rats were allowed to acclimatize to the housing conditions (22 ± 3 °C, 12 h light/dark cycles and about 42% humidity). The rats were given a standard diet (SICO, Sfax, Tunisia) and ad libitum. All experiments involving animals were conducted according to the Ethical Committee Guidelines for the care and use of laboratory animals of our institution (University of Sfax, Tunisia) and approved by the local committee.

3.4.2. Wound Treatment

After anesthesia (intraperitoneal injection of chloral hydrate), an impression by a round seal of 1 cm diameter was made on the dorsal thoracic regions of the rats. The skin of the impressed area (sterilized and shaved before circular wound creation) was superficially excised to the full thickness to create the wound area [50].

Wounds rats were randomly divided into 4 groups of 6 rats each. Group I was treated with sterile saline and designated as negative control. Group II was treated with *Allium subhirsutum* L. extract (ASE), group III was treated with *Allium subhirsutum* L. oil (ASO), and group IV (reference group) was treated with a reference drug "Cytolcentella®" (Ref).

After cleaning the wounds with sterile saline, all treatments using extract and oil of *Allium subhirsutum* L. and the reference drug "Cytolcentella®" were topically applied every two days until sacrifice.

3.4.3. Percentage of Wound Closure Rate

The wound perimeters were traced using transparent paper and the percentage of the healed area was recorded. The percentage of wound closure was calculated using the following formula [51]:

$$\text{Wound closure (\%)} = (\text{Area of wound on day 0} - \text{Area of wound on nth day})/(\text{area of wound on day 0}) \times 100$$

where n represents the number of days, i.e., 3rd, 5th, 7th, 9th and 11th.

The required number of days for complete wound contraction was registered together with the re-epithelialization progress and the infection evolution were evaluated using macroscopic images.

3.4.4. Collection of Blood and Tissue

After sacrifice under chloral hydrate anesthesia, blood samples were collected by cardiac puncture and centrifuged at $2700 \times g$ for 15 min for various biochemical parameters, such as fribrinogen markers. The skin samples were collected, and the dissected wound tissue was used for analysis of oxidative damage markers and the enzymatic antioxidant defense system. For oxidative stress profile studies, each collected wound tissue was homogenized in TBS buffer (Tris-HCl 50 mM and NaCl 150 mM (1:2, w/v)) at pH 7.4 using an Ultra-Turax homogenizer. After centrifugation at 10,000× g for 15 min at 4°C, the supernatant was used to determine the protein content, as described by Lowry et al. [52]

3.4.5. Determination of Inflammatory Markers

Inflammatory markers of treated and control rats were evaluated after the sacrifice by measuring fibrinogen levels in blood samples. The level of fibrinogen was measured using a commercial kit obtained from STA Liquid fibrinogen (diagnostica stago), according to the manufacturer's instructions.

3.5. Determination of Oxidative Stress Markers of Granulation Tissue

3.5.1. Thiobarbituric Acid Reactive Substances (TBARS)

TBARS was assessed after the sacrifice using the spectrophotometric method described by Buege and Aust [53]. A total of 375 μL of extract, 150 μL of TBS and 375 μL of TCA 20% and 1% BHT were mixed to deproteinize the extracts. After centrifugation (1000× g for 10 min), 400 μL of the supernatant were mixed with 80 μL of HCl (0.6 M) and 320 μL of Tris-TBA (26 mMTris, 120 mM thiobarbituric acid). The optical density was measured at 530 nm. The TBARS amount was measured using 0.156 mM^{-1} cm^{-1} as the extinction coefficient.

3.5.2. Conjugated Diene (CD)

Conjugated diene levels were evaluated after the sacrifice by Halliwell and Gutteridge [54]. A total of 25 μL of wound tissue, 3 mL of chloroform and methanol (2:1, v/v) were mixed and then centrifuged at 3000 rpm for 5 min. An amount of 2 mL of the supernatant were taken and dried at 45 °C overnight. The extract obtained is again dissolved in 2 mL of methanol. We read the OD at 190 nm.

3.5.3. Advanced Oxidation of Protein Products Levels (AOPP)

The AOPP level was assessed after the sacrifice using the spectrophotometric method described by Witko et al. [55] Amounts of 200 μL of potassium iodide and 20 μL of acetic acid were placed in the presence of the sample diluted using 800 μL of PBS. AOPP has the capacity to absorb at 340 nm in an acid medium. Chloramine-T (0 to 200 μM) used as standard absorbed at 340 nm in the presence of potassium iodide.

3.5.4. Carbonyl Protein (CP)

The CP was assessed after the sacrifice using the spectrophotometric method described by Reznick and Packer [56]. A solution of TCA (20%) was added to the samples of the homogenate in order to precipitate the proteins. Then, a solution of DNPH (10 mM) was solubilized in HCl (2N) for 1 h at room temperature. The mixture was centrifuged for 15 min at 4 °C at 4000× g. The samples were treated with a guanidine–HCl solution (6 M) and placed in water at a temperature of 37 °C for 15 min. The protein carbonyl content was measured at 370 nm against a guanidine blank using a molar extinction coefficient of 22,000 M 1 cm^{-1}.

3.6. Determination of Enzymatic Antioxidant Profile of the Granulation Tissue
3.6.1. Superoxide Dismutase Activity (SOD)

SOD activity was assessed after the sacrifice using the spectrophotometric method described by Beyer and Fridovich [57]. The reaction mixture containing 50 mM of the tissue homogenates was prepared; then, the absorbance was measured at 560 nm and the SOD activity was expressed as unit per mg of protein (Unit/mg protein).

3.6.2. Glutathione Peroxidase Activity (GPx)

GPx activity was assessed after the sacrifice using the method described by Flohe and Gunzler [58] using 5% TCA. After centrifugation at 1500× g for 10 min, the supernatant was collected. A total of 0.1 mL of the tissue supernatant was mixed with 0.7 mL of 5.50 dithiobis-(2-nitrobenzoic acid) and (DTNB, 0.4 mg/mL) and 0.2 mL of phosphate buffer (0.1 M pH 7.4). The absorbance was measured at 420 nm and the GPx activity was expressed as nmoles of GSH/min/mg protein.

3.6.3. Catalase Activity (CAT)

CAT activity was assessed after the sacrifice using the method described by Aebi [59]. Briefly, 20 µL of tissue homogenate was added to 880 µL of H_2O_2 solution (pH = 7.4), which contains 0.5 mol/L H_2O_2 and 0.1 mol/L of phosphate buffer. The principle of the method is based on monitoring the H_2O_2 decomposition spectrophotometrically at 290 nm via the absorbance decrease. The extinction coefficient was $0.043/\text{mM}^{-1}\text{cm}^{-1}$ and the enzyme activity was expressed as µmol H_2O_2 decomposed/min/mg of protein (µM/min/mg protein).

3.7. Statistical Analysis

All results were expressed as mean ± standard error of the mean (SEM). Differences were considered statistically significant at $p \leq 0.05$. The results were analyzed by one-way analysis of variance (ANOVA) to assess the comparisons between groups using SPSS for Windows (version 18).

4. Conclusions

In conclusion both ASE and ASO possessed interesting amounts of polyphenols. Nevertheless, ASO was shown to contain more flavonoids and polyphenols. These high levels were associated with good antioxidant potential as assessed by DPPH, FRAP, ABTS and total antioxidant capacity and experimental wound healing in rats. They were also associated with better activity in terms of inflammation biomarkers, antioxidant parameters and wound healing activity. The latter revealed significantly accelerated both re-epithelialization and vascularization processes. The polyphenol, flavonoid and tannin contents of AS paralleled the positive effects on wound healing and the inflammatory reduction in the wound-healing treated rats. These results confirmed the ethno-pharmacological potential of *Allium subhirsutum* and encourage its use in the pharmaceutical industry due to its promising activity, particularly the oil fraction.

Supplementary Materials: The following are available online. Figure S1. Calibration curves of total phenolic components, flavonoids and tannins. OD: Optical density.

Author Contributions: Conceptualization, M.S. (Mongi Saoudi) and R.B.; methodology, M.S. (Mongi Saoudi) and A.C.; software, M.S. (Mongi Saoudi); validation, R.B., M.S. (Mohd Saeed) and A.E.F.; investigation, M.S. (Mongi Saoudi); R.B; resources, C.K. and A.E.F.; data curation, J.M.A.; writing—original draft preparation, M.S. (Mongi Saoudi); writing—review and editing, M.S. (Mongi Saoudi) and R.B.; visualization, S.E. and N.B.; supervision, R.B. and A.E.F.; project administration, R.B.; funding acquisition, R.B. All authors have read and agreed to the published version of the manuscript.

Funding: This research was supported by grants from the Deanship of Scientific Research—University of Ha'il (UoH) under a project number RG-20 070.

Institutional Review Board Statement: All animal experiments were conducted according to the Ethical Committee Guidelines for the care and use of laboratory animals of our institution (university of Sfax, Tunisia).

Informed Consent Statement: Not applicable.

Data Availability Statement: All data generated or analyzed during this study are included in this article.

Conflicts of Interest: The authors declare no conflict of interest.

Sample Availability: Samples of the compounds are available from the authors.

References

1. Pastar, I.; Wong, L.L.; Egger, A.N.; Tomic-Canic, M. Descriptive vs mechanistic scientific approach to study wound healing and its inhibition: Is there a value of translational research involving human subjects? *Exp. Dermatol.* **2018**, *27*, 551–562. [CrossRef]
2. Shetty, S.; Udupa, S.; Udupa, L. Evaluation of antioxidant and wound healing effects of alcoholic and aqueous extract of Ocimum sanctum Linn in rats. *Evid. Based Compl. Alt. Med.* **2008**, *5*, 95–101. [CrossRef]
3. Oryan, A.; Alemzadeh, E.; Moshiri, A. Biological properties and therapeutic activities of honey in wound healing: A narrative review and meta-analysis. *J. Tissue Viability* **2016**, *25*, 98–118. [CrossRef] [PubMed]
4. Djemaa, F.G.B.; Bellassoued, K.; Zouari, S.; El Feki, A.; Ammar, E. Antioxidant and wound healing activity of Lavandula aspic L. ointment. *J. Tissue Viability* **2016**, *25*, 193–200. [CrossRef] [PubMed]
5. Zhou, L.; Xu, T.; Yan, J.; Li, X.; Xie, Y.; Chen, H. Fabrication and characterization of matrine-loaded konjacglucomannan/fish gelatin composite hydrogel as antimicrobial wound dressing. *Food Hydrocoll.* **2020**, *104*, 105–702. [CrossRef]
6. Yadav, A.; Verma, S.; Keshri, G.K.; Gupta, A. Role of 904 nm superpulsed laser-mediated photobiomodulation on nitroxidative stress and redox homeostasis in burn wound healing. *Photodermatol. Photoimmunol. Photomed.* **2020**, *36*, 208–218. [CrossRef]
7. Firat, E.T.; Dağ, A.; Günay, A.; Kaya, B.; Karadede, M.İ.; Kanay, B.E.; Ketani, A.; Evliyaoglu, O.; Uysal, E. The effects of low-level laser therapy on palatal mucoperiosteal wound healing and oxidative stress status in experimental diabetic rats. *Photomed. Laser Surg.* **2013**, *31*, 315–321. [CrossRef] [PubMed]
8. Serarslan, G.; Altuğ, E.; Kontas, T.; Atik, E.; Avci, G. Caffeic acid phenetyl ester accelerates cutaneous wound healing in a rat model and decreases oxidative stress. *Clin. Exp. Dermatol.* **2007**, *32*, 709–715. [CrossRef] [PubMed]
9. Badraoui, R.; Sahnoun, Z.; Abdelmoula, N.B.; Hakim, A.; Fki, M.; Rebaï, T. May antioxidant status depletion by Tetradifon induce secondary genotoxicity in female Wistar rats via oxidative stress? *Pestic. Biochem. Physiol.* **2007**, *88*, 149–155. [CrossRef]
10. Badraoui, R.; Alrashedi, M.M.; El-May, M.V.; Bardakci, F. Acute respiratory distress syndrome: A life threatening associated complication of SARS-CoV-2 infection induced COVID-19. *J. Biomol. Struct. Dyn.* **2020**, 1–10. [CrossRef] [PubMed]
11. Zammel, N.; Saeed, M.; Bouali, N.; Elkahoui, S.; Alam, J.M.; Rebai, T.; Kausar, M.A.; Adnan, M.; Siddiqui, A.J.; Badraoui, R. Antioxidant and anti-inflammatory effects of Zingiberofficinaleroscoe and Allium subhirsutum: In Silico, biochemical and histological study. *Foods* **2021**, *10*, 1383. [CrossRef]
12. Bai, Q.; Han, K.; Dong, K.; Zheng, C.; Zhang, Y.; Long, Q.; Lu, T. Potential Applications of Nanomaterials and Technology for Diabetic Wound Healing. *Int. J. Nanomed.* **2020**, *15*, 9717. [CrossRef]
13. Akacha, A.; Badraoui, R.; Rebai, T.; Zourgui, L. Effect of Opuntiaficusindica extract on methotrexate-induced testicular injury: A biochemical, docking and histological study. *J. Biomol. Struct. Dyn.* **2020**, 1–11. [CrossRef]
14. Mzid, M.; Badraoui, R.; Khedir, S.B.; Sahnoun, Z.; Rebai, T. Protective effect of ethanolic extract of Urticaurens L. against the toxicity of imidacloprid on bone remodeling in rats and antioxidant activities. *Biomed. Pharmacother.* **2017**, *91*, 1022–1041. [CrossRef] [PubMed]
15. Sharif, A.; Asif, H.; Younis, W.; Riaz, H.; Bukhari, I.A.; Assiri, A.M. Indigenous medicinal plants of Pakistan used to treat skin diseases: A review. *Chin. Med.* **2018**, *13*, 1–26.
16. Rekik, D.M.; Khedir, S.B.; Daoud, A.; Moalla, K.K.; Rebai, T.; Sahnoun, Z. Wound Healing Effect of Lawsoniainermis. *Skin Pharmacol. Physiol.* **2019**, *32*, 295–306. [CrossRef]
17. Badraoui, R.; Rebai, T.; Elkahoui, S.; Alreshidi, M.; Veettil, V.N.; Noumi, E.; Al-Motair, A.K.; Aouadi, K.; Kadri, A.; De Feo, V.; et al. Allium subhirsutum L. as a Potential Source of Antioxidant and Anticancer Bioactive Molecules: HR-LCMS Phytochemical Profiling, In Vitro and In Vivo Pharmacological Study. *Antioxidants* **2020**, *9*, 1003. [CrossRef]
18. Saoudi, M.; Badraoui, R.; Rahmouni, F.; Jamoussi, K.; El Feki, A. Antioxidant and protective effects of Artemisia campestris essential oil against chlorpyrifos-induced kidney and liver injuries in rats. *Front. Physiol.* **2021**, *12*, 194. [CrossRef] [PubMed]
19. Rahmouni, F.; Saoudi, M.; Amri, N.; El-Feki, A.; Rebai, T.; Badraoui, R. Protective effect of Teucriumpolium on carbon tetrachloride induced genotoxicity and oxidative stress in rats. *Arch. Physiol. Biochem.* **2018**, *124*, 1–9. [CrossRef] [PubMed]
20. Edwards, Q.T.; Colquist, S.; Maradiegue, A. What's cooking with garlic: Is this complementary and alternative medicine for hypertension? *J. Am. Assoc. Nurse Pract.* **2005**, *17*, 381–385. [CrossRef] [PubMed]
21. Sut, S.; Maggi, F.; Bruno, S.; Badalamenti, N.; Quassinti, L.; Bramucci, M.; Beghelli, D.; Lupidi, G.; Dall'Acqua, S. Hairy garlic (Allium subhirsutum) from Sicily (Italy): LC-DAD-MSn analysis of secondary metabolites and in vitro biological properties. *Molecules* **2020**, *25*, 2837. [CrossRef]
22. Sener, G.; Sakarcan, A.; Yeğen, B.Ç. Role of garlic in the prevention of ischemia-reperfusion injury. *Mol. Nutr. Food Res.* **2007**, *51*, 1345–1352. [CrossRef]
23. Kothari, D.; Lee, W.D.; Kim, S.K. Allium Flavonols: Health Benefits, Molecular Targets, and Bioavailability. *Antioxidants* **2020**, *9*, 888. [CrossRef]
24. Khan, M.S.; Qureshi, N.A.; Jabeen, F.; Wajid, M.; Sabri, S.; Shakir, M. The role of garlic oil in the amelioration of oxidative stress and tissue damage in rohuLabeorohita treated with silver nanoparticles. *Fish. Sci.* **2020**, *86*, 255–269. [CrossRef]
25. Juan-García, A.; Agahi, F.; Drakonaki, M.; Tedeschi, P.; Font, G.; Juan, C. Cytoprotection assessment against mycotoxins on HepG2 cells by extracts from Allium sativum L. *Food Chem. Toxicol.* **2021**, *151*, 112–129. [CrossRef] [PubMed]

26. Batiha, G.E.S.; Alkazmi, L.M.; Wasef, L.G.; Beshbishy, A.M.; Nadwa, E.H.; Rashwan, E.K. Syzygiumaromaticum L. (Myrtaceae): Traditional uses, bioactive chemical constituents, pharmacological and toxicological activities. *Biomolecules* **2020**, *10*, 202. [CrossRef] [PubMed]
27. Polerà, N.; Badolato, M.; Perri, F.; Carullo, G.; Aiello, F. Quercetin and its natural sources in wound healing management. *Curr. Med. Chem.* **2019**, *26*, 5825–5848. [CrossRef]
28. Hemmatpor, Z.; Kamali, J.; Mehrabani, M.; Hashemi, S.A.; Marashi, S.M.A.; Pahlevan, S.; Tavakoli-Far, B. Study the Effect of Aqueous Extract of Garlic (*Allium sativum*) on Healing Procedure of Burn Wound on Rat. *Egypt. J. Vet. Sci.* **2020**, *51*, 181–189. [CrossRef]
29. Nagori, B.P.; Solanki, R. Role of medicinal plants in wound healing. *Res. J. Med. Plants* **2011**, *5*, 392–405. [CrossRef]
30. Majumdar, A.; Sangole, P. Alternative approaches to wound healing. Alexandrescu VA. In *Wound Healing: New insights into Ancient Challenges*; IntechOpen: London, UK, 2016; p. 459.
31. Amagase, H.; Petesch, B.L.; Matsuura, H.; Kasuga, S.; Itakura, Y. Intake of garlic and its bioactive components. *J. Nutr.* **2001**, *131*, 955S–962S. [CrossRef]
32. Farhat, Z.; Hershberger, P.A.; Freudenheim, J.L.; Mammen, M.J.; Blair, R.H.; Aga, D.S.; Mu, L. Types of garlic and their anticancer and antioxidant activity: A review of the epidemiologic and experimental evidence. *Eur. J. Nutr.* **2021**, 1–25. [CrossRef]
33. Jantan, I.; Haque, M.A.; Arshad, L.; Harikrishnan, H.; Septama, A.W.; Mohamed-Hussein, Z.A. Dietary polyphenols suppress chronic inflammation by modulation of multiple inflammation-associated cell signaling pathways. *J. Nutr. Biochem.* **2021**, *93*, 108634. [CrossRef]
34. Yadav, E.; Singh, D.; Yadav, P.; Verma, A. Attenuation of dermal wounds via downregulating oxidative stress and inflammatory markers by protocatechuic acid rich n-butanol fraction of Trianthemaportulacastrum Linn. in wistar albino rats. *Biomed. Pharmacother.* **2017**, *96*, 86–97. [CrossRef] [PubMed]
35. Badraoui, R.; Nasr, H.B.; Louati, N.; Ellouze, F.; Rebai, T. Nephrotoxic effect of tetradifon in rats: A biochemical and histomorphometric study. *Exp. Toxicol. Pathol.* **2012**, *64*, 645–650. [CrossRef]
36. Amri, N.; Rahmouni, F.; Chokri, M.A.; Rebai, T.; Badraoui, R. Histological and biochemical biomarkers analysis reveal strong toxicological impacts of pollution in hybrid sparrow (*Passer domesticus* × *Passerhispaniolensis*) in southern Tunisia. *Environ. Sci. Pollut. Res.* **2017**, *24*, 17845–17852. [CrossRef] [PubMed]
37. Ben Nasr, H.; Hammami, S.; Chaker, S.; Badraoui, R.; Sahnoun, Z.; Jamoussi, K.; Rebai, T.; Zeghal, K. Some biological effects of scorpion envenomation in late pregnant rats. *Exp. Toxicol. Pathol.* **2009**, *61*, 573–580. [CrossRef]
38. Cano Sanchez, M.; Lancel, S.; Boulanger, E.; Neviere, R. Targeting oxidative stress and mitochondrial dysfunction in the treatment of impaired wound healing: A systematic review. *Antioxidants* **2018**, *7*, 98. [CrossRef] [PubMed]
39. Yadav, E.; Singh, D.; Yadav, P.; Verma, A. Antioxidant and anti-inflammatory properties of *Prosopis cineraria* based phenolic rich ointment in wound healing. *Biomed. Pharmacother.* **2018**, *108*, 1572–1583. [CrossRef] [PubMed]
40. Ansary, J.; Forbes-Hernández, T.Y.; Gil, E.; Cianciosi, D.; Zhang, J.; Elexpuru-Zabaleta, M.; Simal-Gandara, J.; Giampieri, F.; Battino, M. Potential health benefit of garlic based on human intervention studies: A brief overview. *Antioxidants* **2020**, *9*, 619. [CrossRef]
41. Li, B.; Cheng, Z.; Sun, X.; Si, X.; Gong, E.; Wang, Y.; Tian, J.; Shu, C.; Ma, F.; Li, D.; et al. Lonicera caerulea L. polyphenols alleviate oxidative stress-induced intestinal environment imbalance and lipopolysaccharide-induced liver injury in HFD-fed rats by regulating the Nrf2/HO-1/NQO1 and MAPK pathways. *Mol. Nutr. Food Res.* **2020**, *64*, 1901315. [CrossRef]
42. Arișanu, A.O.; Rus, F. Current techniques and processes for vegetable oil extraction from oilseed crops. *Bull. Transilv. Univ. Bras.* **2017**, *10*, 65–70.
43. Wolfe, K.; Wu, X.; Liu, R.H. Antioxidant activity of apple peels. *J. Agric. Food Chem.* **2003**, *51*, 609–614. [CrossRef] [PubMed]
44. Chang, C.C.; Yang, M.H.; Wen, H.M.; Chern, J.C. Estimation of total flavonoid content in propolis by two complementary colorimetric methods. *J. Food Drug Anal.* **2002**, *10*, 178–182.
45. Broadhurst, R.B.; Jones, W.T. Analysis of condensed tannins using acidified vanillin. *J. Sci. Food Agric.* **1978**, *29*, 788–794. [CrossRef]
46. Kirby, A.J.; Schmidt, R.J. The antioxidant activity of Chinese herbs for eczema and of placebo herbs. *J. Ethnopharmacol.* **1997**, *56*, 103–108. [CrossRef]
47. Oyaizu, M. Studies on products of browning reactions: Antioxidative activities of browning reaction prepared from glucosamine. *Jpn. J. Nutr.* **1986**, *44*, 307–315. [CrossRef]
48. Re, R.; Pellegrini, N.; Proteggente, A.; Pannala, A.; Yang, M.; Rice-Evans, C. Antioxidant activity applying an improved ABTS radical cation decolorization assay. *Free Radic. Biol. Med.* **1999**, *26*, 1231–1237. [CrossRef]
49. Prieto, P.; Pineda, M.; Aguilar, M. Spectrophotometric quantitation of antioxidant capacity through the formation of a phosphomolybdenum complex: Specific application to the determination of vitamin E. *Anal. Biochem.* **1999**, *269*, 337–341. [CrossRef]
50. Suguna, L.; Singh, S.; Sivakumar, P.; Sampath, P.; Chandrakasan, G. Influence of *Terminalia chebula* on dermal wound healing in rats. *Phytother. Res.* **2002**, *16*, 227–231. [CrossRef]
51. Jridi, M.; Sellimi, S.; Lassoued, K.B.; Beltaief, S.; Souissi, N.; Mora, L.; Toldra, F.; Elfeki, A.; Nasri, M.; Nasri, R. Wound healing activity of cuttlefish gelatin gels and films enriched by henna (Lawsoniainermis) extract. *Colloid Surf. A Physicochem. Eng. Asp.* **2017**, *512*, 71–79. [CrossRef]

52. Lowry, O.H.; Rosebrough, N.J.; Farr, A.L.; Randall, R.J. Protein measurement with Folin phenol reagent. *J. Biol. Chem.* **1951**, *193*, 265–275. [CrossRef]
53. Buege, J.A.; Aust, S.D. Microsomal lipid peroxidation. *Methods Enzymol.* **1972**, *51*, 302–310.
54. Halliwell, B.; Gutteridge, J.C. Lipid peroxidation, oxygen radicals, cell damage, and antioxidant therapy. *Lancet (Br. Ed.)* **1984**, *8391*, 1396–1397. [CrossRef]
55. Witko-Sarsat, V.; Friedlander, M.; Capeillère-Blandin, C.; Nguyen- Khoa, T.; Nguyen, A.T.; Zingraff, J.; Jungers, P.; Descamps-Latscha, B. Advanced oxidation protein products as a novel marker of oxidative stress in uremia. *Kidney Int.* **1996**, *49*, 1304–1313. [CrossRef]
56. Reznick, A.Z.; Packer, L. Oxidative damage to proteins: Spectrophotometric method for carbonyl assay. *Methods Enzymol.* **1994**, *233*, 357–363. [PubMed]
57. Beyer, W.F.; Fridovich, I. Assaying for superoxide dismutase activity: Some large consequences of minor changes in conditions. *Anal. Biochem.* **1987**, *161*, 559–566. [CrossRef]
58. Floche, L.; Gunzler, W.A. Analysis of glutathione peroxidase. *Methods Enzymol.* **1984**, *105*, 114–121.
59. Aebi, H. Catalase in vitro. *Methods Enzymol.* **1974**, *105*, 121–126.

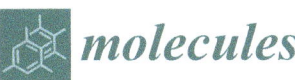

Correction

Correction: Saoudi et al. The Role of *Allium subhirsutum* L. in the Attenuation of Dermal Wounds by Modulating Oxidative Stress and Inflammation in *Wistar* Albino Rats. *Molecules* 2021, 26, 4875

Mongi Saoudi [1,*], Riadh Badraoui [2,3,*], Ahlem Chira [1], Mohd Saeed [2], Nouha Bouali [2], Salem Elkahoui [2], Jahoor M. Alam [2], Choumous Kallel [4] and Abdelfattah El Feki [1]

1. Animal Ecophysiology Laboratory, Sciences Faculty of Sfax, University of Sfax, Sfax 3054, Tunisia
2. Laboratory of General Biology, Department of Biology, University of Ha'il, Ha'il 81451, Saudi Arabia
3. Section of Histology and Cytology, Medicine Faculty of Tunis, University of Tunis El Manar, La Rabta, Tunis 1007, Tunisia
4. Hematology Laboratory, Hospital Habib Bourguiba, Sfax 3029, Tunisia
* Correspondence: mongifss@yahoo.fr (M.S.); riadh.badraoui@fmt.utm.tn (R.B.); Tel.: +216-99740205 (M.S.)

The authors wish to make the following change to their paper [1]. We realized that, unfortunately, the selection of the corresponding photos for the different groups in Figure 1 was not completely correct. Therefore, after careful verifications, the authors want to publish a corrected version of Figure 1.

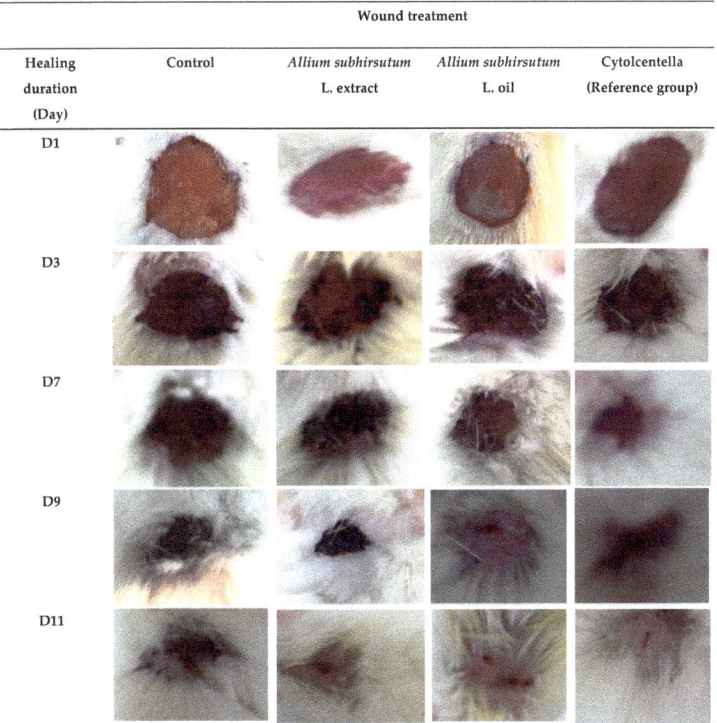

Figure 1. Photographic illustrations of wound healing process in the different experimental groups on 1, 3, 7, 9 and 11 days post-wounding.

The authors apologize for any inconvenience caused and state that the change does not affect the results of the study and the conclusions drawn from it. The original publication has also been updated.

Reference

1. Saoudi, M.; Badraoui, R.; Chira, A.; Saeed, M.; Bouali, N.; Elkahoui, S.; Alam, J.M.; Kallel, C.; El Feki, A. The Role of *Allium subhirsutum* L. in the Attenuation of Dermal Wounds by Modulating Oxidative Stress and Inflammation in *Wistar* Albino Rats. *Molecules* **2021**, *26*, 4875. [CrossRef] [PubMed]

molecules

Article

HPLC Analysis and the Antioxidant and Preventive Actions of *Opuntia stricta* Juice Extract against Hepato-Nephrotoxicity and Testicular Injury Induced by Cadmium Exposure

Xiaoli Zhu [1,2,3] and Khaled Athmouni [4,*]

1. College of Food Science & Institute of Food Biotechnology, South China Agricultural University, Guangzhou 510642, China
2. College of Food and Biotechnology, Guangdong Industry Polytechnic, Guangzhou 510300, China
3. Research Center for Micro-Ecological Agent Engineering and Technology of Guangdong Province, Guangzhou 510642, China
4. Laboratory of Animal Ecophysiology, Faculty of Sciences of Sfax, University of Sfax, Sfax 3000, Tunisia
* Correspondence: athmounikhaled1989@gmail.com; Tel.: +216-93242084

Abstract: *Opuntia stricta* is a rich source of phenolic compounds. This species generally has strong antioxidant activities in vitro and in vivo. This study aimed to analyze the antioxidant properties of phenolic compounds isolated from *Opuntia stricta*, including its radical scavenging activities and preventive action against Cd-induced oxidative stress in rats. To assess the protection of prickly pear juice extract (PPJE) against Cd-induced hepato-nephrotoxicity and testicular damage, male albino rats received PPJE (250 mg kg^{-1}) and/or Cd (1 mg kg^{-1}) by oral administration and injection, respectively, for five consecutive weeks. The preventive action of PPJE was estimated using biochemical markers of kidney and liver tissues, antioxidant status, and histological examinations. In the present study, the lipid peroxidation, protein carbonyls, antioxidant status, and metallothionein levels were determined in different tissues. The chromatographic analysis indicated that PPJE extract is very rich in phenolic compounds such as verbascoside, catechin hydrate, and oleuropein. Our results showed that PPJE-treated rats had significantly ($p < 0.05$) decreased Cd levels in liver and kidney tissues. In addition, the administration of PPJE induced a significant ($p < 0.05$) decrease in lipid peroxidation of 30.5, 54.54, and 40.8 in the liver, kidney, and testicle, respectively, and an increase in antioxidant status in these tissues. Additionally, PPJE showed a strong ability to protect renal, hepatic, and testicular architectures against Cd exposure. This study revealed that PPJE protects against the toxic effects of Cd, possibly through its free radical scavenging and antioxidant activities.

Keywords: antioxidant activity; hepato-nephrotoxicity; HPLC analysis; *O. stricta*; testicular damage

1. Introduction

Cadmium exposure can enhance oxidative stress in several organs, including kidney and hepatic tissues [1]. Heavy metals are known to induce carcinogenic toxicity [2] and adverse effects in humans, causing public health risks. However, they act as a threat to living organisms since they are highly toxic and accumulate in their body tissues [1]. Nevertheless, liver and kidney tissues perform detoxification and excretion actions. Among these metals, cadmium (Cd) is a very toxic metal that causes several alterations in human and animal tissues. Cd toxicity arises from its wide distribution in fertilizer, and consequently foods, and tobacco smoke [3] and is commonly used in industry development [4]. Usually, accumulation and intoxication phenomena occur in both liver and kidney tissues. Cd exposure can cause many alterations in kidney cells [2]. In addition, during Cd exposure, this metal accumulates predominantly in the liver, kidneys, reproductive organs, and tissues [5]. Principally, this heavy metal accumulation increases in both kidney and liver tissues [6]. Several studies have indicated that the mechanisms of toxicity of Cd exposure are: a reduction in glutathione levels (GSH), alterations in antioxidant enzymes, and enhanced ROS production in exposed tissues [7]. This unnatural level of ROS induces lipid peroxidation and oxidative DNA damage in cells [8]. Moreover, this metal causes several complications, such as liver and kidney injuries, respiratory diseases, neurological disorders, and testicular damage [9].

Medicinal plants generally have various preventive actions against several diseases [10]. In addition, the phenolic extracts of medicinal plants can reduce ROS levels in tissues [10]. Additionally, the preventive actions of natural antioxidant molecules against metal that cause several alterations are usually studied [8]. In recent years, studies on the antioxidant activities of medicinal plants have increased remarkably due to increased interest in their potential use as a rich and natural source of antioxidants. Many medicinal plants contain large amounts of antioxidants such as polyphenols, which can play an important role in absorbing and neutralizing free radicals, quenching singlet and triplet oxygen, or decomposing peroxides. The beneficial health effects of plants are attributed to flavonoids, a class of secondary metabolites that protect the plant against ultraviolet light and even herbivores.

In addition, cladode juice contains various compounds with high antioxidant potentials, including phenolic compounds, vitamins C and E, b-carotene (provitamin A), glutathione, etc. [11]. Moreover, several authors have reported that cladode juice exerts preventive actions against various alterations and enhanced Cd exposure [12]. This preventive action may be explained by the presence of the flavonoid compound quercetin 3-methyl ether in cladode extracts, which minimizes ROS levels in cells [13].

In the present study, the preventive action of prickly pear plant extract was evaluated against Cd toxicity. The prickly pear *Opuntia stricta*, a member of the Cactaceae family, is widespread in Mexico, much of Latin America, South Africa, and the Mediterranean area [14]. Accordingly, several authors have found that prickly pear has various pharmacological activities, including anti-proliferative and anti-viral [15], anti-inflammatory [16], and anti-hyperlipidemic properties [17] and analgesic action [18]. These data make prickly pear fruits and cladodes perfect candidates for cytoprotective investigations.

Interestingly, there are data in the literature showing that Opuntia extracts can be considered reliable and safe since no toxicity or only low toxicity has been found in animal models. An in vivo toxicity study suggests that the oral administration of *Opuntia ficus indica* extract at levels up to 2000 mg/kg/day does not cause adverse effects in male and female rats [19]. In an oral toxicity study, Sharma et al. [20] found that rats given the crude drug at doses up to 50 mL/kg exhibited no symptoms of toxicity. The crude extracts of *Opuntia* genus cladodes showed low toxicity in animal models [21,22].

The present study aimed to evaluate the hepato-nephro and testicular protective effects of the phenolic extract isolated from *O. stricta* cladode juice against Cd exposure by determining kidney, liver, and testicular biomarkers in male Wistar rats.

2. Results

2.1. Phytochemical Determination and Antioxidant Potentials

The amounts of phenolic and flavonoid contents in PPJE are presented in Table 1. The juice extract of this Cactaceae showed high phenolic (24.71 ± 3.93 mg GAE/g DW) and flavonoid contents (8.84 ± 0.41 mg QE g^{-1} extract).

Table 1. Total phenolic content and total flavonoids of juice extract of *O. stricta* cladode.

	Juice Extract of *O. stricta* Cladode
Total phenol (mg GAE/g DW)	24.71 ± 3.93
Flavonoids (mg QE/g DW)	8.48 ± 0.43
ABTS (µM TE/g DW)	0.061 ± 0.001

Data expressed as average ± SD (n = 3) standard deviations. GAE: gallic acid equivalent; QE: quercetin equivalent; TE: Trolox equivalent; DW: dry weight.

In the present work, the antioxidant activity of *O. stricta* was estimated by DPPH and ABTS methods. As shown in Figure 1, the values of DPPH radical scavenging activity varied between 20 and 83%. Concerning the ABTS radical scavenging capacity, the juice extract showed high antioxidant capacity (0.061 µM TE g^{-1} DW) (Table 1).

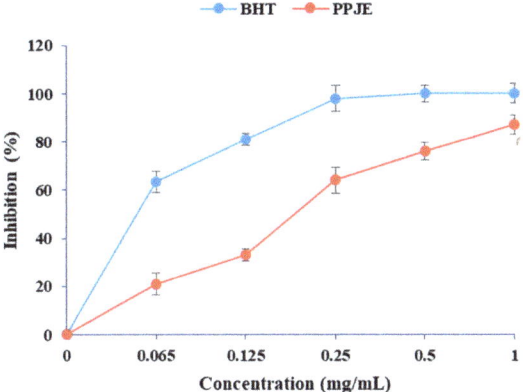

Figure 1. Effects of extracts of *O. stricta* on *in vitro* free radicals (DPPH).

2.2. HPLC Analysis of PPJE

The phenolic profile of PPJE is presented in Figure 2. Catechin hydrate, tyrosol, 4HOBenz, verbascoside, rutin, apigenin 7Glu, oleuropein, quercetin, pinoresinol and apigenin were found in *O. stricta*. Verbascoside was the major component (3.12 µg g^{-1}), followed by catechin hydrate (1.43 µg g^{-1}) and oleuropein (1.39 µg g^{-1}). Minor phenolic compounds included pinoresinol, quercetin, and apigenin (Table 2).

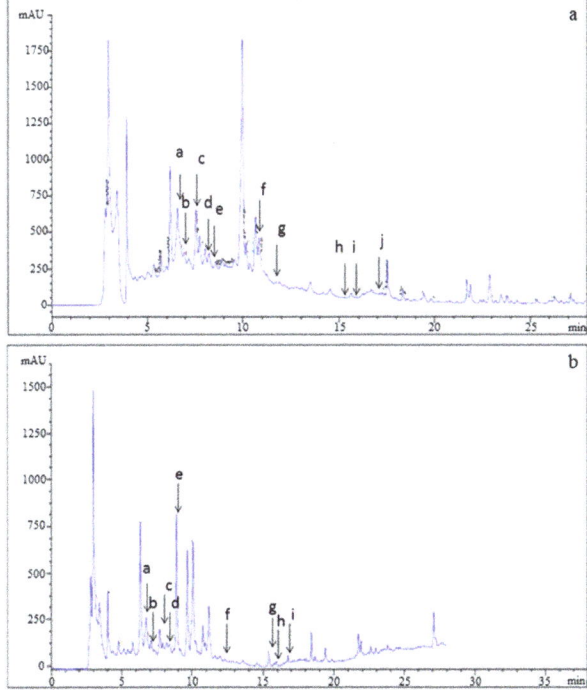

Figure 2. HPLC analysis of (a) standards and (b) juice extract of *O. stricta* cladode.

Table 2. Chemical composition of ethanol extracts from *O. stricta* cladode juice by HPLC analysis.

Short Name	Retention Time (min)	Composition (µg/g)
Catechin hydrate	6.71	1.43
Tyrosol	7.06	1.10
4-Hydroxybenzoic acid	7.67	1.34
Verbascoside	8.88	3.12
Rutin	8.15	1.29
Apigenin 7glucoside	10.75	1.10
Oleuropein	11.95	1.39
Quercetin	15.40	0.21
Pinoresinol	15.90	0.11
Apigenin	16.74	0.27
Luteolin-7-Glu	Nd	Nd

Nd: not detected.

2.3. Effects of PPJE Cd-Induced Damage in Rats

2.3.1. Markers of Hepatic and Nephrotoxicity Toxicity

Cd administration significantly decreased (by 40%) the levels of ALT, AST, and bilirubin in the liver compared with the control group after 5 weeks (Table 3). The Cd-treated rats had significantly ($p < 0.05$) enhanced plasma levels of creatinine and urea in kidney tissue as compared to the normal rats. Treatments of rats with PPJE decreased the levels of AST, ALT, and bilirubin in the liver and creatinine and urea in the kidney compared with the Cd group.

Table 3. Serum ALT, AST, bilirubin, urea, and creatinine of the studied groups. Control group. Juice extract (250 mg/kg)-treated rat kidney showing normal appearance of glomeruli. $CdCl_2$ (1 mg/kg)-treated rat kidney showing tubule glomerular degeneration. $CdCl_2$ + juice extract (250 mg/kg)-treated rat.

Group	ALT	AST	Bilirubin (µmol/L)			Creatinine	Urea
	(IU/L)	(IU/L)	Total	Conjugated	Unconjugated	(mmol/L)	(mmol/L)
Control	22.31 ± 2.31 [a]	112.42 ± 9.65 [a]	0.43 ± 0.08 [a]	0.41 ± 0.07 [a]	0.02 ± 0.00 [a]	8.51 ± 0.54 [a]	38.65 ± 4.65 [a]
PPJE extract	21.54 ± 1.46 [a]	114.54 ± 7.64 [a]	0.38 ± 0.09 [a]	0.36 ± 0.02 [a]	0.02 ± 0.00 [a]	11.31 ± 1.32 [a]	41.32 ± 7.34 [a]
$CdCl_2$	43.54 ± 2.14 [c]	135.76 ± 5.74 [c]	1.46 ± 0.21 [c]	1.14 ± 0.06 [b]	0.32 ± 0.04 [c]	17.64 ± 2.21 [b]	65.81 ± 5.67 [c]
$CdCl_2$ + PPJE extract	28.64 ± 1.65 [b]	123.54 ± 5.82 [b]	1.08 ± 0.13 [b]	0.94 ± 0.07 [b]	0.14 ± 0.06 [b]	11.32 ± 1.57 [a]	51.64 ± 7.07 [b]

[a–c] Values having different letters on the same line showed significant differences ($p < 0.05$).

2.3.2. Enzymatic Antioxidants

The levels of the antioxidant enzymes SOD, CAT, and GPx in the liver, kidney, and testicular tissues of the experimental animals are given in Tables 4–6. Cd treatment led to a significant decrease in hepatic SOD, CAT, and GPx (−48.44%, −48.29%, and −6.9%, respectively) compared to those of the control group. After five weeks of Cd exposure, levels of enzymatic activity such as SOD, CAT, and GPx in kidney and testicular tissues were significantly increased compared to the normal group ($p < 0.05$). Our results indicated that PPJE-treated rats were able to protect the antioxidant status from Cd toxicity.

Table 4. Antioxidant enzyme activities and stress biomarkers levels in liver tissue of the studied groups. Control rats. PPJE extract (250 mg/kg)-treated rats. CdCl$_2$ (1 mg/kg)-treated rats. CdCl$_2$ + PPJE extract (250 mg/kg)-treated rats. α: U mg^{-1} protein; β: μmoles/H$_2$O$_2$ consumed min^{-1} mg^{-1} of protein; γ: nmoles GSH min^{-1} mg^{-1} of protein; δ: nmoles of MDA g^{-1} of tissue; ε: nmoles mg^{-1} of protein.

	Control	PPJE Extract	CdCl$_2$	CdCl$_2$ + PPJE Extract
SOD α	28.28 ± 3.41 [d]	27.37 ± 1.74 [cd]	14.58 ± 2.54 [a]	23.07 ± 2.04 [b]
CAT β	37.64 ± 2.45 [d]	36.85 ± 1.75 [c]	19.46 ± 1.82 [a]	31.25 ± 3.05 [b]
GPx γ	362.33 ± 7.84 [d]	361.05 ± 7.42 [c]	337.32 ± 9.64 [a]	353.61 ± 6.54 [b]
LPO δ	0.74 ± 0.11 [b]	0.72 ± 0.08 [a]	1.34 ± 0.42 [d]	0.93 ± 0.21 [c]
Protein carbonyl ε	1.81 ± 0.13 [b]	1.78 ± 0.21 [a]	4.37 ± 0.37 [d]	2.36 ± 0.17 [c]

[a-d]—Values having different letters on the same line showed significant differences ($p < 0.05$).

Table 5. Antioxidant enzyme activities and stress biomarkers levels in kidney tissue of the studied groups. Control rats. PPJE extract (250 mg/kg)-treated rats. CdCl$_2$ (1 mg/kg)-treated rats. CdCl$_2$ + PPJE extract (250 mg/kg)-treated rats. α: U mg^{-1} protein; β: μmoles/H$_2$O$_2$ consumed min^{-1} mg^{-1} of protein; γ: nmoles GSH min^{-1} mg^{-1} of protein; δ: nmoles of MDA g^{-1} of tissue; ε: nmoles mg^{-1} of protein.

	Control	PPJE Extract	CdCl$_2$	CdCl$_2$ + PPJE Extract
SOD α	41.44 ± 1.47 [c]	42.24 ± 2.45 [c]	18.07 ± 1.65 [a]	34.51 ± 1.84 [b]
CAT β	51.31 ± 3.14 [c]	52.62 ± 1.84 [c]	28.21 ± 2.74 [a]	41.21 ± 1.87 [b]
GPx γ	375.31 ± 3.24 [d]	373.34 ± 5.62 [c]	342.27 ± 6.04 [a]	361.07 ± 7.86 [b]
LPO δ	0.71 ± 0.12 [b]	0.68 ± 0.08 [a]	2.31 ± 0.32 [d]	1.05 ± 0.11 [c]
Protein carbonyl ε	1.85 ± 0.23 [b]	1.77 ± 0.32 [a]	6.34 ± 0.63 [d]	2.74 ± 0.14 [c]

[a-d]—Values having different letters on the same line showed significant differences ($p < 0.05$).

Table 6. Antioxidant enzyme activities and stress biomarkers levels in testicular tissue of the studied groups. Control rats. PPJE extract (250 mg/kg)-treated rats. CdCl$_2$ (1 mg/kg)-treated rats. CdCl$_2$ + PPJE extract (250 mg/kg)-treated rats. α: U mg^{-1} protein; β: μmoles/H$_2$O$_2$ consumed min^{-1} mg^{-1} of protein; γ: nmoles GSH min^{-1} mg^{-1} of protein; δ: nmoles of MDA g^{-1} of tissue; ε: nmoles mg^{-1} of protein.

	Control	PPJE Extract	CdCl$_2$	CdCl$_2$ + PPJE Extract
SOD α	38.51 ± 2.07 [c]	37.65 ± 1.67 [c]	15.32 ± 0.84 [a]	27.84 ± 2.23 [b]
CAT β	47.21 ± 2.54 [c]	48.74 ± 1.67 [c]	24.82 ± 3.75 [a]	38.74 ± 2.34 [b]
GPx γ	365.31 ± 2.31 [c]	364.43 ± 4.08 [c]	338.72 ± 5.72 [a]	357.63 ± 3.65 [b]
LPO δ	0.65 ± 0.42 [a]	0.66 ± 0.11 [a]	2.23 ± 0.22 [c]	1.32 ± 0.08 [b]
Protein carbonyl ε	1.64 ± 0.34 [a]	1.63 ± 0.21 [a]	5.54 ± 0.37 [c]	2.86 ± 0.42 [b]

[a-c]—Values having different letters on the same line showed significant differences ($p < 0.05$).

2.3.3. Lipid Peroxidation and Protein Oxidation Indices

Cd exposure induced increases in lipid peroxidation (LPO) of 30.5%, 54.54%, and 40.8% in the liver, kidney, and testicle, respectively, compared with the Cd-treated group (Tables 4–6). In addition, the protein carbonyl contents in the liver, kidney, and testicle were significantly higher in the Cd-treated group compared with control rats, as shown in Tables 4–6, respectively. In addition, the administration of ethanolic PPJE (250 mg kg^{-1}) alone to rats caused a significant reduction in LPO and protein carbonyl levels in these different organs.

2.3.4. Effects of Cd Exposure on MT Concentration in Rat Liver and Kidney

Metallothionein is widely considered a sensitive marker of oxidative stress. The metallothionein concentrations in the liver and kidney tissues were enhanced in the Cd-treated group compared with untreated rats (Figure 3a,b). Additionally, the present study indicated that the treatments of ethanolic PPJE (250 mg kg^{-1}) significantly decreased the MT concentration in both organs when compared with Cd-treated rats.

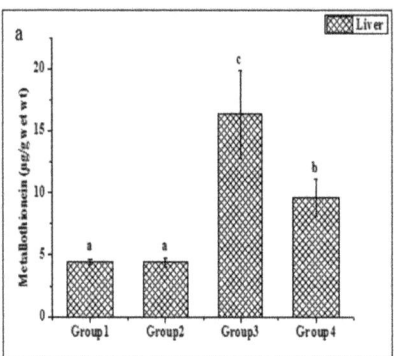
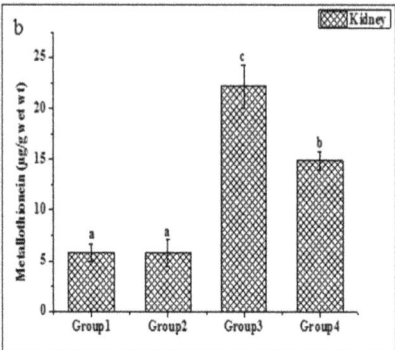

Figure 3. Effect of juice extract of *O. stricta* on Cd-induced changes in the levels of metallothionein in the liver (**a**) and kidney (**b**) of control and experimental rats. Group 1: Normal rats. Group 2: Juice extract (250 mg/kg)-treated rats. Group 3: CdCl$_2$ (1 mg/kg)-treated rats. Group 4: CdCl$_2$ + juice extract (250 mg/kg)-treated rats. Values are mean ± SD for 6 rats in each group. Bars not sharing a common superscript letter (a, b, c) differ significantly at $p < 0.05$ (Duncan).

2.3.5. Cadmium Estimation

The Cd concentrations in hepatic and kidney tissues are given in Table 7. The results of the ANOVA test showed that Cd content in these organs was significantly higher ($p < 0.05$) than that in normal rats. The amount of Cd content varied among different groups and ranged from 0.01 to 0.46 µg g^{-1} w.t.w in the liver, whereas this metal varied between 0.01 and 1.34 µg g^{-1} w.t.w in kidney tissue. The highest Cd concentration was measured in the Cd group. In contrast, the administration of PPJE extract (250 mg kg^{-1}) decreased the concentrations of Cd in liver and kidney tissues when compared to the Cd-treated group.

Table 7. Effect of *O. stricta* juice extract on Cd content in liver and kidney tissues. Control rats. PPJE extract (250 mg/kg)-treated rats. CdCl$_2$ (1 mg/kg)-treated rats. CdCl$_2$ + PPJE extract (250 mg/kg)-treated rats.

Groups	Cd Concentration µg g^{-1} Dry Mass	
	Liver	Kidney
Control	0.01 ± 0.00 [a]	0.01 ± 0.00 [a]
PPJE extract	0.01 ± 0.00 [a]	0.01 ± 0.01 [a]
CdCl$_2$	0.46 ± 0.05 [c]	1.34 ± 0.08 [c]
CdCl$_2$ + PPJE extract	0.24 ± 0.03 [b]	0.97 ± 0.07 [b]

[a–c]—Values having different letters on the same line showed significant differences ($p < 0.05$).

2.4. Effects on Histopathological Changes

The histopathological changes in the liver and kidneys are presented in Figures 4 and 5, respectively. The liver and kidneys of controls showed normal morphologies (Figures 4a and 5a, respectively). In contrast, treatment with Cd alone produced focal hepatocyte swelling, vacuolation and inflammation (leukocyte infiltration), focal proximal tubule degeneration (Figure 4c), and glomerular swelling (Figure 5c) in the kidneys. Administration of PPJE

(250 mg kg^{-1}) preserved the morphology and also restored the architectures of the liver and kidney tissues (Figures 4d and 5d, respectively).

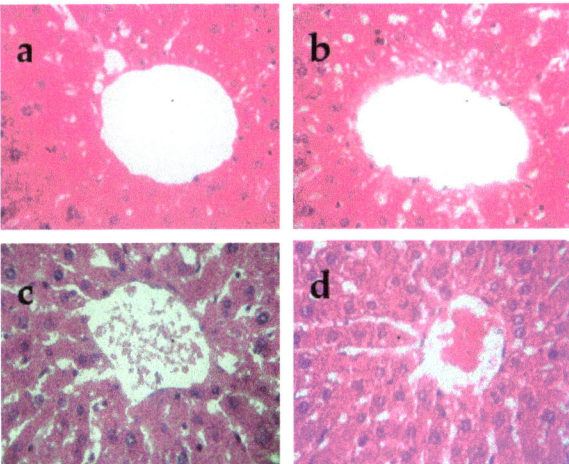

Figure 4. Representative photographs from the liver showing the protective effect of juice extract against Cd-induced hepatic damage in rats (H&E 40×). (**a**) Normal rat liver showing normal hepatic parenchyma and intact central vein. (**b**) Juice extract (250 mg/kg)-treated rat liver showing normal appearance of hepatocytes around the central vein. (**c**) CdCl$_2$ (1 mg/kg)-treated rat liver showing extensive degeneration of hepatocytes with focal necrosis, vacuolated cytoplasm, inflammatory cell infiltration, and damaged central vein. (**d**) CdCl$_2$ + juice extract (250 mg/kg)-treated rat liver showing near-normal hepatic architecture and normal histological features.

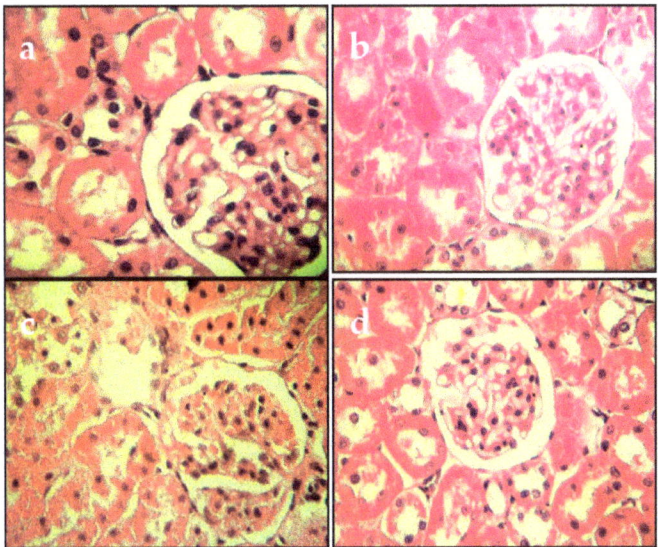

Figure 5. Representative photomicrographs of section from kidney. (**a**) Control group. (**b**) Juice extract (250 mg/kg)-treated rat kidney showing normal appearance of glomeruli. (**c**) CdCl$_2$ (1 mg/kg)-treated rat kidney showing tubule glomerular degeneration. (**d**) CdCl$_2$ + juice extract (250 mg/kg)-treated rat kidney showing near-normal kidney architecture and normal histological features. All sections were stained with hematoxylin/eosin; 400× for all panels.

After 5 weeks of Cd exposure, the histopathological examination of testicular tissues showed testicular alterations comprising edematous vasculitis and stromal hemorrhage. Many seminiferous tubules were edematous and undergoing degeneration. Spermatogenesis was almost absent (Figure 6c). In the control and juice extract alone groups, the histology was similar (Figure 6a,b). In rats co-treated with Cd and juice extract, a significant reduction in the restoration of spermatogenesis in most of the seminiferous tubules was observed (Figure 6d).

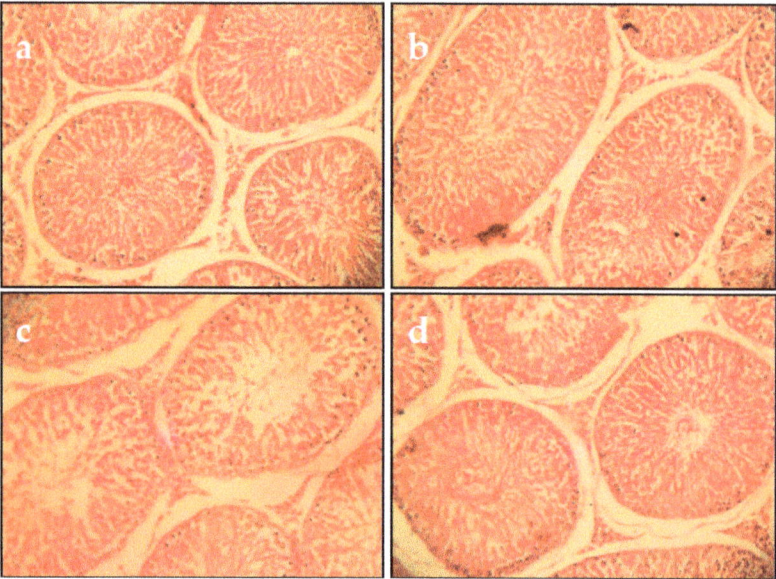

Figure 6. Microscopic evaluation of testicular tissue from juice extract of *O. stricta* alone, Cd and juice co-treated groups at 5 weeks (H&E 400): (**a**) Control group. (**b**) Juice extract (250 mg/kg)-treated group showing that the seminiferous tubular cells and interstitial tissue were normal. (**c**) Section of testes from rats treated with Cd (1 mg/kg, for 5 weeks); interstitial tissues showed edema, hemorrhage, and vacuolation, and seminiferous tubules were edematous with intact germinal layer and undergoing degeneration along with loss of spermatogenesis. (**d**) Section of testes from rats treated with Cd (5 weeks) and juice extract of *O. stricta* (250 mg/kg).

3. Discussion

Polyphenol compounds have attracted considerable attention because of their various biological activities, including: antioxidant, antimutagenic, antitumor, and anti-inflammatory activities [23]. Our results showed that the PPJE extract exhibited a high content of phenolic compounds and flavonoids. This is similar to the results reported by another study [12]. Concerning the qualitative analysis of the phenolic extract, major phenolic compounds were isolated and identified from many Tunisian medicinal plants, such as *O. stricta*. The major types and representative components of natural compounds (catechin hydrate, tyrosol, 4-hydroxybenzoic acid (4HOBenz), verbascoside, rutin, apigenin 7glucoside (apigenin 7Glu), oleuropein, quercetin, pinoresinol, and apigenin) were found in *Opuntia stricta*. Verbascoside was the major component, followed by catechin hydrate and oleuropein. Minor phenolic compounds included pinoresinol, quercetin, and apigenin. Several studies have found that these natural compounds have anti-inflammatory, analgesic, and antioxidant effects [12,24].

Extracts of active compounds from natural plants provide potent protection to the biological system against the damaging effect of natural oxidation processes in the organism.

In this investigation, the antioxidant capacity of PPJE extract was evaluated by two assays. Each antioxidant assay possesses its own unique mechanism to evaluate the antioxidant activity in the sample. Our results in this study showed that ethanolic PPJE exhibited high antioxidant capacity. It is worth noting that the extract produced with ethanol presented high antioxidant potential and also a high content of total phenols.

The present study is the first to investigate and reveal the protective impact of juice extract on liver and kidney metabolism under Cd exposure. Our results indicated a significant increase in serum ALT, AST, unconjugated bilirubin, creatinine, and urea after Cd administration to rats. The highest levels of these enzymes in plasma represent biomarkers of hepato-nephrotoxicity [25]. Moreover, Cd exposure significantly elevated serum hepatic and kidney marker enzymes [26]. The highest levels of these enzymes are a marker of cell damage [26]. Indeed, these radicals adversely affect the antioxidant system of the organism [27]. The important enzymes of this system are SOD, CAT, and GPx, which protect cells against reactive oxygen species (ROS). Cd toxicity is associated with the elevation of ROS levels, DNA damage, and lipid peroxidation in vitro. In the current study, the levels of oxidative stress in these three organs were significantly decreased compared to levels in the control group, which indicated that Cd was able to induce serious oxidative stress. Cd induces the accumulation of superoxide anion in cells, which is why we studied the effects of this metal on SOD activity. Concerning these enzymes, the inhibitory action of Cd on SOD may be due to competition between Cd and Zn or Cu (cofactors of SOD activity) [28]. In addition, this heavy metal altered the transport systems of calcium (Ca), Fe, Zn, Cu, and Mg [29]. These elements represent cofactors of the antioxidant system. In addition, in vivo administration of Cd altered the SOD activity. Nguyen et al. [30] found that Cd exposure induced the subcellular accumulation of hydrogen peroxide. Indeed, a higher H_2O_2 concentration might be implicated in the induction of catalase activity. The reduction in catalase activity in this investigation may be explained by the Cd-catalyzed oxidation of peroxisomal proteins, inducing carbonylation, particularly of the CAT enzyme [31]. In the present investigation, the decrease in antioxidant status due to Cd was accompanied by an elevation of hepatic protein carbonyls. The decrease in catalase activity by Cd may be explained by a decrease in iron absorption, an essential trace element required for CAT activity [32]. The effect of Cd exposure on glutathione peroxidase (GPx), which plays an important role in the detoxification of xenobiotics, was studied in the liver and kidney of Wistar rats. Our results indicate that the Cd-induced decrease in glutathione peroxidase activity may arise as a consequence of Se-mediated detoxification of Cd, where the Se level is insufficient to maintain optimal GPx activity [33]. Moreover, the administration of PPJE ameliorated the SOD, CAT, and GPx activities in Cd-treated rats. Accordingly, Eneman et al. [34] indicated that phenolic compounds were able to modulate the transcription and expression of proteins related to antioxidant enzymes. In addition, Cd exposure induced the peroxidation of membrane lipids of cells in various organs by stimulating reactive oxygen species. These free radicals bind to cellular macromolecules and stimulate lipid peroxidation and protein oxidation. In the present work, the marker of lipid peroxidation and protein destruction (protein carbonyl contents) decreased in the PPJE-treated group compared to the control. Several studies found that hepato-nephrotoxicity induced by Cd may be prevented by antioxidant supplementation, which are present in medicinal plants [35]. In general, polyphenols are known to be able to protect cell membrane integrity, protecting cells from death. Phenolic compounds are reported to be potent antioxidants and protect tissues from the toxic effects of Cd exposure [36]. The effect of Cd was also detected on the metallothionein (MT) levels. The present findings indicated that MT levels significantly increased in Cd-treated rats. This protein has been implicated in the scavenging of heavy metals by forming trimercaptide linkages [37]. The binding of Cd to MT is considered a mechanism of cell defense as MT sequesters, transports, and inactivates metal ions. The administration of juice extract decreased the concentration of MT in liver and kidney tissues compared with untreated rats. This diminution of Cd-induced alteration in Mt expression is connected with the ability of these compounds to chelate Cd [38].

4. Materials and Methods

4.1. Preparation and Extraction of Opuntia Stricta Cladode Powder

Fresh cladodes from *Opuntia stricta* were collected from the area of Sidi Bouzid (Tunisia) (latitude 35°2′25″ N, longitude 9°29′37″ E; elevation: 41 m) throughout February 2015. Experts of the Plant Biology Department of the University of Sfax confirmed plant identity. Voucher specimens were deposited in the National Gene Bank of Tunisia. After sample preparation, cladode juice (500 mL) was extracted using ethanol (75%) at room temperature for 48 h. Finally, the homogenate was condensed under reduced pressure by a rotary evaporator, and the yield of this extract was calculated.

4.2. Phytochemical Properties of O. stricta Juice Extract

4.2.1. Determination of Total Phenolic Content

The total phenols of cladode juice of this plant sample were determined using Folin–Ciocalteu's phenol reagent [39]. The results were determined at 765 nm using a colorimetric assay. The total phenolic content was expressed as mg gallic acid equivalent (GAE) mg^{-1} of dry weight. All analyses were performed in triplicate.

4.2.2. Determination of Total Flavonoids

Aluminum chloride ($AlCl_3$) was used to evaluate the flavonoid content in *O. stricta* [40]. Catechin was used as a standard. The results were expressed as mg catechin equivalents g^{-1} of dry weight. All analyses were performed in triplicate.

4.3. Antioxidant Properties of O. stricta

4.3.1. Diphenyl–2-Picrylhydrazyl (DPPH) Radical Scavenging Activity

The DPPH radical scavenging activity of the samples was determined using the method described by Ozturk et al. [41]. The optical density was measured spectrophotometrically at 515 nm. The percent of inhibition (PI) was measured according to the following formula:

$$\text{Inhibition (\%)} = [(A_{control} - A_{test})/A_{control}] \times 100 \qquad (1)$$

where $A_{control}$ is the absorbance of the control, and A_{test} is the absorbance of the juice extract. All samples were measured in triplicate.

4.3.2. Free Radical Scavenging Ability with the Use of ABTS Radical Cation (ABTS Assay)

The antioxidant potential of the cladode juice extract of *O. stricta* (PPJE) was also evaluated by determining their capacity to minimize the $ABTS^{\bullet+}$ free radical using the method reported by Ozgen et al. [42]. The final result was expressed as μM of Trolox equivalents (TE) per g of dry weight.

4.4. High-Performance Liquid Chromatography Analysis (HPLC) of PPJE

The PPJE samples were subjected to HPLC analysis using a Varian Prostar HPLC equipped with a C 18 reverse phase column (Varian, 250 mm × 4.6 mm, particle size 5 μm), a ternary pump (model Prostar 230), and a Prostar 330 diode array detector with gradient elution. Phenolic compounds in the sample were quantified using standard curves of standard solutions injected into the HPLC. The flow rate was 1 mL min^{-1}, and the injection volume was 20 μL at 30 °C. The identifications were performed at 290 nm for phenolic acids and at 365 nm for flavonoids based on the comparison with the retention times of standards and by co-injection. The quantification of these compounds was carried out by comparing the areas of the peaks with an internal standard (resorcinol). The result was expressed as μg of phenols g^{-1} of dry weight.

4.5. Experimental Design

Albino male Wistar rats aged 3–4 months, weighing 180 ± 20 g, and purchased from the Central Pharmacy (SIPHAT, Ben Arous, Tunisia) were used in the present study. They were housed at room temperature (37 °C) in a light/dark cycle of 12 h and a relative humidity below 40%. They had free access to a commercial pellet diet (SNA, Sfax, Tunisia) and tap water. The Committee of Animal Ethics of Sfax approved the experimental protocols. In our experiment, we used 24 rats. The Tunisian ethics committee for the care and use of laboratory animals approved the handling of the animals. Three weeks after acclimation to laboratory conditions, rats were randomly divided into four groups, each with six rats.

Group 1 (control group) received normal saline for 5 weeks.

Group 2 (Opuntia stricta only) received cladode juice extract (250 mg kg^{-1} body wt/day) orally by gavage for 5 weeks.

Group 3 (cadmium chloride (CdCl$_2$)-treated group) received CdCl$_2$ (1 mg kg^{-1} body wt/day.p.i.) for 5 weeks.

Group 4 (cadmium chloride/Opuntia stricta juice co-administration) received CdCl$_2$ (1 mg kg^{-1} body wt/day) orally by gavage concurrently with cladode juice extract (250 mg kg^{-1} body wt day^{-1}) for 5 weeks.

Five weeks later, the rats were sacrificed by decapitation, and their trunk blood was collected in EDTA tubes. The serum was prepared by centrifugation (3500× g, 15 min, 4 °C). Other blood samples were immediately used for the determination of serum enzymes and other biochemical indices.

All samples were stored at −80 °C until used. For histological studies, sections of the liver, kidney, and testicle were stored in 4% formalin solution. Sections of 5 µm thickness were stained with hematoxylin–eosin.

4.6. Biochemical Biomarker Assays

The serum urea, creatinine, alanine, and aspartate aminotransferase activities (ALT and AST) were measured using commercial kits (from Biolabo, Maizy, France) on an automatic biochemistry analyzer (Vitalab Flexor E, Irvine, CA, USA).

4.7. Enzymatic Antioxidant Status

Liver, kidney, and testicle homogenates were used for the evaluation of enzymatic status: superoxide dismutase was determined by the method of Beauchamp and Fridovich [43], catalase was measured as described by Aebi [44], and glutathione peroxidase (GPx) was determined using the method developed by Flohé and Günzler [45].

4.8. Oxidative Stress Biomarkers

Lipid peroxidation was estimated calorimetrically by measuring thiobarbituric acid-reactive substances (TBARS), as developed by Niehaus [46]. The protein oxidation level was detected in the liver and kidney by determining the total protein carbonyl content using a technique developed by Levine [47] and expressed as nmol/mg protein.

4.9. Determination of MT Concentration

Metallothionein (MT) levels in liver and kidney tissues were evaluated using Ellman's reagent [0.4 mM 5,5′-dithiobis-(2-nitrobenzoic acid) (DTNB) in 100 mM KH$_2$PO$_4$] at pH 8.5. This reagent was mixed with NaCl (2 M) and 1 mM EDTA. Then, aliquots of homogenate of each organ were homogenized in three volumes of 0.5 M sucrose and 20 mM Tris–HCl buffer (pH 8.6) with the addition of 0.006 mM leupeptin, 0.5 mM phenyl methylsulfonyl fluoride (PMSF), and 0.01% 2-mercaptoethanol. The homogenate was then centrifuged at 15,000× g for 30 min at 4 °C. The obtained supernatant was treated with ethanol/chloroform as described by Viarengo et al. [48] in order to obtain the MT-enriched pellet. The MT pellet was resuspended in HCl/EDTA in order to remove metal ions still bound to the MT. Finally, the interaction between thiol and DTNB reagent was detected in NaCl solution (2 M).

4.10. Cadmium Estimation

After acid digestion, the Cd content in the liver and kidney was estimated by atomic absorption spectrometry (Perkin-Elmer, model: 370, Waltham, MA, USA). The results are expressed as micrograms of Cd per gram of wet tissue weight (µg/g w.t.w).

4.11. Histopathological Studies

Sections of the kidney, liver, and testicle were fixed in 4% formalin solution and embedded in paraffin. Finally, tissue preparations were examined and photographed using an Olympus CX41 microscope (Tokyo, Japan).

4.12. Statistical Analysis

Mean values of different assays were used in variance (ANOVA) analysis with IBM SPSS Statistics version 20. The significance level was determined ($p < 0.05$), and significant differences were measured according to Duncan's Multiple Range Test (DMRT) with a confidence level of 95%.

5. Conclusions

In summary, these findings clearly show that *O. stricta* juice extract exhibited a high amount of phenolic and flavonoid contents, as well as antioxidant capacity. The juice extract of *O. stricta* could protect the hepatic and kidney tissues of rats from Cd-induced oxidative damage. The faithful mechanisms of protection offered by the investigated juice extract may involve the scavenging of free radicals generated during Cd metabolism in vivo and/or the induction of antioxidative enzymes. In addition, juice extract containing certain phenolic compounds has a strong ability to scavenge free radicals and stimulate the antioxidant system of rats. Moreover, studies are required to explain the detailed molecular mechanism of protection of this juice extract against Cd-induced toxicity.

Author Contributions: X.Z. was responsible for the conception and design, testing, and data acquisition. K.A. was responsible for the analysis and data interpretation, drafted the manuscript, and approved the final manuscript. All authors have read and agreed to the published version of the manuscript.

Funding: This research received no external funding.

Institutional Review Board Statement: The experimental protocols were conducted in accordance with the guide for the care and use of laboratory animals issued by the University of Sfax, Tunisia, and approved by the Committee of Animal Ethics of Sfax.

Informed Consent Statement: Not applicable.

Data Availability Statement: The authors declare that all data supporting the findings of this study are available within the paper.

Acknowledgments: This work was jointly supported by the Projects of National Natural Science Foundation of China (Grant Nos. 31772373, 31801918, and 31901693) and the Project of Guangdong Province Innovation Team Construction Program on Modern Agriculture Industrial Technology System (The Edible Fungus) (Grant No. 2020KJ103).

Conflicts of Interest: The authors declare that they have no competing interest and non-financial competing interest.

Abbreviations

ALT: alanine aminotransferase; AST: aspartate aminotransferase; CAT: catalase; Cd: cadmium; FAs: fatty acids; GPx: glutathione peroxidase; HDL: high-density lipoprotein; H_2O_2: hydrogen peroxide; LD: lethal dose; LDL: low-density lipoprotein; LNA: linoleic acid; LPO: lipid peroxidation; MDA: malondialdehyde; NBT: nitro blue tetrazolium; $O_2^{\bullet-}$: superoxide; $OH^\bullet$: hydroxyl; PPJE: prickly pear juice extract; ROS: reactive oxygen species; SOD: superoxide dismutase; TBARS: thiobarbituric acid-reactive substances.

References

1. Rehman, A.U.; Nazir, S.; Irshad, R.; Tahir, K.; ur Rehman, K.; Islam, R.U.; Wahab, Z. Toxicity of Heavy Metals in Plants and Animals and Their Uptake by Magnetic Iron Oxide Nanoparticles. *J. Mol. Liq.* **2021**, *321*, 114455. [CrossRef]
2. Adaramoye, O.A.; Akanni, O.O. Modulatory Effects of Methanol Extract of Artocarpus Altilis (Moraceae) on Cadmium-Induced Hepatic and Renal Toxicity in Male Wistar Rats. *Pathophysiology* **2016**, *23*, 1–9. [CrossRef] [PubMed]
3. Dkhil, M.A.; Al-Quraishy, S.; Diab, M.M.S.; Othman, M.S.; Aref, A.M.; Abdel Moneim, A.E. The Potential Protective Role of *Physalis peruviana* L. Fruit in Cadmium-Induced Hepatotoxicity and Nephrotoxicity. *Food Chem. Toxicol.* **2014**, *74*, 98–106. [CrossRef] [PubMed]
4. Klaassen, C.D.; Liu, J.; Diwan, B.A. Metallothionein Protection of Cadmium Toxicity. *Toxicol. Appl. Pharmacol.* **2009**, *238*, 215–220. [CrossRef]
5. Jihen, E.H.; Fatima, H.; Nouha, A.; Baati, T.; Imed, M.; Abdelhamid, K. Cadmium Retention Increase: A Probable Key Mechanism of the Protective Effect of Zinc on Cadmium-Induced Toxicity in the Kidney. *Toxicol. Lett.* **2010**, *196*, 104–109. [CrossRef] [PubMed]
6. Buraimoh, A.; Bako, I.; Ibrahim, F.B. Hepatoprotective Effect of Ethanolic Leave Extract of Moringa Oleifera on the Histology of Paracetamol Induced Liver Damage in Wistar Rats. *Int. J. Anim. Vet. Adv.* **2011**, *3*, 10–13.
7. Ognjanović, B.I.; Marković, S.D.; Ethordević, N.Z.; Trbojević, I.S.; Stajn, A.S.; Saićić, Z.S. Cadmium-Induced Lipid Peroxidation and Changes in Antioxidant Defense System in the Rat Testes: Protective Role of Coenzyme Q(10) and Vitamin E. *Reprod. Toxicol.* **2010**, *29*, 191–197. [CrossRef]
8. Thijssen, S.; Cuypers, A.; Maringwa, J.; Smeets, K.; Horemans, N.; Lambrichts, I.; Van Kerkhove, E. Low Cadmium Exposure Triggers a Biphasic Oxidative Stress Response in Mice Kidneys. *Toxicology* **2007**, *236*, 29–41. [CrossRef]
9. Schöpfer, J.; Drasch, G.; Schrauzer, G.N. Selenium and Cadmium Levels and Ratios in Prostates, Livers, and Kidneys of Nonsmokers and Smokers. *Biol. Trace Elem. Res.* **2010**, *134*, 180–187. [CrossRef]
10. Heeba, G.H.; Abd-Elghany, M.I. Effect of Combined Administration of Ginger (Zingiber Officinale Roscoe) and Atorvastatin on the Liver of Rats. *Phytomedicine* **2010**, *17*, 1076–1081. [CrossRef]
11. Tesoriere, L.; Allegra, M.; Butera, D.; Livrea, M.A. Absorption, Excretion, and Distribution of Dietary Antioxidant Betalains in LDLs: Potential Health Effects of Betalains in Humans. *Am. J. Clin. Nutr.* **2004**, *80*, 941–945. [CrossRef] [PubMed]
12. Ncibi, S.; Ben Othman, M.; Akacha, A.; Krifi, M.N.; Zourgui, L. Opuntia Ficus Indica Extract Protects against Chlorpyrifos-Induced Damage on Mice Liver. *Food Chem. Toxicol.* **2008**, *46*, 797–802. [CrossRef] [PubMed]
13. Dok-Go, H.; Lee, K.H.; Kim, H.J.; Lee, E.H.; Lee, J.; Song, Y.S.; Lee, Y.-H.; Jin, C.; Lee, Y.S.; Cho, J. Neuroprotective Effects of Antioxidative Flavonoids, Quercetin, (+)-Dihydroquercetin and Quercetin 3-Methyl Ether, Isolated from Opuntia Ficus-Indica Var. Saboten. *Brain Res.* **2003**, *965*, 130–136. [CrossRef]
14. Zou, D.; Brewer, M.; Garcia, F.; Feugang, J.M.; Wang, J.; Zang, R.; Liu, H.; Zou, C. Cactus Pear: A Natural Product in Cancer Chemoprevention. *Nutr. J.* **2005**, *4*, 25. [CrossRef]
15. Ahmad, A.; Viljoen, A. The in Vitro Antimicrobial Activity of Cymbopogon Essential Oil (Lemon Grass) and Its Interaction with Silver Ions. *Phytomedicine* **2015**, *22*, 657–665. [CrossRef]
16. Park, E.H.; Kahng, J.H.; Lee, S.H.; Shin, K.H. An Anti-Inflammatory Principle from Cactus. *Fitoterapia* **2001**, *72*, 288–290. [CrossRef]
17. Gentile, C.; Tesoriere, L.; Allegra, M.; Livrea, M.A.; D'Alessio, P. Antioxidant Betalains from Cactus Pear (*Opuntia Ficus-Indica*) Inhibit Endothelial ICAM-1 Expression. *Ann. N. Y. Acad. Sci.* **2004**, *1028*, 481–486. [CrossRef]
18. Park, E.H.; Kahng, J.H.; Paek, E.A. Studies on the Pharmacological Action of Cactus: Identification of Its Anti-Inflammatory Effect. *Arch. Pharm. Res.* **1998**, *21*, 30–34. [CrossRef]
19. Han, E.H.; Lim, M.K.; Lee, S.H.; Rahman, M.M.; Lim, Y.H. An oral toxicity test in rats and a genotoxicity study of extracts from the stems of *Opuntia ficus-indica* var. saboten. *BMC Complement. Altern. Med.* **2019**, *19*, 31. [CrossRef]
20. Sharma, C.; Rani, S.; Kumar, B.; Kumar, A.; Raj, V. Plant *opuntia dillenii*: A review on its traditional uses, phytochemical and pharmacological properties. *EC Pharm. Sci.* **2015**, *1*, 29–43.
21. Chahdoura, H.; Adouni, K.; Khlifi, A.; Dridi, I.; Haouas, Z.; Neffati, F.; Flamini, G.; Mosbah, H.; Achour, L. Hepatoprotective effect of *Opuntia microdasys* (Lehm.) Pfeiff flowers against diabetes type II induced in rats. *Biomed. Pharmacother.* **2017**, *94*, 79–87. [CrossRef] [PubMed]
22. Attanzio, A.; Tesoriere, L.; Vasto, S.; Pintaudi, A.M.; Livrea, M.A.; Allegra, M. Short-term cactus pear [*Opuntia ficus-indica* (L.) Mill] fruit supplementation ameliorates the inflammatory profile and is associated with improved antioxidant status among healthy humans. *Food Nutr. Res.* **2018**, *20*, 62. [CrossRef] [PubMed]
23. Yoshida, Y.; Kiso, M.; Goto, T. Efficiency of the Extraction of Catechins from Green Tea. *Food Chem.* **1999**, *67*, 429–433. [CrossRef]
24. Grace, M.H.; Esposito, D.; Timmers, M.A.; Xiong, J.; Yousef, G.; Komarnytsky, S.; Lila, M.A. Chemical Composition, Antioxidant and Anti-Inflammatory Properties of Pistachio Hull Extracts. *Food Chem.* **2016**, *210*, 85–95. [CrossRef] [PubMed]
25. Amamou, F.; Nemmiche, S.; Meziane, R.K.; Didi, A.; Yazit, S.M.; Chabane-Sari, D. Protective Effect of Olive Oil and Colocynth Oil against Cadmium-Induced Oxidative Stress in the Liver of Wistar Rats. *Food Chem. Toxicol.* **2015**, *78*, 177–184. [CrossRef] [PubMed]
26. Firdaus, S.B.; Ghosh, D.; Chattyopadhyay, A.; Dutta, M.; Paul, S.; Jana, J.; Basu, A.; Bose, G.; Lahiri, H.; Banerjee, B.; et al. Protective Effect of Antioxidant Rich Aqueous Curry Leaf (Murraya Koenigii) Extract against Gastro-Toxic Effects of Piroxicam in Male Wistar Rats. *Toxicol. Rep.* **2014**, *1*, 987–1003. [CrossRef]

27. Zhang, H.; Lei, Y.; Yuan, P.; Li, L.; Luo, C.; Gao, R.; Tian, J.; Feng, Z.; Nice, E.C.; Sun, J. ROS-Mediated Autophagy Induced by Dysregulation of Lipid Metabolism Plays a Protective Role in Colorectal Cancer Cells Treated with Gambogic Acid. *PLoS ONE* **2014**, *9*, e96418. [CrossRef]
28. Huang, Y.-H.; Shih, C.-M.; Huang, C.-J.; Lin, C.-M.; Chou, C.-M.; Tsai, M.-L.; Liu, T.P.; Chiu, J.-F.; Chen, C.-T. Effects of Cadmium on Structure and Enzymatic Activity of Cu, Zn-SOD and Oxidative Status in Neural Cells. *J. Cell Biochem.* **2006**, *98*, 577–589. [CrossRef]
29. Kippler, M.; Lönnerdal, B.; Goessler, W.; Ekström, E.-C.; Arifeen, S.E.; Vahter, M. Cadmium Interacts with the Transport of Essential Micronutrients in the Mammary Gland—A Study in Rural Bangladeshi Women. *Toxicology* **2009**, *257*, 64–69. [CrossRef]
30. Romero-Puertas, M.C.; Rodríguez-Serrano, M.; Corpas, F.J.; Gómez, M.; Del Río, L.A.; Sandalio, L.M. Cadmium-Induced Subcellular Accumulation of O_2- and H_2O_2 in Pea Leaves. *Plant Cell Environ.* **2004**, *27*, 1122–1134. [CrossRef]
31. Nguyen, A.T.; Donaldson, R.P. Metal-Catalyzed Oxidation Induces Carbonylation of Peroxisomal Proteins and Loss of Enzymatic Activities. *Arch. Biochem. Biophys.* **2005**, *439*, 25–31. [CrossRef] [PubMed]
32. Trabelsi, H.; Azzouz, I.; Ferchichi, S.; Tebourbi, O.; Sakly, M.; Abdelmelek, H. Nanotoxicological Evaluation of Oxidative Responses in Rat Nephrocytes Induced by Cadmium. *Int. J. Nanomed.* **2013**, *8*, 3447–3453. [CrossRef]
33. Othman, M.S.; Nada, A.; Zaki, H.S.; Abdel Moneim, A.E. Effect of *Physalis peruviana* L. on Cadmium-Induced Testicular Toxicity in Rats. *Biol. Trace Elem. Res.* **2014**, *159*, 278–287. [CrossRef] [PubMed]
34. Eneman, J.D.; Potts, R.J.; Osier, M.; Shukla, G.S.; Lee, C.H.; Chiu, J.F.; Hart, B.A. Suppressed Oxidant-Induced Apoptosis in Cadmium Adapted Alveolar Epithelial Cells and Its Potential Involvement in Cadmium Carcinogenesis. *Toxicology* **2000**, *147*, 215–228. [CrossRef]
35. Chang, J.C.; Lin, C.C.; Wu, S.J.; Lin, D.L.; Wang, S.S.; Miaw, C.L.; Ng, L.T. Antioxidative and Hepatoprotective Effects of Physalis Peruviana Extract against Acetaminophen-Induced Liver Injury in Rats. *Pharm. Biol.* **2008**, *46*, 724–731. [CrossRef]
36. Hermenean, A.; Ardelean, A.; Stan, M.; Herman, H.; Mihali, C.-V.; Costache, M.; Dinischiotu, A. Protective Effects of Naringenin on Carbon Tetrachloride-Induced Acute Nephrotoxicity in Mouse Kidney. *Chem. Biol. Interact.* **2013**, *205*, 138–147. [CrossRef]
37. Kondoh, M.; Kamada, K.; Kuronaga, M.; Higashimoto, M.; Takiguchi, M.; Watanabe, Y.; Sato, M. Antioxidant Property of Metallothionein in Fasted Mice. *Toxicol. Lett.* **2003**, *143*, 301–306. [CrossRef]
38. Morales, A.I.; Vicente-Sánchez, C.; Jerkic, M.; Santiago, J.M.; Sánchez-González, P.D.; Pérez-Barriocanal, F.; López-Novoa, J.M. Effect of Quercetin on Metallothionein, Nitric Oxide Synthases and Cyclooxygenase-2 Expression on Experimental Chronic Cadmium Nephrotoxicity in Rats. *Toxicol. Appl. Pharmacol.* **2006**, *210*, 128–135. [CrossRef]
39. Kim, D.-O.; Jeong, S.W.; Lee, C.Y. Antioxidant Capacity of Phenolic Phytochemicals from Various Cultivars of Plums. *Food Chem.* **2003**, *81*, 321–326. [CrossRef]
40. Zhishen, J.; Mengcheng, T.; Jianming, W. The Determination of Flavonoid Contents in Mulberry and Their Scavenging Effects on Superoxide Radicals. *Food Chem.* **1999**, *64*, 555–559. [CrossRef]
41. Ozturk, H.; Kolak, U.; Meriç, Ç. Antioxidant, Anticholinesterase and Antibacterial Activities of Jurinea Consanguinea DC. *Rec. Nat. Prod.* **2011**, *5*, 43–51.
42. Ozgen, M.; Reese, R.N.; Tulio, A.Z.; Scheerens, J.C.; Miller, A.R. Modified 2,2-Azino-Bis-3-Ethylbenzothiazoline-6-Sulfonic Acid (Abts) Method to Measure Antioxidant Capacity of Selected Small Fruits and Comparison to Ferric Reducing Antioxidant Power (FRAP) and 2,2′-Diphenyl-1-Picrylhydrazyl (DPPH) Methods. *J. Agric. Food Chem.* **2006**, *54*, 1151–1157. [CrossRef] [PubMed]
43. Beauchamp, C.; Fridovich, I. Superoxide Dismutase: Improved Assays and an Assay Applicable to Acrylamide Gels. *Anal. Biochem.* **1971**, *44*, 276–287. [CrossRef]
44. Aebi, H. Catalase in Vitro. *Methods Enzymol.* **1984**, *105*, 121–126. [CrossRef]
45. Flohé, L.; Günzler, W.A. Assays of Glutathione Peroxidase. *Methods Enzymol.* **1984**, *105*, 114–121. [CrossRef]
46. Niehaus, W.G.; Samuelsson, B. Formation of Malonaldehyde from Phospholipid Arachidonate during Microsomal Lipid Peroxidation. *Eur. J. Biochem.* **1968**, *6*, 126–130. [CrossRef]
47. Levine, R.L.; Garland, D.; Oliver, C.N.; Amici, A.; Climent, I.; Lenz, A.G.; Ahn, B.W.; Shaltiel, S.; Stadtman, E.R. Determination of Carbonyl Content in Oxidatively Modified Proteins. *Methods Enzymol.* **1990**, *186*, 464–478. [CrossRef]
48. Viarengo, A.; Ponzano, E.; Dondero, F.; Fabbri, R. A simple spectrophotometric method for metallothionein evaluation in marine organisms: An application to Mediterranean and Antarctic molluscs. *Mar. Environ. Res.* **1997**, *44*, 69–84. [CrossRef]

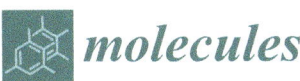

Article

Solid Lipid Nanoparticles Administering Antioxidant Grape Seed-Derived Polyphenol Compounds: A Potential Application in Aquaculture †

Adriana Trapani [1], María Ángeles Esteban [2,*], Francesca Curci [1], Daniela Erminia Manno [3], Antonio Serra [3], Giuseppe Fracchiolla [1], Cristóbal Espinosa-Ruiz [2], Stefano Castellani [4] and Massimo Conese [5]

1. Department of Pharmacy-Drug Sciences, University of Bari "Aldo Moro", Via Orabona 4, 70125 Bari, Italy; adriana.trapani@uniba.it (A.T.); francesca.curci@uniba.it (F.C.); giuseppe.fracchiolla@uniba.it (G.F.)
2. Department of Cell Biology and Histology, Faculty of Biology, Regional Campus of International Excellence "Campus Mare Nostrum", University of Murcia, 30100 Murcia, Spain; cespinosa31416@gmail.com
3. Dipartimento di Matematica e Fisica "E. De Giorgi", University of Salento, 73100 Lecce, Italy; daniela.manno@unisalento.it (D.E.M.); antonio.serra@unisalento.it (A.S.)
4. Department of Biomedical Sciences and Human Oncology, University of Bari "Aldo Moro", 70124 Bari, Italy; stefano.castellani@uniba.it
5. Department of Medical and Surgical Sciences, University of Foggia, 71122 Foggia, Italy; massimo.conese@unifg.it
* Correspondence: aesteban@um.es
† This work is dedicated to Carlo Franchini on the occasion of his retirement.

Abstract: The supply of nutrients, such as antioxidant agents, to fish cells still represents a challenge in aquaculture. In this context, we investigated solid lipid nanoparticles (SLN) composed of a combination of Gelucire® 50/13 and Precirol® ATO5 to administer a grape seed extract (GSE) mixture containing several antioxidant compounds. The combination of the two lipids for the SLN formation resulted in colloids exhibiting mean particle sizes in the range 139–283 nm and zeta potential values in the range +25.6–43.4 mV. Raman spectra and X-ray diffraction evidenced structural differences between the free GSE and GSE-loaded SLN, leading to the conclusion that GSE alters the structure of the lipid nanocarriers. From a biological viewpoint, cell lines from gilthead seabream and European sea bass were exposed to different concentrations of GSE-SLN for 24 h. In general, at appropriate concentrations, GSE-SLN increased the viability of the fish cells. Furthermore, regarding the gene expression in those cells, the expression of antioxidant genes was upregulated, whereas the expression of *hsp70* and other genes related to the cytoskeleton was downregulated. Hence, an SLN formulation containing Gelucire® 50/13/Precirol® ATO5 and GSE may represent a compelling platform for improving the viability and antioxidant properties of fish cells.

Keywords: solid lipid nanoparticles; grape seed–derived extract; drug delivery; X-ray diffraction; antioxidant activity; fish cells

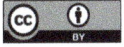

1. Introduction

To improve fish nutrition, to date, different diet protocols have been proposed, and in each of them, the presence of antioxidant substances has been crucial to ensure optimal fundamental metabolic processes. Apart from single antioxidant molecules such as vitamin E and glutathione, which are already included in fish diet protocols, natural mixtures that include antioxidant compounds can also be of interest for fish nutrition if they are adopted as an entire extract without any separation of the active principles. In this context, we previously studied a mixture based on Apulian grape seed extract (GSE) for its favorable antioxidant and anti-inflammatory effects in human cells due to the relevant pro-anthocyanidin and polyphenol content (Figure 1; in [1,2]). With regard to pro-anthocyanidins contained in GSE, previous studies in the area of fish immunology elucidated that, once excessive fat accumulation takes place in fish, with consequent hepatic lipid metabolism disorder, then GSE allows hypolipidemic and potential anti-inflammatory effects in the liver, as occurred, for instance, in grass carp [3]. Moreover, the antioxidant effects of GSE were recently evaluated in a zebrafish embryo model [4]. However, to the best of our knowledge, no attention has been paid to investigating which type of pharmaceutical dosage form can enhance the administration of GSE using fish cell lines.

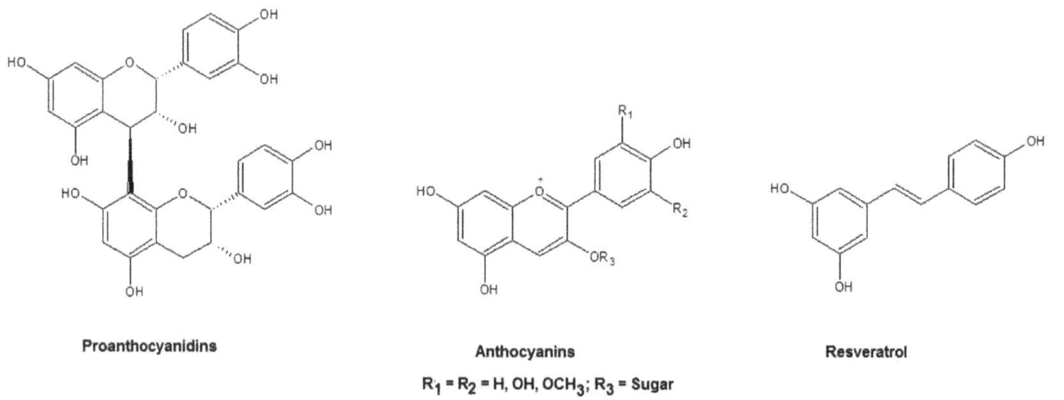

Figure 1. Chemical structures of the main compounds found in grape seed extract (GSE).

In this context, different approaches for the delivery of antioxidant agents were reviewed, evidencing the relevance and the feasibility of the production of colloidal carriers, such as nanoparticles, liposomes, and nanosized lipid particles, for this purpose [5,6]. Among the colloidal carriers, solid lipid nanoparticles (SLN) have been shown to have several benefits, including enhanced safety and stability, and controlled drug release, and can be prepared on a large scale according to scale-up industrial guidelines. In our laboratory, we have already investigated SLNs made of a single lipid, namely Gelucire® 50/13, for uptake in fish cell lines in order to ascertain the possible immunological applications, and by ex vivo investigations, the biocompatibility of such a synthetic lipid was assessed [7–9]. From a chemical viewpoint, it could be assumed that using two or more lipids may be better than using only one. In this sense, Precirol® ATO5 is a suitable candidate to be assayed with another lipid. In the literature, Precirol® ATO5 has been combined with other lipids, such as the liquid Transcutol® for paediatric drug administration [10], and it was blended with Compritol® 888 ATO to achieve an SLN for lycopene vectorization [11]. Precirol® ATO5 is based on mono-, di-, and triglycerides of palmitostearic acids (C16 or C18), and the diester fraction accounts for 40–60% of the total mass; whereas Gelucire® 50/13 is composed of mono-, di-, and triglycerides with polyethylene glycol(PEG) residues. According to the manufacturer's instructions, both in veterinary and human medicine, Precirol® ATO5 and Gelucire® 50/13 are approved, and, indeed, from an excipient regulatory status, Precirol® ATO5 is recognized as GRAS degree and it belongs to the Japanese Standard of Food Additives; whereas Gelucire® 50/13 is approved as a US Food Additive [12,13].

To gain insight into the vector comprising Precirol® ATO5 and Gelucire® 50/13, several studies of the solid state were carried out, namely FT-IR spectroscopy, differential scanning calorimetry (DSC), X-ray diffraction, and Raman spectroscopy.

On the basis of this knowledge, the aim of this study was to assess if GSE administered via modified drug delivery systems, such as nanoparticles rather than conventional dosage forms, could achieve an immunomodulation role in two fish cell lines obtained from gilthead seabream and European sea bass. In the present work, we have attempted to formulate SLN using a lipid mixture, rather than one single lipid, i.e., forming the lipid matrix structure in the presence of Precirol® ATO5 and Gelucire® 50/13. Finally, concerning the biological evaluation of GSE-SLN, the cell viability and the expression of different selected gene codes for the structural proteins involved in cell movement were determined in SAF-1 and DBL-1 cell lines. The results arising from these investigations are reported and discussed below.

2. Results

2.1. Physico-Chemical Properties of SLN

Table 1 shows the main physico-chemical properties of GSE-SLN. In detail, the particle size of all types of GSE-SLN was found in the range 139–283 nm, with a slightly broader size distribution, as shown by the PDI range values (0.44–0.59). All types of GSE-SLN were smaller than unloaded SLN, whose mean diameter was 486 ± 5 nm. The largest particles herein studied are GSE-SLN$_{(6mg)}$-adsorbing GSE, but their zeta potential value is similar to the that of GSE-SLN$_{(6mg)}$, perhaps because the adsorption layer of GSE, instead of shielding the negative charges of the lipid matrix, induces some structural modifications in the SLN, leading to the exposure on the surface of a higher number of such charges. As for the zeta potential of these nanocarriers, they resulted in the range −25.6–−43.4 mV indicative of a good colloidal stability.

Table 1. Physicochemical properties of GSE containing SLN. Mean ± standard deviations. are reported, n = 6. SLN without GSE (Unloaded SLN) were used as control for formulations. (**) $p \leq 0.001$.

Formulation	Size (nm)	PDI	Zeta Potential (mV)	Association Efficiency (AE) (%)
Unloaded SLN	486(±5)	0.42–0.48	−32.7(±1.1)	–
GSE-SLN$_{(6mg)}$	208(±21) **	0.44–0.49	−43.4(±1.8) **	49.7(±3.2)
GSE-SLN$_{(12mg)}$	139(±15) **	0.44–0.48	−25.6(±2.8) **	64.9(±1.0)
GSE-SLN$_{(6mg)}$-adsorbing GSE	283(±32) **	0.50–0.59	−43.0(±1.3) **	74.6(±0.2)

Furthermore, from the data reported in Table 1, high percentages of GSE entrapment were obtained (i.e., 49.7–74.6%) via the use of a lipid matrix where Gelucire® 50/13 and Precirol® ATO5 were combined and, notably, the GSE-SLN$_{(6mg)}$-adsorbing GSE formulation was found to be the one loading the highest amount of the GSE mixture in comparison with our previous work [2]. As shown in Figure 2, to visualize SLN administering GSE, transmission electron spectroscopy (TEM) morphology was examined (Figure 2), and in the case of GSE-SLN$_{(6mg)}$, an oval shape (Figure 2a) was detected rather than the spherical shape of GSE-SLN$_{(6mg)}$-adsorbing GSE (Figure 2b). Moreover, GSE-SLN$_{(6mg)}$ and GSE-SLN$_{(6mg)}$-adsorbing GSE showed a bimodal particle distribution (Figure 2c,d). Importantly, GSE-SLN$_{(6mg)}$ showed a very pronounced bimodal distribution with a clear separation between smaller diameter SLN (<Standard deviation> = 240 nm, S.D. = 70 nm) and larger diameter SLN (<Standard deviation> = 700 nm, s = 200 nm). GSE-SLN$_{(6mg)}$-adsorbing GSE showed a less evident bimodal distribution; in this case, the difference between smaller diameter SLN (<Standard deviation> = 260 nm, S.D. = 80 nm) and larger diameter SLN (<Standard deviation> = 390 nm, S.D. = 80 nm) were much less pronounced, perhaps suggesting a stabilizing action due to the adsorbed GSE.

2.2. Solid-State Studies

Multiple studies of the solid-state of GSE-SLN were carried out to gain a deeper insight into their organization. With regard to FT-IR spectra (Figure 3), the peaks at 3435 cm^{-1} and 1738–1739 cm^{-1} (Figure 3a–c), and 1732–1737 cm^{-1} (Figure 3b,d) could be assigned to partially hydrated Gelucire® 50/13 [14,15], evidencing the external localization of such lipids in the SLN structure.

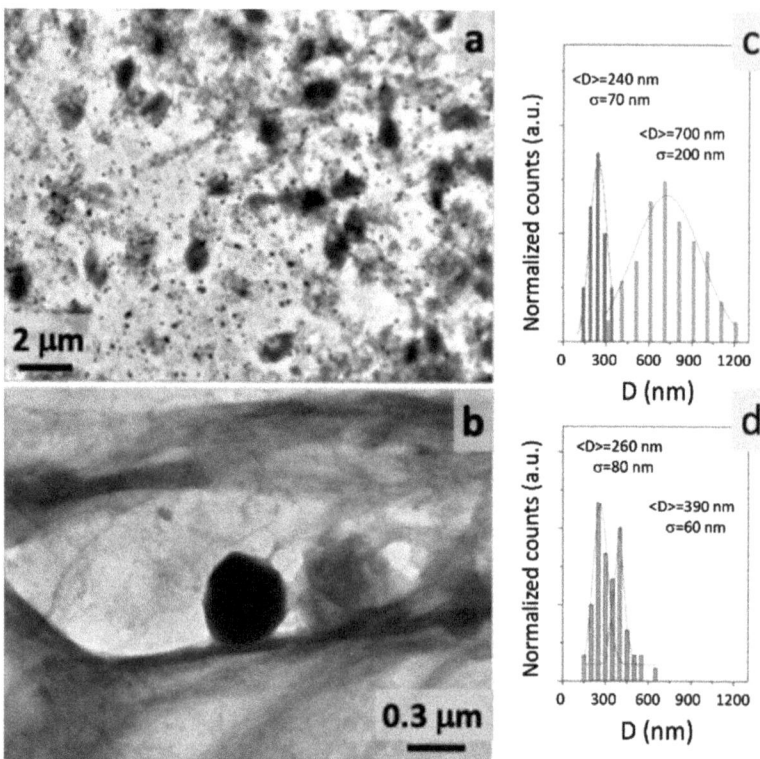

Figure 2. Transmission electron spectroscopy (TEM) images of: GSE-SLN$_{(6mg)}$ (**a**); GSE-SLN$_{(6mg)}$-adsorbing GSE (**b**); and related particle diameter distribution (**c**,**d**). Feret diameters were measured for each sample.

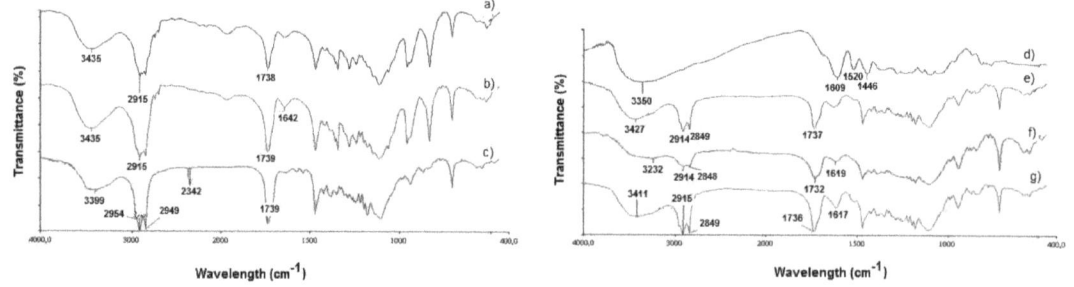

Figure 3. Left panel: FT-IR spectra of pure Gelucire® 50/13 (**a**); Gelucire® 50/13/Precirol® ATO5 blend (**b**); and unloaded SLN (**c**). **Right panel**: FT-IR spectra of pure GSE (**d**); GSE-SLN$_{(6mg)}$ (**e**); GSE-SLN$_{(12mg)}$ (**f**); and GSE-SLN$_{(6mg)}$-adsorbing GSE (**g**).

Indeed, when the FT-IR spectra of GSE-SLN were examined (as seen in Figure 3a), the characteristic band attributable to GSE at 1609 cm^{-1} was shifted at 1619 cm^{-1} and 1617 cm^{-1} for GSE-SLN$_{(12mg)}$ and GSE-SLN-adsorbing GSE, respectively (Figure 3c,d).

Regarding DSC thermograms (Figure 4a), the GSE-SLN$_{(6mg)}$-adsorbing GSE thermogram is the only one where small endothermic peaks at 114 °C and 118 °C are shown, and as pure GSE melting point is at 160 °C, they can be attributed to the shift of the endothermal peak of the extract because the esothermal peak at 160 °C resembles one of the Gelucire®

50/13/Precirol® ATO5 blends. Furthermore, as previously seen for the SLN containing GSE based on pure Gelucire® 50/13 [2], in the DSC thermograms of GSE-SLN$_{(6mg)}$ and GSE-SLN$_{(12mg)}$, no peak ascribable to GSE was detected (Figure 4b,d), suggesting that the molecular encapsulation of the extract occurred in these formulations. In the range 47–56 °C, either in the unloaded SLN or in GSE-containing SLN, endothermal signals were recorded, and they can be attributed to the Gelucire® 50/13/Precirol® ATO5 mixture. This assessment is based on the DSC peaks recorded when the Gelucire® 50/13/Precirol® ATO5 blend underwent a calorimetric run (Figure 4b), and it is also corroborated by the fact that the drop point of Precirol® ATO5 is well known to be in the range 53–57 °C, according to the manufacturer instructions.

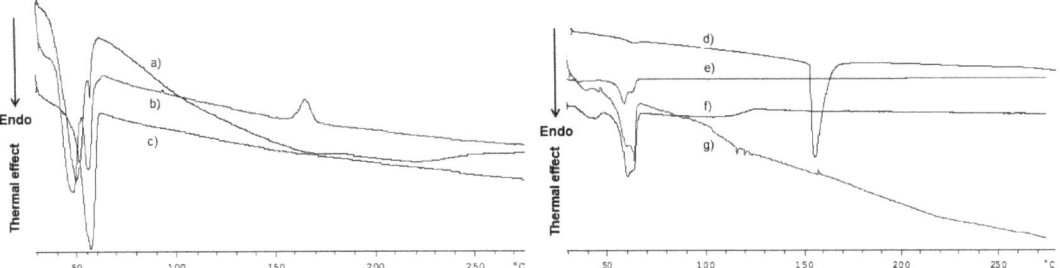

Figure 4. Left panel: DSC thermograms of pure Gelucire® 50/13 (**a**); Gelucire® 50/13/Precirol® ATO5 blend (**b**); and unloaded SLN (**c**). **Right panel**: DSC thermograms of pure GSE (**d**); GSE-SLN$_{(6mg)}$ (**e**); GSE-SLN$_{(6mg)}$-adsorbing GSE (**f**); and GSE-SLN$_{(12mg)}$ (**g**).

2.3. X-ray Diffraction and Raman Spectroscopy

To gain insight into the structural characterization of SLN, the X-ray diffraction patterns of Precirol® ATO5, Gelucire® 50/13, GSE, GSE-SLN$_{(6mg)}$, and GSE-SLN$_{(6mg)}$-adsorbing GSE are shown in Figure 5. The diffraction patterns of Gelucire® 50/13 revealed diffraction maxima at 2q = 19.2, 21.2, and 23.4 deg. These peaks correspond to the lattice spacing 0.46, 0.42, and 0.38 nm, respectively, and are indicative of the crystalline nature of the substance. The X-ray diffractograms of Precirol® ATO5 show large peaks in the small-angle range at 2q = 2.16, 5.25 deg (5 and 6 in Figure 5(right panel)), and 21.2 deg (2 in Figure 5). These reflections correspond to the lattice spacings 4.18, 1.69, and 0.42 nm, respectively. According to the literature [16], the main polymorphic forms of triacylglycerols are α, β', and β. The α-form is a hexagonal sub-cell with a short spacing of 0.42 nm, the β'-form [17] is an orthorhombic perpendicular sub-cell with short spacings of 0.42–0.43 and 0.37–0.40 nm, and the β-form is a triclinic parallel sub-cell with a short spacing of 0.46 nm [18]. The peaks observed at small angles (0° < θ < 5°) allow us to measure the thickness of the lamellar structures, which corresponds to the longitudinal stacking, and it is possible to deduce whether the stackings correspond to 2 L or 3 L organizations (Figure 5).

The peak at 2q = 2.5 deg corresponds to the stacking 3L$_{002}$ of α phase [19] and leads to a distance of approximately d = 3.5 nm; the peak at 2q = 2.2 deg corresponds to the stacking 2L$_{002}$ of β' phase and leads to a distance of about d = 4.0 nm [20]. Moving from these measurements, GSE-SLN$_{(6mg)}$ shows a faint peak at 19.2, 21.2, and 23.4 deg superimposed to a large band due to very short-range crystallinity material, together with a faint peak at 2q = 2.2 deg and strong peaks at 2q = 2.5 deg (stacking α + β' polymorphic form), and GSE-SLN$_{(6mg)}$-adsorbing GSE, with the exception of a peak at 2q = 2.2 deg (stacking 3L$_{002}$ of β' phase), completely loses any ordered contribution.

Figure 6 and Table 2 display a survey of Raman spectra for the analysed bulk materials and SLN. The spectral region relative to the 1000–1200 cm^{-1} is primarily related to C-C stretching motions [21]. Both frequency differences and relative intensity changes for these vibrational modes can be used to monitor specific conformational changes in the hydrocarbon chains. The 1100 cm^{-1} region, in particular, has been shown to be a superposition of the C-C stretching modes for segments of all-trans hydrocarbon conformations. An increase in the intensity of the 1115 cm^{-1} band relative to the intensities of the 1050 cm^{-1} transitions is indicative of a greater fluidity within the hydrocarbon chains, so the increase in the 1115 cm^{-1} band originates from the increased intramolecular disorder in the systems.

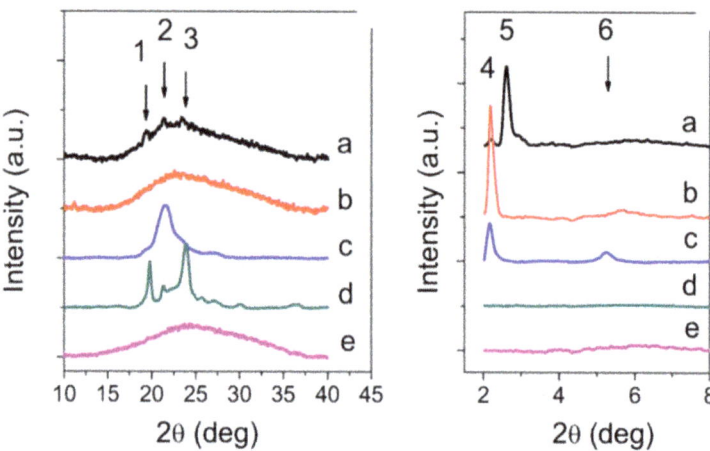

Figure 5. X-ray diffraction spectra of: GSE-SLN$_{(6mg)}$ (**a**); GSE-SLN$_{(6mg)}$-adsorbing GSE (**b**); Precirol® ATO5 (**c**); Gelucire® 50/13 (**d**); and GSE (**e**), in the wide angle range 10–40 deg (**left panel**) and in the small angle range 2–5 deg (**right panel**).

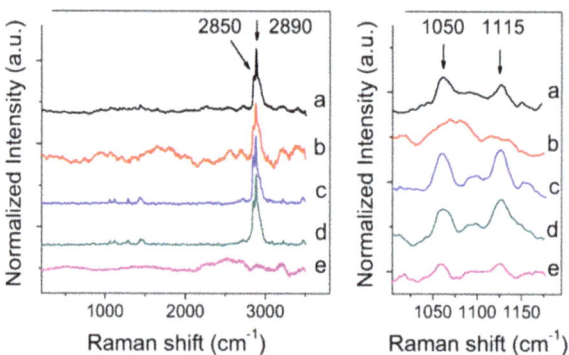

Figure 6. Survey of Raman spectra acquired from: GSE-SLN$_{(6mg)}$ (**a**); GSE-SLN$_{(6mg)}$-adsorbing GSE (**b**); Precirol® ATO5 (**c**); Gelucire® 50/13 (**d**); and GSE (**e**), from different systems (**left panel**) and an enlargement relative to the 1000–1200 cm^{-1} spectral region (**right panel**).

Table 2. Raman intensity ratios related to C-C stretching vibrational bands and to C-H stretching vibrational bands of analysed systems.

Sample	I_{1115}/I_{1050}	I_{2890}/I_{2850}
Precirol® ATO5	1	1.4
Gelucire® 50/13	1.02	1.67
Pure GSE	0.968	1.51
GSE-SLN$_{(6mg)}$	0.867	1.83
GSE-SLN$_{(6mg)}$-adsorbing GSE	0.562	1.84

The region around 3000 cm^{-1} of the Raman spectrum consists of a large number of overlapping peaks, containing both fundamental CH-stretch vibrations and Fermi resonance bands.

The CH$_3$ symmetric stretching modes appear in the 2870–2880 cm^{-1} spectral region, with a Fermi resonance (FR) component in the 2930–2940 cm^{-1} region. The peaks in the 2950–2970 cm^{-1} spectral region are the CH$_3$ out-of-plane and in-plane methyl antisymmetric stretches [22].

The methylene vibrations at approximately 2850, 2880, 2900, and 2930 cm^{-1} are sensitive to conformational changes as well as intermolecular interactions of the alkyl chains of lipids. The ν_a(CH$_2$) antisymmetric stretch is coupled to rigid rotations–torsional vibrations so that it broadens considerably with temperature, and increases continuously in frequency from 2880 cm^{-1} to 2900 cm^{-1} as gauche conformers are introduced. The ν_s(CH$_2$) symmetric stretch contains three components, centred at 2852 cm^{-1}, 2900 cm^{-1}, and 2928 cm^{-1}, due to extensive Fermi resonance interactions with overtones of the bending modes and is affected by intra- and intermolecular interactions [23].

The relative intensities of these peaks change notably with changes in hydration state, packing, and conformational order. To utilize this spectral sensitivity toward the lipid environment, several spectral parameters have been used in the literature that empirically describe the order of the lipid layers. The peak height ratio I_{2890}/I_{2850} has been used as a marker for chain packing and conformational disorder, where higher values indicate a higher ordering of the chains [24].

2.4. Antioxidant Activity of GSE-SLN

The antioxidant activity of GSE-SLN was determined and the data are summarized in Table 2. GSE-SLN$_{(12mg)}$ showed higher values of antioxidant activity than GSE-SLN$_{(6mg)}$ or GSE-SLN$_{(6mg)}$-adsorbing GSE. Furthermore, the total antioxidant values for GSE-SLN$_{(6mg)}$-adsorbing GSE were slightly lower than those observed for GSE-SLN$_{(6mg)}$ (Table 3).

Table 3. Total antioxidant activity of GSE-SLN.

Formulation	Total Antioxidant Activity (TAA) (eq Asc.) mM/mg Nanoparticles
GSE-SLN$_{(6mg)}$	1.735 ± 0.327
GSE-SLN$_{(12mg)}$	2.202 ± 0.321
GSE-SLN$_{(6mg)}$-adsorbing GSE	1.411 ± 0.200

2.5. Viability Assay

The effects of GSE-SLN$_{(6mg)}$, GSE-SLN$_{(12mg)}$, and GSE-SLN$_{(6mg)}$-adsorbing GSE on the viability of SAF-1 and DLB-1 cells were evaluated by 3-(4,5-dimethylthiazol-2-yl)-2,5-diphenyltetrazolium bromide(MTT) (Figure 7). Results from the cytotoxicity test showed that incubation of DLB-1 cells with the highest concentration (20 µg mL^{-1}) of GSE-SLN$_{(6mg)}$, GSE-SLN$_{(12mg)}$, and GSE-SLN$_{(6mg)}$-adsorbing GSE significantly increased the cell viability (164.6 ± 27.2%; 142.5 ± 8.4%; and 520.5 ± 27.9%, respectively, $p < 0.05$). These results are in agreement with previous reports describing that cell viability could increase after exposure to plant extracts rich in antioxidant compounds. For example, SAF-1 cells showed increased viability after oregano aqueous extracts, which are demonstrated to have a rich antioxidant profile [25–27]. Moreover, incubation with 10 µg mL^{-1} of GSE-SLN$_{(6mg)}$-adsorbing GSE significantly increased the cell viability (321.6 ± 27.3%, $p < 0.05$), meaning that, with a lower concentration of GSE (namely GSE-SLN$_{(6mg)}$), cell viability is reached to a higher degree than GSE-SLN$_{(12mg)}$. The viability results seem to indicate that the SLN antioxidants present in GSE-SLN$_{(6mg)}$-adsorbing GSE particles arrived at cells in higher concentrations than when the cells were incubated with GSE-SLN$_{(12mg)}$.

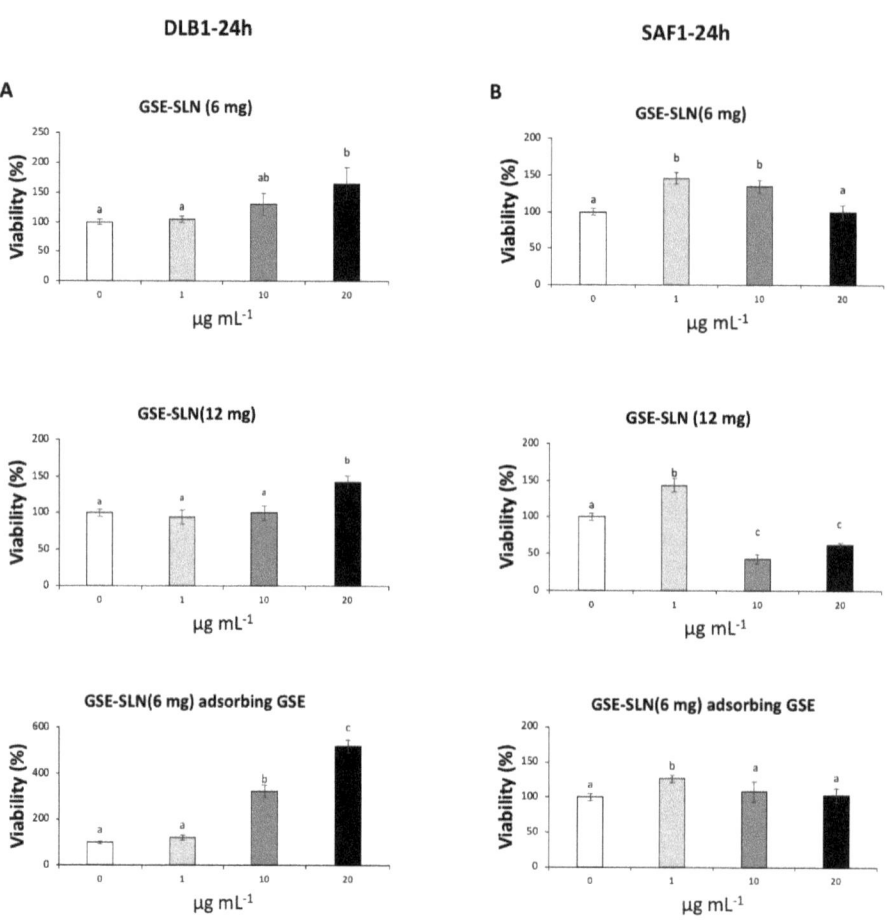

Figure 7. Cytotoxicity of DLB-1 (**A**) and SAF-1 cells (**B**) exposed to different concentrations of GSE-SLN (0, 1, 10, and 20 µg mL^{-1}) for 24 h. Bars represent the mean ± SEM (n = 6). Statistically significant differences (ANOVA; $p < 0.05$) were denoted using different letters.

On the other hand, the lowest concentration (1 µg mL^{-1}) of GSE-SLN$_{(6mg)}$, GSE-SLN$_{(12mg)}$, and GSE-SLN$_{(6mg)}$-adsorbing GSE significantly increased the SAF-1 viability (146.0 ± 7.9%; 143.6 ± 14.7%; and 126.8 ± 5.2%, respectively, $p < 0.05$). These results seem to indicate that SAF-1 cells are more sensitive to these kinds of molecules than DLB-1 cells. In fact, higher concentrations of GSE, such as 10 and 20 µg mL^{-1} of GSE-SLN$_{(12mg)}$ significantly decreased the viability of SAF-1 cells (42.6 ± 6.1% and 61.5 ± 3.2%, respectively, $p < 0.05$). These results are also consistent with previous studies that demonstrated that exposure to extracts with a high antioxidant profile could increase or decrease the viability of SAF-1 cells depending on their concentrations and nature [25,26].

2.6. Gene Expression

The expression of genes related to antioxidant defence (*Nrf2*, *cat*, and *sod*), stress (*Hsp70*), apoptosis (*bax* and *casp3*), detoxification and antioxidant defence (*mt*), and the cytoskeleton (*vim* and *tub-a*) was evaluated on SAF-1 and DLB1 cells after GSE-SLN$_{(6mg)}$, GSE-SLN$_{(12mg)}$, and GSE-SLN$_{(6mg)}$-adsorbing GSE incubation for 24 h (Figures 8 and 9, Tables 4 and 5).

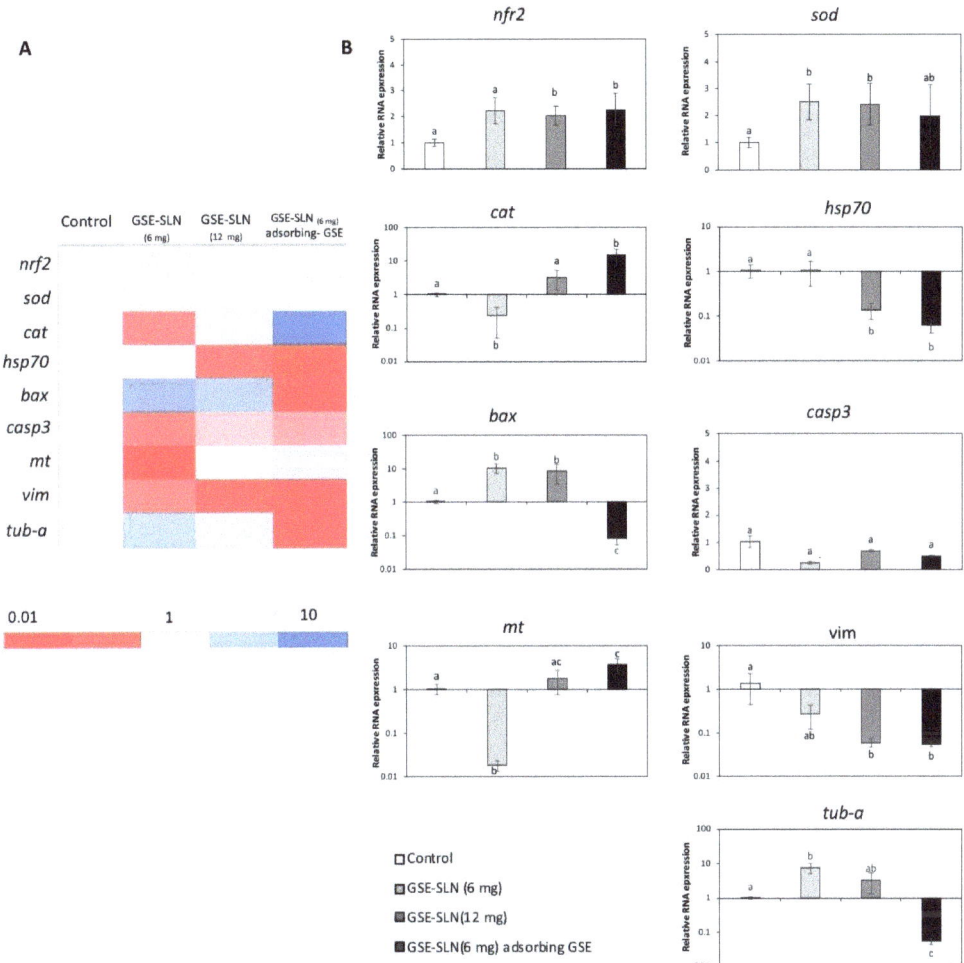

Figure 8. (**A**) Heat-map of the nine differentially expressed genes on DLB-1 cells after GSE-SLN incubation for 24 h. Dark blue: upregulation; red: downregulation. (**B**) Relative gene expression of nine genes (*Nrf2*, *sod*, *cat*, *Hsp70*, *bax*, *casp3*, *mt*, *vim*, and *tubulin α* (*tub-a*)) from DLB-1 cells exposed to 0 (control) or 20 µg mL^{-1} of loaded particles (SLN and SLN-adsorbing GSE) for 24 h. Bars represent the mean ± SEM (n = 5). Statistically significant differences (ANOVA; $p < 0.05$) were denoted using different letters.

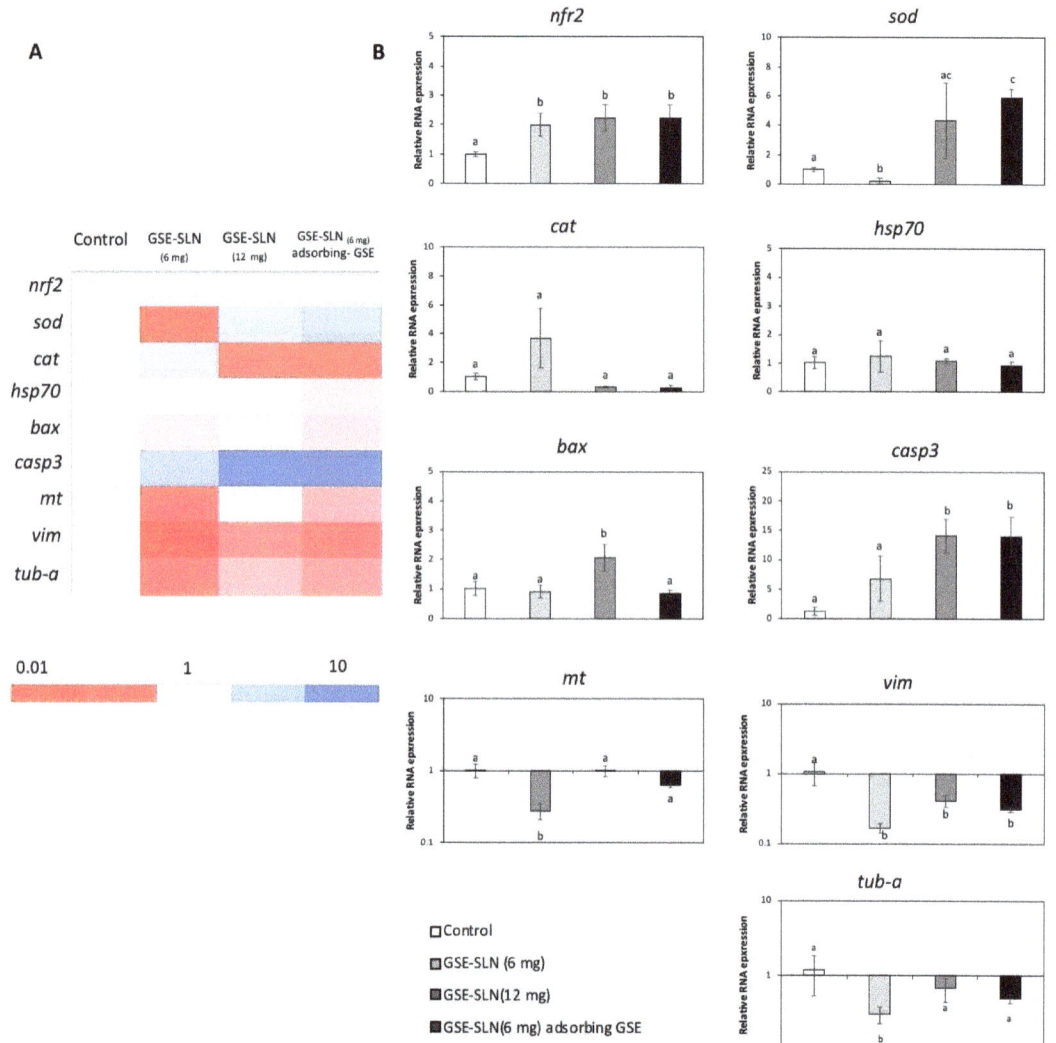

Figure 9. (**A**) Heat-map of the nine differentially expressed genes on SAF-1 cells after GSE-SLN incubation for 24 h. Dark blue: upregulation; red: downregulation. (**B**) Relative gene expression of nine genes (*Nrf2, sod, cat, Hsp70, bax, casp3, mt, vim, tubulin α (tub-a)*) from SAF-1 cells exposed to 0 (control) or 20 µg mL^{-1} of loaded particles (SLN and SLN-adsorbing GSE) for 24 h. Bars represent the mean ± SEM (n = 5). Statistically significant differences (ANOVA; $p < 0.05$) were denoted using different letters.

Table 4. Gilthead seabream primer sequences used for real-time PCR.

Gene	Accession Number	F/R Primer Sequence (5′–3′)
nrf-2	FP335773	F: GTTCAGTCGGTGCTTTGACA R: CTCTGATGTGCGTCTCTCCA
sod	AJ937872	F: CCATGGTAAGAATCATGGCGG R: CGTGGATCACCATGGTTCTG
cat	FG264808	F: TTCCCGTCCTTCATTCACTC R: CTCCAGAAGTCCCACACCAT
hsp70	EU805481	F: AATGTTCTGCGCATCATCAA R: GCCTCCACCAAGATCAAAGA
bax	AM963390	F: CAACAAGATGGCATCACACC R: TGAACCCGCTCGTATATGAAA
casp3	EU722334	F: CTGATCTGGATGGAGGCATT R: AGTAGTAGCCTGGGGCTGTG
mt	X97276	F: ACAAACTGCTCCTGCACCTC R: CAGCTAGTGTCGCACGTCTT
vim	FM155527	F: CGCTTACCTGTGAGGTGGAT R: GTGTCTTGGTAACCGCCTGT
tub-a	AY326430	F: AAGATGTGAACTCCGCCATC R: CTGGTAGTTGATGCCCACCT
act-β	X89920	F: GGCACCACACCTTCTACAATG R: GTGGTGGTGAAGCTGTAGCC
18S	AM490061	F: CTTCAACGCTCAGGTCATCAT R: AGTTGGCACCGTTTATGGTC

Table 5. European sea bass primer sequences used for real-time PCR.

Gene	Accession Number	F/R Primer Sequence (5′–3′)
nrf2	DLAgn_00051120	F: AACTAAGCCTCCCCTCACAC R: GTTGTGGTCCATCTCCTCCA
sod	FJ860004	F: TGTTGGAGACCTGGGAGATG R: ATTGGGCCTGTGAGAGTGAG
cat	FJ860003	F: GAGGTTTGCCTGATGGCTAC R: TGCAGTAGAAACGCTCACCA
hsp70	AY423555	F: CTGCTAAGAATGGCCTGGAG R: CTCGTTGCACTTGTCCAGAA
bax	FM011848	F: TGTCGACTCGTCATCAAAGC R: CACATGTTCCCGGAGGTAGT
casp3	DQ345773	F: AATTCACCAGGCTTCAATGC R: CTACGGCAGAGACGACATCA
mt	AF199014	F: GCACCACCTGCAAGAAGACT R: AGCTGGTGTCGCACGTCT
vim	FM018579	F: AGCGCCAGATTAGAGAGCTG R: GCCATCTCGTCCTTCATGTT
tub-a	AY326429	F: ACGAGGCCATCTACGACATC R: GGCCGTTATGGACGAGACTA
act-β	AJ537421	F: TCCCTGGAGAAGAGCTACGA R: AGGAAGGAAGGCTGGAAAAG
18S	AY831388	F: TTCCTTTGATCGCTCTTAACG R: TCTGATAAATGCACGCATCC

3. Discussion

Searching for orally approved delivery systems such as solid dispersions [28] and cyclodextrins [29], capable to supply micro and macronutrients for fish growth is still a challenge for fish immunology researchers as. The reason is that, once administered *in vivo*, some of them can fail, leading to the loss of their cargo prior to target immunocompetent fish cells [30,31]. Among antioxidant agents, the whole GSE mixture has been studied for its beneficial effects on fish cells [3,4], Moreover, even the isolated polyphenols arising from GSE; namely, resveratrol was found to inhibit both lipopolysaccharide-induced and endogenous eicosanoid production [32], and polyphenol-enriched extract was seen to decrease the oxidative stress and extend the life span of medaka fish [33].

The safe and effective use of nanoparticles in biology and medicine requires in-depth knowledge, down to the molecular level, of how nanoparticles interact with cells in a physiological environment [34]. Until now, the relevance of GSE nanoparticles for administration to gilthead seabream and European sea bass cell lines has never been investigated. These two model cell lines were herein selected as they were obtained from two of the most important marine fish species farmed in the Mediterranean area. In fact, cell cultures are considered as a feasible approach to implementing the "3R principle": replacement, reduction, and refinement of animal usage. For the purpose of designing nanoparticles for GSE supply to fish cells, three different types of SLN containing GSE were prepared to employ the Gelucire® 50/13/Precirol® ATO5 blend. From a technological viewpoint, Precirol® ATO5 is well recommended as an excipient for taste masking, offering excellent anti-friction properties, and is ideal for capsule filling. On the other hand, Gelucire® 50/13 acts as a water-dispersible surfactant, forming fine (micro)emulsions and, as is the case with Precirol® ATO5, high biocompatibility is ensured both in the human and veterinary fields. Two of the three formulations of SLN herein presented were conceived with different starting amounts of GSE (i.e., GSE-SLN$_{(6mg)}$ and GSE-SLN$_{(12mg)}$). Furthermore, the loading of GSE at two different doses (i.e., 6 and 12 mg of GSE) was thought to increase the vectorization of the mixture due to the SLN carrier, while, at the same time, increasing the GSE loading from 6 to 12 initial milligrams in the cargo seemed to be a way to reduce the frequency of administration of the particulate SLN delivery system to the fish cells. The relatively large dimensions of the control SLN could depend on the adoption of two lipids forming the matrix (i.e., Gelucire® 50/13 and Precirol® ATO5). On the other hand, when SLN were loaded with GSE, a reduced mean diameter of these nanocarriers was noted, particularly for those charged with 12 mg of GSE where a size of 139 ± 15 nm was observed. It may be due to the encapsulated GSE, which induces some structural modifications in the SLN structure such as a conformational modification of the PEG moieties occurring in Gelucire® 50/13, leading to SLN shrinkage and exposure of negative charges on the surface of SLN. An intermediate mean diameter between unloaded SLN and GSE-loaded SLN was observed for GSE-SLN$_{(6mg)}$ adsorbing GSE (i.e., 283 ± 32 nm) which causes an increase of mean diameter from 208 ± 21 nm to 283 ± 32 nm. It may be ascribed to the adsorption layer of GSE surrounding SLN. To understand the zeta potential values of observed for GSE-SLN, it is also possible to invoke the lipid composition based on the combination of Gelucire® 50/13 with Precirol® ATO5 taking into account that SLN containing GSE, and only Gelucire® 50/13 as lipid matrix exhibited an external surface charge equal to −14.5 ± 2.0 mV [1]. As previously pointed out, the biggest particles are GSE-SLN adsorbing GSE, but their zeta potential value is similar to the one of GSE-SLN$_{(6mg)}$. It may suggest that in the case of GSE-SLN$_{(6mg)}$ the negative charges on the surface of SLN are more densely located on the surface while, in the case of GSE-SLN$_{(12mg)}$, they are looser and the negative charge density on the surface of these particles is lower. Finally, from TEM observations, indirect information on adsorption was also provided as the nanoparticles were seen to cling to form cluster-shaped complexes.

To understand how the solid-state organization can influence the behavior of the nano-system SLN once incubated with gilthead seabream and European sea bass, first FT-IR spectra and DSC thermograms were acquired. The external localization of Gelucire®

50/13 as derived by FT-IR spectra in our study is in good agreement with the interpretation by Jeon et al. [35], who proposed that the molecular assembly between Precirol® ATO5 and Gelucire 50/13® when the Gelucire® 50/13 to Precirol® ATO5 mass ratio is lower than in our case leads to the fact that Gelucire® 50/13 polar molecules might be located over the surfaces of Precirol® ATO5 molecules, and the lipophilic moieties of Gelucire® 50/13 intercalate between the molecules of Precirol® ATO5. From the FT-IR spectrum of GSE-SLN$_{(6mg)}$-adsorbing GSE, it could be deduced that the adsorption process as described in Section 4.2 also determines, to some extent, the external localization of GSE and, indeed, the corresponding DSC thermogram could reinforce such a hypothesis. Hence, the molecular encapsulation of GSE in the SLN arising from the DSC thermograms of SLN (where no endothermic peak ascribable to GSE is detected) also helps us to understand the high percentages of association efficiency (AE) found for these carriers. Notably, for the GSE-SLN herein described, the molecular distribution of GSE in the lipid matrix derived from DSC thermograms is also consistent with X-ray analysis and is also in agreement with the concept that the amorphous state could contribute to the increased carrying capacity of the active ingredient in the SLN [36]. In parallel, the decrease in the crystalline state of the lipids detected by X-ray diffraction in the SLN has often been observed and indicates the incorporation of the active principles in the SLN [37]. Finally, when Raman spectra were acquired, the intensity ratios of the Raman peaks analysed showed a strengthening of the intermolecular bonds in the layer and between the layers, which is also associated with a more pronounced decrease in long-range crystallinity in GSE-SLN$_{(6mg)}$-adsorbing GSE than in GSE-SLN$_{(6mg)}$.

Furthermore, the exposure of GSE-SLN to DLB-1 and SAF-1 cells allowed us to clarify the genetic processes involved in cell viability and cell defence. First, the expression of antioxidant genes such as *Nrf2*, *cat*, and *sod* was significantly affected by the SLN exposure. NRF2 is a transcription factor that is activated in response to a wide range of oxidative and electrophilic stimulations, including radical oxygen species (ROS) and some chemical agents [38], and it promotes the expression of the antioxidant gene response (such as catalase or superoxide dismutase, which codify the antioxidant enzymes involved in the detoxification of free radicals) and phase II enzymes [39]. In our experiment, *Nrf2* expression was upregulated with respect to the control on DLB-1 and SAF-1 cells after GSE-SLN exposure. These results indicated that GSE-SLN exposure activated the antioxidant response elements that prepared cells against pro-oxidative future events. Increments of *Nrf2* expression after antioxidant exposure both in vivo [40,41] and in vitro [42] have been described. Interestingly, *cat* and *sod* expression in the cells trend to be upregulated with respect to the control after GSE-SLN exposure, although the response depends on the cell type used in the assays (SAF-1 or DLB-1 cells), as was also observed in the viability results.

The management of *Hsp70* expression is an optimal example of a cellular defence mechanism developed to protect the organisms against diverse categories of damages (e.g., high temperature, toxins, and ROS) [43]. Since *HSP70* is considered as a stress marker [44], the decrease in *Hsp70* expression in DLB-1 cells seems to indicate an improvement in the cell welfare parameters, as it has been suggested in vitro [45]. However, no significant changes in *Hsp70* expression were observed on the SAF-1 cells after being incubated with the particles, with respect to the values observed for control samples.

We also monitored the Bax protein trend, where the Bax protein is a member of the Bcl-2 family that promotes apoptosis [46]. The incubation with GSE-SLN significantly affected *bax* expression on the DLB-1 and SAF-1 cells. In fact, the DLB-1 cells showed significant upregulation induced by GSE-SLN$_{(6mg)}$ and GSE-SLN$_{(12mg)}$ exposure ($p < 0.05$), while *bax* expression was significantly downregulated after GSE-SLN$_{(6mg)}$-adsorbing GSE incubation for 24 h ($p < 0.05$). On the other hand, the SAF-1 cells showed the *bax* expression to be downregulated compared with the control group after GSE-SLN$_{(12mg)}$ exposure ($p < 0.05$). Interestingly, the *bax* expression increases on the DLB-1 and SAF-1 cells were not perfectly correlated with the cell viability, except in the case of the SAF-1 cells exposed to GSE-SLN$_{(12mg)}$. Concomitantly, caspase-3 is an executioner protease that stimulates the death receptor extrinsic and mitochondrial intrinsic apoptosis pathways [47]. The *casp3* expression was increased on the SAF-1 cells exposed to GSE-SLN$_{(12mg)}$ and GSE-SLN$_{(6mg)}$-adsorbing GSE, which could be correlated with the decrease in viability observed on the SAF-1 cells after GSE-SLN$_{(12mg)}$ exposure. No significant changes were observed in the *casp3* expression on the DLB-1 cells.

In addition to other antioxidants systems (such as catalase, superoxide dismutase, glutathione, and Zinc ions), metallothionein plays a key role against heavy metal toxicity [48], although it has been proposed to have other functions, such as the sequestration of ROS, radical nitrogen species (RNS), or electrophiles [49]. Both the DLB-1 and SAF-1 cells exposed to GSE-SLN$_{(6mg)}$ showed a decreased *mt* expression, compared with the control cells ($p < 0.05$). However, contrarily, the DLB-1 cells exposed to GSE-SLN$_{(6mg)}$-adsorbing GSE showed a significantly up-regulated *mt* expression ($p < 0.05$). These results are also consistent with the hypothesis that the GSE-SLN$_{(6mg)}$-adsorbing GSE increase antioxidant defence, as described above. Overall, the amount of GSE entrapped in the SLN, once slowly released, elicits a biological effect as was observed for the other SLNs with the same or a higher amount of GSE. These observations, again, point to the acquisition of the same or higher biological effects with lower amounts of GSE, including improvements in skin wound healing, keeping in mind that the SAF-1 cells were obtained from fins [50].

Finally, we also focused on cytoskeleton function, as it is well known that it plays an important role in many cellular processes, including apoptosis, considering that both vimentin and tubulin have been located in apoptotic body formation [51,52]. In general, herein, both vimentin and tubulin gene expression was downregulated on the DLB-1 and SAF-1 cells after exposure to GSE-SLN$_{(6mg)}$, GSE-SLN$_{(12mg)}$, and GSE-SLN$_{(6mg)}$-adsorbing GSE. Overall, although only an in vitro study was performed in the present work, future in vivo studies are planned to investigate the pharmacokinetic properties of the bioactive compounds.

4. Materials and Methods

4.1. Materials

The grape seed extract was kindly provided by Farmalabor (Canosa di Puglia, Italy). It was obtained after the acetone/water extraction of artificially dried seeds of *Vitis vinifera* L., leading to the final content of pro-anthocyanidins ≥95.0%. According to the manufacturer's instructions, the grape seed extract also contained 13–19% as total percentage of catechin and epicatechin. Tween®85 and the salts used for buffer preparation were purchased from Sigma-Aldrich (Milan, Italy). Gelucire® 50/13 and Precirol® ATO5 were gifted by Gattefossè (Milan, Italy). Throughout this work, double-distilled water was used. All other chemicals were of reagent grade and the different companies are detailed together with the methodology.

4.2. Preparation of SLN

The SLNs were prepared from Precirol® ATO5 and Gelucire® 50/13, adopting the melt homogenization procedure, following Jeon et al.'s method with slight modifications [53]. The association of GSE to the SLNs containing Gelucire® 50/13/Precirol® ATO5 followed different procedures: (i) Gelucire® 50/13 (20 mg) and Precirol® ATO5 (50 mg) were co-melted at 80 °C (higher than the melting points of all the lipids) and, in a separate vial, the surfactant (Tween®85, 22 mg) and 1.37 mL of double-distilled water were also heated at 80 °C. In the aqueous phase, 6 mg (or 12 mg) of GSE was dispersed under homogenization at 12,300 rpm for 2 min with an UltraTurrax model T25 apparatus (Janke and Kunkel, Germany) and let to equilibrate for 30 min at 80 °C. Afterwards, the aqueous phase was mixed with melted Gelucire®/Precirol® ATO5, and the emulsion was homogenized at 12,300 rpm for 2 min by UltraTurrax prior to carrying out centrifugation at 16,000× g, for 45 min (Eppendorf 5415D, Germany). The SLN prepared to start from 6 mg and 12 mg of GSE were herein indicated as GSE-SLN$_{(6mg)}$ and GSE-SLN$_{(12mg)}$, respectively; and (ii) a suspension of GSE-SLN$_{(6mg)}$ (0.5 mL), obtained as reported above in (i), was incubated with

1 mL of GSE aqueous solution (concentration of 1 mg/mL) at room temperature for 3 h under light protection and mild stirring (50 oscillations/min). When the incubation time was over, the mixture was then centrifuged at 16,000× g, for 45 min and the supernatant was discarded. The SLNs prepared to start from 6 mg of GSE were herein indicated as GSE-SLN$_{(6mg)}$-adsorbing GSE. All pellets resulting from centrifugation were used for the following studies. Unloaded SLNs were prepared following the same procedure described above in (i) without any addition of any GSE to the aqueous phase [8,9,54].

4.3. Physic-Chemical Characterization of SLN

Particle size and polydispersion index (PDI) for the SLNs were evaluated using a Zetasizer Nano ZS (ZEN 3600, Malvern, UK) apparatus following photon correlation spectroscopy (PCS) mode. Particle size and PDI were measured after dilution 1:1 (v/v) with double-distilled water, while the zeta-potential value was determined after dilution of sample 1:20 (v/v) with KCl (1 mM, pH 7) described in [55]. GSE quantification was assessed by HPLC analysis as previously reported in [2] using an HPLC apparatus consisting of a Waters Model 600 pump (Waters Corp., Milford, MA, USA), a Waters 2996 photodiode array detector, and a 20 μL loop injection autosampler (Waters 717 plus). A Synergy Hydro-RP (25 cm × 4.6 mm, 4 μm particles; Phenomenex, Torrance, CA, USA) column in conjunction with a precolumn C18 insert as a stationary phase was used for the analyses, and the elution of the column in isocratic mode took place at a flow rate of 0.7 mL/min. The mobile phase was composed adopting 0.02 M potassium phosphate buffer, pH 2.8: CH$_3$OH 70:30 (v/v), providing a GSE retention time equal to 12 min. For the GSE, calibration curve linearity ($R^2 > 0.999$) was checked over the range of concentrations equal to 100–50 mg/mL, and for concentrations lower than 50 mg/mL, a fluorometer apparatus (Varian Cary Eclipse, Mulgrave, Australia, excitation wavelength: 560 nm; emission wavelength: 583 nm; slits: 2.5 nm) was used. When a fluorometric assay was employed, the linearity was checked over the range of concentrations equal to 50–2.5 mg/mL.

To determine the GSE association efficiency (AE) in the SLN, freeze-dried particles were cleaved upon enzymatic digestion operated by carboxyl ester hydrolase as previously described [2,37]. The enzyme was dissolved at 12 I.U./mL in phosphate buffer (pH 5) and aliquots of lyophilized SLN in the range 1–2 mg were incubated with 1 mL of the enzyme solution for 30 min in an agitated (40 rpm/min) water bath set at 37 °C (Julabo, Milan, Italy). The samples were then centrifuged (16,000× g, 45 min, Eppendorf 5415D) and the resulting supernatant was injected in HPLC for GSE content evaluation. The AE% of GSE in the SLN was calculated as follows:

AE% = GSE in the supernatant after enzymatic assay with esterase/Total GSE × 100

where the total GSE is intended as the initial amount of GSE used for the SLN preparation. Each measurement was performed in triplicate.

4.4. Transmission Electron Spectroscopy (TEM)

For the GSE containing SLN, TEM observations were also carried out. The morphology and dimensions of the SLNs were determined by cryogenic transmission electron microscopy (Cryo-TEM). All observations were performed using a Hitachi 7700 electron microscope, at a temperature of 105 K and an acceleration voltage of 100 kV. The procedure for vitrifying the samples (as previously described in [56]) can be summarized as follows. A drop of suspension containing the nanocarriers was deposited on copper grids covered with an amorphous carbon film. After removing the excess solution with buffer paper, the sample was vitrified by immersion in liquid ethane maintained just above its freezing point. The sample was then transferred to the Gatan 626 cryo holder. The sample was protected against atmospheric conditions during the entire procedure to prevent the formation of ice crystals. The digital images were acquired with an AMT-XR-81 camera and processed with the EMIP software. Counting and size distribution of the nanoparticles were obtained by processing the obtained TEM images. Twenty fields, randomly chosen, were taken into consideration for each sample, and the morphology and particle size of the particles present in randomly selected areas on the basis of the count of 500 particles for each sample was determined.

4.5. Solid State Studies

FT-IR spectroscopy: FT-IR spectra were obtained using powders of 2–5 mg of lyophilized SLN (Lio Pascal 5P, Milan, Italy). Such powders were milled with KBr discs prior to acquire spectra from a Perkin Elmer 1600 FT-IR spectrometer (Perkin Elmer, Milan, Italy). The analysis was carried out at room temperature (r.t.) in the range of 4000–400 cm^{-1} at a resolution of 1 cm^{-1} [57].

DSC: for bulk lipids, unloaded SLN, and GSE-SLN, DSC runs were performed on a Mettler Toledo DSC 822e. The instrument was calibrated with indium for melting point and heat of fusion, and in each run, the heating rate of 5 °C/min was used in the range of 25–275 °C. About 5 mg of lyophilized samples were taken in the standard aluminum sample pans for analysis, and an empty pan was used as reference in each case. The analyses were performed under nitrogen purge; triple runs were carried out on each sample [28,58].

X-ray diffraction: X-ray diffraction spectra were acquired with a MiniFlex Rigaku diffractometer, operating in step-scan mode and equipped with a Cu Kα source (wavelength λ = 0.154 nm) at 30 kV and 100 mA. The X-ray diffraction data were collected in the Bragg-Brentano geometry, from 2 to 8 deg and from 10 to 40 deg, at a scanning speed of 0.02 deg/s.

Raman Spectroscopy: Raman scattering measurements were obtained by a Renishaw spectrometer equipped with a Leica metallographic microscope. The instrumentation included a 514.5 nm air-cooled Argon ions laser source and 1800 lines/mm lattice/monochromator with a RenCam CCD detector that assured a resolution of 1 cm^{-1}. The analysis of the obtained data was performed using Renishaw Wire 2.0 software.

4.6. Total Antioxidant Activity

The total antioxidant activity (TAA) was evaluated in the SLNs using a method based on the ability of the antioxidants in the sample to reduce the radical cation of 2,20-azino-bis-3-(ethylbenzothiazoline-6-sulphonic acid) (ABTS), determined by the decoloration of ABTS$^+$, and measuring the quenching of the absorbance at the wavelength of 730 nm (BMG Labtech, Fluostar Omega, UK) [59]. This activity was calculated by comparing the values of the sample with a standard curve of ascorbic acid, and expressed as ascorbic acid equivalents (mmol) per milligram of SLN.

4.7. Cell Lines Culture

Two cell lines, SAF-1 from gilthead seabream and DLB-1 from European sea bass, were used throughout the study. The established SAF-1 cell line [60] was seeded in 75-cm^2 plastic tissue culture flasks (Nunc, Denmark) and cultured at 25 °C in an atmosphere with 85% relative humidity using a L-15 Leibowitz medium supplemented with 10% foetal bovine serum (FBS, Sigma–Aldrich), 2 mM L-glutamine, 100 µg/mL streptomycin, and 100 U/mL penicillin. The subculture was carried out according to standard trypsinization methods (0.25% trypsin/0.53 mM EDTA, Sigma–Aldrich). The cells were centrifuged (200× g, 10 min) and the viability determined using the trypan blue exclusion test. The SAF-1cells were plated in 48-well plates at 2.5 × 10^5 cell/well and cultured overnight at 25 °C with 85% relative humidity and 5% CO$_2$ in the incubator chamber.

4.7.1. Cell Monolayers DLB-1

The DLB-1 cells were grown at 25 °C in a L-15 Leibovitz medium containing 0.16% NaCl, 15% foetal bovine serum (FBS), 20 mM HEPES, 2 mM glutamine, penicillin (100 IU/mL), and streptomycin (100 µg/mL) and subcultured by trypsinization every week. The cells were centrifuged (200× g, 10 min) and the viability determined using the trypan blue exclusion test [61,62]. The cells were plated in 48-well plates at 2.5 × 10^5 cell/well and cultured overnight at 25 °C with 85% relative humidity and 5% CO$_2$ in the incubator chamber.

4.7.2. In Vitro Incubation of Fish Cell Lines with Particles

To determine whether GSE-SLN affected the viability of the SAF-1 and DLB-1 cells, the cells were incubated without (control) or with different concentrations of loaded particles (GSE-SLN$_{(6mg)}$, GSE-SLN$_{(12mg)}$, and GSE-SLN$_{(6mg)}$-adsorbing GSE) (1, 10, and 20 µg/mL of culture medium, respectively) at 25 °C with 85% relative humidity for 24 h. All the trials were performed using six replicates.

4.8. Viability Assay

The cell viability was evaluated using the MTT (3-(4,5-dimethylthiazol-2-yl)-2,5-diphenyltetrazolium bromide; Sigma-Aldrich) colorimetric assay based on the reduction of the yellow soluble tetrazolium salt into a blue, insoluble formazan product by the mitochondrial succinate dehydrogenase [1]. For this, the SAF-1 and DLB-1 cells were washed and incubated with 200 µL/well of culture medium containing 1 mg/mL of MTT. After 4 h of incubation at 25 °C, the wells were washed, the formazan solubilized, and the absorbance at 570 nm and 690 nm was determined in a microplate reader (BMG Labtech, Fluostar Omega, UK). Blanks consisted of wells without cells.

4.9. Gene Expression

The SAF-1 and DLB1 cells were plated on uncoated 12-well culture dishes at a density of 5×10^5 cells/well and incubated until 100% confluence. The cells were exposed in culture medium to 0 (control) or 20 µg mL^{-1} of loaded particles (SLN and SLN-adsorbing GSE) using 3 wells for each one and incubated for 24 h. The relative gene expression on the cells was then evaluated using real-time PCR and the $2^{-\Delta\Delta CT}$ method [63].

Total RNA was extracted from the cells using TRIzol reagent (Invitrogen; Berlin, Germany) following the manufacturer's instructions. The RNA was then treated with DNase I (Invitrogen) to remove genomic DNA contamination. Complementary DNA (cDNA) was synthesized from 1 mg of total RNA using the SuperScriptIV reverse transcriptase (Invitrogen; Berlin, Germany) with an oligo-dT18 primer. The expression of 14 selected genes was analysed by real-time PCR, performed with an ABI PRISM 7500 instrument (Applied Biosystems; Waltham, CA, USA) using SYBRGreen PCR Core Reagents (Applied Biosystems; Waltham, CA, USA), as previously described [64]. These genes code for structural proteins involved in antioxidant response, cell stress, apoptosis, and cell movement (nuclear factor erythroid 2-related factor 2 (*nrf2*), superoxide dismutase (*sod*), catalase (*cat*), heat-shock protein 70 (*hsp70*), BCL2 Associated X, apoptosis regulator (*bax*), caspase 3 (*casp3*), metallothionein (*mt*), vimentin (*vim*), and tubulin alpha (*tub-a*)). For each mRNA, the gene expression was corrected by the median of the β-actin and 18-S expression content in each sample. The primers used are shown in Tables 4 and 5. In all cases, each PCR was performed with triplicate samples.

4.10. Statistical Analyses

For physic-chemical properties and size stability studies, statistical analyses were carried out using Prism Version 4, GraphPad Software Inc. (San Diego, CA, USA). Data were expressed as either mean ± SD. Multiple comparisons were based on one-way analysis of variance (ANOVA) with either Bonferroni's or Tukey's post hoc test, and differences were considered significant when $p < 0.05$.

For biological studies, statistical differences among the groups were assessed by one-way ANOVA analyses, followed by the Bonferroni or Games–Howell test, depending on the homogeneity of the variables. The normality of the variables was confirmed by the Shapiro–Wilk test and the homogeneity of variance by the Levene test. The significance level was 95% in all cases ($p < 0.05$). All the data were analysed by the computer application SPSS for Windows® (version 15.0, SPSS Inc., Chicago, IL, USA).

5. Conclusions

For aquaculture application, we formulated a novel Gelucire® 50/13/Precirol® ATO5-based SLN intended as a colloidal vector for the administration of the antioxidant GSE to immunocompetent fish cells. The mild melt-emulsification technique provided particles that combined high AE% of GSE with a reduced crystallinity level regarding the organization of the solid state, as evidenced by X-ray diffraction and Raman spectra. From the biological evaluation of the SLNs, it was deduced, firstly, that both cell lines (SAF-1 and DLB-1) had different sensitivities to the exposure to the different GSE-SLNs at the concentrations and incubation times tested in the present study. Furthermore, our results demonstrated an important increase in antioxidant response (up-regulated expression of *Nrf2*, *cat*, *sod*, and *mt*) in the cells after being incubated with the GSE-SLN. The concentration of GSE, as well as the method of loading the GSE into the SLN, played crucial roles in the physiological effects on the SAF-1 and DLB-1 cell lines, as was demonstrated by the cytotoxicity assays and the gene expression of different apoptosis markers (*casp3* and *bax*). Finally, GSE-SLN affected the expression of different proteins related to the cytoskeleton and apoptosis, which evidenced that GSE-SLN can be considered as a compelling and valuable tool for use in different disease treatments. Moving on from good physicochemical characteristics, ex vivo results in terms of cell viability and the expression of different genes related to antioxidant defense, viability, and the cytoskeleton could be addressed in future studies to evaluate if SLNs containing GSE could be a candidate for in vivo trials in nutraceutical industries.

Author Contributions: A.T.: supervision, project conceptualization, and administration, writing—review and editing; M.Á.E.: supervision, project conceptualization, and administration; writing—review and editing; F.C.: data curation; D.E.M.: methodology; A.S.: data curation; G.F.: data curation; C.E.-R.: investigation and data curation; writing—review and editing; S.C.: methodology, writing—review and editing; M.C.: data curation, writing—review and editing. All authors have read and agreed to the published version of the manuscript.

Funding: This work was supported by the *Fundación Seneca de la Región de Murcia (Grupo de Excelencia* grant no. 19883/GERM/15).

Institutional Review Board Statement: Not applicable.

Informed Consent Statement: Not applicable.

Data Availability Statement: The datasets generated during the current study will be available upon request.

Acknowledgments: A.T. would acknowledge Gennaro Agrimi (University of Bari, Italy), Lucia Catucci, and Vincenzo De Leo (University of Bari, Italy) for their valuable technical assistance.

Conflicts of Interest: The authors declare no conflict of interest.

Sample Availability: Samples are not available from the authors.

References

1. Castellani, S.; Trapani, A.; Spagnoletta, A.; di Toma, L.; Magrone, T.; Di Gioia, S.; Mandracchia, D.; Trapani, G.; Jirillo, E.; Conese, M. Nanoparticle delivery of grape seed-derived proanthocyanidins to airway epithelial cells dampens oxidative stress and inflammation. *J. Transl. Med.* **2018**, *16*, 140. [CrossRef] [PubMed]
2. Trapani, A.; Guerra, L.; Corbo, F.; Castellani, S.; Sanna, E.; Capobianco, L.; Monteduro, A.G.; Manno, D.E.; Mandracchia, D.; Di Gioia, S.; et al. Cyto/Biocompatibility of Dopamine Combined with the Antioxidant Grape Seed-Derived Polyphenol Compounds in Solid Lipid Nanoparticles. *Molecules* **2021**, *26*, 916. [CrossRef]
3. Lu, R.H.; Qin, C.B.; Yang, F.; Zhang, W.Y.; Zhang, Y.R.; Yang, G.K.; Yang, L.P.; Meng, X.L.; Yan, X.; Nie, G.X. Grape seed proanthocyanidin extract ameliorates hepatic lipid accumulation and inflammation in grass carp (*Ctenopharyngodon idella*). *Fish Physiol. Biochem.* **2020**, *46*, 1665–1677. [CrossRef]
4. Cerbaro, A.F.; Rodrigues, V.S.B.; Rigotti, M.; Branco, C.S.; Rech, G.; de Oliveira, D.L.; Salvador, M. Grape seed proanthocyanidins improves mitochondrial function and reduces oxidative stress through an increase in sirtuin 3 expression in EA. hy926 cells in high glucose condition. *Mol. Biol. Rep.* **2020**, *47*, 3319–3330. [CrossRef]

5. Esposito, E.; Drechsler, M.; Puglia, C.; Cortesi, R. New Strategies for the Delivery of Some Natural Anti-oxidants with Therapeutic Properties. *Mini Rev. Med. Chem.* **2019**, *19*, 1030–1039. [CrossRef] [PubMed]
6. Esposito, E.; Sguizzato, M.; Drechsler, M.; Mariani, P.; Carducci, F.; Nastruzzi, C.; Valacchi, G.; Cortesi, R. Lipid nanostructures for antioxidant delivery: A comparative preformulation study. *Beilstein J. Nanotechnol.* **2019**, *10*, 1789–1801. [CrossRef] [PubMed]
7. Trapani, A.; Mandracchia, D.; Di Franco, C.; Cordero, H.; Morcillo, P.; Comparelli, R.; Cuesta, A.; Esteban, M.A. In vitro characterization of 6-Coumarin loaded solid lipid nanoparticles and their uptake by immunocompetent fish cells. *Colloids Surf. B Biointerfaces* **2015**, *127*, 79–88. [CrossRef] [PubMed]
8. Trapani, A.; Tripodo, G.; Mandracchia, D.; Cioffi, N.; Ditaranto, N.; De Leo, V.; Cordero, H.; Esteban, M.A. Glutathione-loaded solid lipid nanoparticles based on Gelucire® 50/13: Spectroscopic characterization and interactions with fish cells. *J. Drug Deliv. Sci. Technol.* **2018**, *47*, 359–366. [CrossRef]
9. Trapani, A.; Tripodo, G.; Mandracchia, D.; Cioffi, N.; Ditaranto, N.; Cerezuela, R.; Esteban, M.A. Glutathione loaded solid lipid nanoparticles: Preparation and in vitro evaluation as delivery systems of the antioxidant peptide to immunocompetent fish cells. *J. Cell. Biotechnol.* **2016**, *2*, 1–14. [CrossRef]
10. Mura, P.; Maestrelli, F.; D'Ambrosio, M.; Luceri, C.; Cirri, M. Evaluation and Comparison of Solid Lipid Nanoparticles (SLNs) and Nanostructured Lipid Carriers (NLCs) as Vectors to Develop Hydrochlorothiazide Effective and Safe Pediatric Oral Liquid Formulations. *Pharmaceutics* **2021**, *13*, 437. [CrossRef]
11. Nazemiyeh, E.; Eskandani, M.; Sheikhloie, H.; Nazemiyeh, H. Formulation and Physicochemical Characterization of Lycopene-Loaded Solid Lipid Nanoparticles. *Adv. Pharm. Bull.* **2016**, *6*, 235–241. [CrossRef]
12. Vaassen, J.; Bartscher, K.; Breitkreutz, J. Taste masked lipid pellets with enhanced release of hydrophobic active ingredient. *Int. J. Pharm.* **2012**, *429*, 99–103. [CrossRef] [PubMed]
13. Wilson, M.; Williams, M.A.; Jones, D.S.; Andrews, G.P. Hot-melt extrusion technology and pharmaceutical application. *Ther. Deliv.* **2012**, *3*, 787–797. [CrossRef]
14. El Hadri, M.; Achahbar, A.; El Khamkhami, J.; Khelifa, B.; Faivre, V.; Abbas, O.; Bresson, S. Lyotropic behavior of Gelucire 50/13 by XRD, Raman and IR spectroscopies according to hydration. *Chem. Phys. Lipids* **2016**, *200*, 11–23. [CrossRef]
15. Perteghella, S.; Mandracchia, D.; Torre, M.L.; Tamma, R.; Ribatti, D.; Trapani, A.; Tripodo, G. Anti-angiogenic activity of N,O-carboxymethyl-chitosan surface modified solid lipid nanoparticles for oral delivery of curcumin. *J. Drug Deliv. Sci. Technol.* **2020**, *56*, 101494. [CrossRef]
16. Souto, E.B.; Mehnert, W.; Müller, R.H. Polymorphic behaviour of Compritol®888 ATO as bulk lipid and as SLN and NLC. *J. Microencapsul* **2006**, *23*, 417–433. [CrossRef] [PubMed]
17. Larsson, K.; Cyvin, S.J.; Rymo, L.; Bowie, J.H.; Williams, D.H.; Bunnenberg, E.; Djerassi, C.; Records, R. Classification of glyceride crystal forms. *Acta Chem. Scand.* **1966**, *20*, 2255–2260. [CrossRef] [PubMed]
18. Himawan, C.; Starov, V.M.; Stapley, A.G. Thermodynamic and kinetic aspects of fat crystallization. *Adv. Colloid Interface Sci.* **2006**, *122*, 3–33. [CrossRef] [PubMed]
19. Bugeat, S.; Perez, J.; Briard-Bion, V.; Pradel, P.; Ferlay, A.; Bourgaux, C.; Lopez, C. Unsaturated fatty acid enriched vs. control milk triacylglycerols:S olid and liquid TAG phases examined by synchrotron radiation X-ray diffraction coupled with DSC. *Food Res. Int.* **2015**, *67*, 91–101. [CrossRef]
20. Takeguchi, S.; Sato, A.; Hondoh, H.; Aoki, M.; Uehara, H.; Ueno, S. Multiple beta Forms of Saturated Monoacid Triacylglycerol Crystals. *Molecules* **2020**, *25*, 5086. [CrossRef]
21. Spiker, R.C.; Levin, I.W. Effect of bilayer curvature on vibrational Raman spectroscopic behavior of phospholipid-water assemblies. *Biochim. Biophys. Acta-Biomembr.* **1976**, *455*, 560–575. [CrossRef]
22. de Lange, M.J.; Bonn, M.; Müller, M. Direct measurement of phase coexistence in DPPC/cholesterol vesicles using Raman spectroscopy. *Chem. Phys. Lipids* **2007**, *146*, 76–84. [CrossRef]
23. Schultz, Z.D.; Levin, I.W. Vibrational spectroscopy of biomembranes. *Annu Rev. Anal. Chem.* **2011**, *4*, 343–366. [CrossRef]
24. Nordgreen, A.; Yúfera, M.; Hamre, K. Evaluation of changes in nutrient composition during production of crosslinked protein microencapsulated diets for marine fish larvae and suspension feeders. *Aquaculture* **2008**, *285*, 159–166. [CrossRef]
25. Bejar, J.; Borrego, J.J.; Alvarez, M.C. A continuous cell line from the cultured marine fish gilt-head seabream (*Sparus aurata* L.). *Aquaculture* **1997**, *150*, 143–153. [CrossRef]
26. Beltrán, J.M.G.; Espinosa, C.; Guardiola, F.A.; Esteban, M.A. In vitro effects of Origanum vulgare leaf extracts on gilthead seabream (*Sparus aurata* L.) leucocytes, cytotoxic, bactericidal and antioxidant activities. *Fish Shellfish Immunol.* **2018**, *79*, 1–10. [CrossRef] [PubMed]
27. Li, X.; Yao, Y.; Wang, S.; Xu, S. Resveratrol relieves chlorothalonil-induced apoptosis and necroptosis through miR-15a/Bcl2-A20 axis in fish kidney cells. *Fish Shellfish Immunol.* **2020**, *107*, 427–434. [CrossRef] [PubMed]
28. Trapani, A.; Catalano, A.; Carocci, A.; Carrieri, A.; Mercurio, A.; Rosato, A.; Mandracchia, D.; Tripodo, G.; Schiavone, B.I.P.; Franchini, C.; et al. Effect of Methyl-beta-Cyclodextrin on the antimicrobial activity of a new series of poorly water-soluble benzothiazoles. *Carbohydr. Polym.* **2019**, *207*, 720–728. [CrossRef] [PubMed]
29. Trapani, A.; Laquintana, V.; Lopedota, A.; Franco, M.; Latrofa, A.; Talani, G.; Sanna, E.; Trapani, G.; Liso, G. Evaluation of new propofol aqueous solutions for intravenous anesthesia. *Int. J. Pharm.* **2004**, *278*, 91–98. [CrossRef] [PubMed]

30. Partridge, G.J.; Rao, S.; Woolley, L.D.; Pilmer, L.; Lymbery, A.J.; Prestidge, C.A. Bioavailability and palatability of praziquantel incorporated into solid-lipid nanoparticles fed to yellowtail kingfish *Seriola lalandi*. *Comp. Biochem. Physiol. C Toxicol. Pharmacol.* **2019**, *218*, 14–20. [CrossRef] [PubMed]
31. Wurpel, G.W.H.; Schins, J.M.; Müller, M. Direct Measurement of Chain Order in Single Phospholipid Mono- and Bilayers with Multiplex CARS. *J. Phys. Chem. B* **2004**, *108*, 3400–3403. [CrossRef]
32. Holen, E.; Araujo, P.; Xie, S.; Søfteland, L.; Espe, M. Resveratrol inhibited LPS induced transcription of immune genes and secretion of eicosanoids in Atlantic salmon (*Salmo salar*), comparing mono-, co- and a novel triple cell culture model of head kidney leukocytes, liver cells and visceral adipocyte tissue. *Comp. Biochem. Physiol. C Toxicol. Pharmacol.* **2019**, *224*, 108560. [CrossRef] [PubMed]
33. Sánchez-Sánchez, A.V.; Leal-Tassias, A.; Rodríguez-Sánchez, N.; Gil, M.P.; Martorell, P.; Genovés, S.; Acosta, C.; Burks, D.; Ramón, D.; Mullor, J.L. Use of Medaka Fish as Vertebrate Model to Study the Effect of Cocoa Polyphenols in the Resistance to Oxidative Stress and Life Span Extension. *Rejuvenation Res.* **2018**, *21*, 323–332. [CrossRef] [PubMed]
34. Cristallini, C.; Barbani, N.; Bianchi, S.; Maltinti, S.; Baldassare, A.; Ishak, R.; Onor, M.; Ambrosio, L.; Castelvetro, V.; Cascone, M.G. Assessing two-way interactions between cells and inorganic nanoparticles. *J. Mater. Sci. Mater. Med.* **2019**, *31*, 1–13. [CrossRef] [PubMed]
35. Jeon, H.S.; Seo, J.E.; Kim, M.S.; Kang, M.H.; Oh, D.H.; Jeon, S.O.; Seong Hoon, J.; Choi, Y.W.; Lee, S. A retinyl palmitate-loaded solid lipid nanoparticle system: Effect of surface modification with dicetyl phosphate on skin permeation in vitro and anti-wrinkle effect in vivo. *Int. J. Pharm.* **2013**, *452*, 311–320. [CrossRef] [PubMed]
36. de Souza Guedes, L.; Martinez, R.M.; Bou-Chacra, N.A.; Velasco, M.V.R.; Rosado, C.; Baby, A.R. An Overview on Topical Administration of Carotenoids and Coenzyme Q10 Loaded in Lipid Nanoparticles. *Antioxidants* **2021**, *10*, 1034. [CrossRef]
37. Ghanbarzadeh, S.; Hariri, R.; Kouhsoltani, M.; Shokri, J.; Javadzadeh, Y.; Hamishehkar, H. Enhanced stability and dermal delivery of hydroquinone using solid lipid nanoparticles. *Colloids Surf. B Biointerfaces* **2015**, *136*, 1004–1010. [CrossRef]
38. Brum, G.; Carbone, T.; Still, E.; Correia, V.; Szulak, K.; Calianese, D.; Best, C.; Cammarata, G.; Higgins, K.; Ji, F.; et al. N-acetylcysteine potentiates doxorubicin-induced ATM and p53 activation in ovarian cancer cells. *Int. J. Oncol.* **2013**, *42*, 211–218. [CrossRef]
39. Dimitriadis, V.K.; Gougoula, C.; Anestis, A.; Pörtner, H.O.; Michaelidis, B. Monitoring the biochemical and cellular responses of marine bivalves during thermal stress by using biomarkers. *Mar. Environ. Res.* **2012**, *73*, 70–77. [CrossRef]
40. Espinosa, C.; Beltrán, J.M.G.; Messina, C.M.; Esteban, M. Effect of Jasonia glutinosa on immune and oxidative status of gilthead seabream (*Sparus aurata* L.). *Fish Shellfish Immunol.* **2020**, *100*, 58–69. [CrossRef]
41. Fazio, A.; Cerezuela, R.; Panuccio, M.R.; Cuesta, A.; Esteban, M.A. In vitro effects of Italian Lavandula multifida L. leaf extracts on gilthead seabream (*Sparus aurata*) leucocytes and SAF-1 cells. *Fish Shellfish Immunol.* **2017**, *66*, 334–344. [CrossRef] [PubMed]
42. Formigari, A.; Irato, P.; Santon, A. Zinc, antioxidant systems and metallothionein in metal mediated-apoptosis: Biochemical and cytochemical aspects. *Comp. Biochem. Physiol. C Toxicol. Pharmacol.* **2007**, *146*, 443–459. [CrossRef]
43. Giudice, A.; Arra, C.; Turco, M.C. Review of molecular mechanisms involved in the activation of the Nrf2-ARE signaling pathway by chemopreventive agents. *Transcr. Factors* **2010**, *647*, 37–74.
44. Heydari, A.R.; Wu, B.; Takahashi, R.; Strong, R.; Richardson, A. Expression of heat shock protein 70 is altered by age and diet at the level of transcription. *Mol. Cell Biol.* **1993**, *13*, 2909–2918. [PubMed]
45. Kim, E.N.; Lim, J.H.; Kim, M.Y.; Ban, T.H.; Jang, I.A.; Yoon, H.E.; Park, C.W.; Chang, Y.S.; Choi, B.S. Resveratrol, an Nrf2 activator, ameliorates aging-related progressive renal injury. *Aging* **2018**, *10*, 83–99. [CrossRef]
46. Messina, C.M.; Pizzo, F.; Santulli, A.; Buselic, I.; Boban, M.; Orhanovic, S.; Mladineo, I. Anisakis pegreffii (Nematoda: Anisakidae) products modulate oxidative stress and apoptosis-related biomarkers in human cell lines. *Parasit. Vectors* **2016**, *9*, 607. [CrossRef] [PubMed]
47. Oltval, Z.N.; Milliman, C.L.; Korsmeyer, S.J. Bcl-2 heterodimerizes in vivo with a conserved homolog, Bax, that accelerates programed cell death. *Cell* **1993**, *74*, 609–619. [CrossRef]
48. Yoshida, M.; Saegusa, Y.; Fukuda, A.; Akama, Y.; Owada, S. Measurement of radical-scavenging ability in hepatic metallothionein of rat using in vivo electron spin resonance spectroscopy. *Toxicology* **2005**, *213*, 74–80. [CrossRef]
49. Yuksel, Y.; Yuksel, R.; Yagmurca, M.; Haltas, H.; Erdamar, H.; Toktas, M.; Ozcan, O. Effects of quercetin on methotrexate-induced nephrotoxicity in rats. *Hum. Exp. Toxicol.* **2017**, *36*, 51–61. [CrossRef] [PubMed]
50. Bichat, F.; Mouawad, R.; Solis-Recendez, G.; Khayat, D.; Bastian, G. Cytoskeleton alteration in MCF7R cells, a multidrug resistant human breast cancer cell line. *Anticancer Res.* **1997**, *17*, 3393–3401.
51. Zhang, D.D. Mechanistic studies of the Nrf2-Keap1 signaling pathway. *Drug Metab. Rev.* **2006**, *38*, 769–789. [CrossRef]
52. Zhuang, Y.; Wu, H.; Wang, X.; He, J.; He, S.; Yin, Y. Resveratrol Attenuates Oxidative Stress-Induced Intestinal Barrier Injury through PI3K/Akt-Mediated Nrf2 Signaling Pathway. *Oxidative Med. Cell. Longev.* **2019**, *2019*, 7591840. [CrossRef] [PubMed]
53. Trapani, A.; Mandracchia, D.; Tripodo, G.; Di Gioia, S.; Castellani, S.; Cioffi, N.; Ditaranto, N.; Esteban, M.A.; Conese, M. Solid lipid nanoparticles made of self-emulsifying lipids for efficient encapsulation of hydrophilic substances. *AIP Conf. Proc.* **2019**, *2145*, 020004.
54. Mandracchia, D.; Trapani, A.; Perteghella, S.; Sorrenti, M.; Catenacci, L.; Torre, M.L.; Trapani, G.; Tripodo, G. pH-sensitive inulin-based nanomicelles for intestinal site-specific and controlled release of celecoxib. *Carbohydr. Polym.* **2018**, *181*, 570–578. [CrossRef] [PubMed]

55. Cometa, S.; Bonifacio, M.A.; Trapani, G.; Di Gioia, S.; Dazzi, L.; De Giglio, E.; Trapani, A. In vitro investigations on dopamine loaded Solid Lipid Nanoparticles. *J. Pharm. BioMed. Anal.* **2020**, *185*, 113257. [CrossRef]
56. Carbone, C.; Caddeo, C.; Grimaudo, M.A.; Manno, D.E.; Serra, A.; Musumeci, T. Ferulic Acid-NLC with Lavandula Essential Oil: A Possible Strategy for Wound-Healing? *Nanomaterials* **2020**, *10*, 898. [CrossRef] [PubMed]
57. Mandracchia, D.; Trapani, A.; Tripodo, G.; Perrone, M.G.; Giammona, G.; Trapani, G.; Colabufo, N.A. In vitro evaluation of glycol chitosan based formulations as oral delivery systems for efflux pump inhibition. *Carbohydr. Polym.* **2017**, *166*, 73–82. [CrossRef]
58. Tripodo, G.; Trapani, A.; Rosato, A.; Di Franco, C.; Tamma, R.; Trapani, G.; Ribatti, D.; Mandracchia, D. Hydrogels for biomedical applications from glycol chitosan and PEG diglycidyl ether exhibit pro-angiogenic and antibacterial activity. *Carbohydr. Polym.* **2018**, *198*, 124–130. [CrossRef] [PubMed]
59. Arnao, M.B.; Cano, A.; Acosta, M. Methods to measure the antioxidant activity in plant material. A comparative discussion. *Free Radic. Res.* **1999**, *31*, 89–96. [CrossRef] [PubMed]
60. Béjar, J.; Porta, J.; Borrego, J.J.; Alvarez, M.C. The piscine SAF-1 cell line: Genetic stability and labeling. *Mar. Biotechnol.* **2005**, *7*, 389–395. [CrossRef]
61. Cerezuela, R.; Meseguer, J.; Esteban, M.A. Effects of dietary inulin, Bacillus subtilis and microalgae on intestinal gene expression in gilthead seabream (*Sparus aurata* L.). *Fish Shellfish Immunol.* **2013**, *34*, 843–848. [CrossRef]
62. Mosmann, T. Rapid colorimetric assay for cellular growth and survival: Application to proliferation and cytotoxicity assays. *J. Immunol. Methods* **1983**, *65*, 55–63. [CrossRef]
63. Livak, K.J.; Schmittgen, T.D. Analysis of relative gene expression data using real-time quantitative PCR and the 2(-Delta Delta C(T)) Method. *Methods* **2001**, *25*, 402–408. [CrossRef]
64. Morcillo, P.; Chaves-Pozo, E.; Meseguer, J.; Esteban, M.Á.; Cuesta, A. Establishment of a new teleost brain cell line (DLB-1) from the European sea bass and its use to study metal toxicology. *Toxicol. Vitr.* **2017**, *38*, 91–100. [CrossRef]

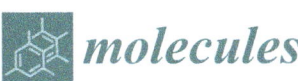

Article

Antioxidant Activity and Anti-Apoptotic Effect of the Small Molecule Procyanidin B1 in Early Mouse Embryonic Development Produced by Somatic Cell Nuclear Transfer

Wei Gao [1,2,†], Tingting Yu [2,†], Guomeng Li [2,†], Wei Shu [2], Yongxun Jin [1], Mingjun Zhang [1] and Xianfeng Yu [1,*]

1. Jilin Provincial Key Laboratory of Animal Model, College of Animal Science, Jilin University, Changchun 130062, China; wellkao@163.com (W.G.); jyx0429@126.com (Y.J.); mjzhang@jlu.edu.cn (M.Z.)
2. Group of Non-Human Primates of Reproductive and Stem Cell, Kunming Institute of Zoology, CAS, Kunming 650203, China; yutingting@mail.kiz.ac.cn (T.Y.); liguomeng@mail.kiz.ac.cn (G.L.); wishsjh@126.com (W.S.)
* Correspondence: xianfeng79@jlu.edu.cn; Tel.: +86-431-8783-6536
† These authors contributed equally to this work.

Abstract: As an antioxidant, procyanidin B1(PB1) can improve the development of somatic cell nuclear transfer (SCNT) embryos; PB1 reduces the level of oxidative stress (OS) during the in vitro development of SCNT embryos by decreasing the level of reactive oxygen species (ROS) and increasing the level of glutathione (GSH) and mitochondrial membrane potential (MMP). Metabolite hydrogen peroxide (H_2O_2) produces OS. Catalase (CAT) can degrade hydrogen peroxide so that it produces less toxic water (H_2O) and oxygen (O_2) in order to reduce the harm caused by H_2O_2. Therefore, we tested the CAT level in the in vitro development of SCNT embryos; it was found that PB1 can increase the expression of CAT, indicating that PB1 can offset the harm caused by oxidative stress by increasing the level of CAT. Moreover, if H_2O_2 accumulates excessively, it produces radical-(HO-) through $Fe^{2+/3+}$ and damage to DNA. The damage caused to the DNA is mainly repaired by the protein encoded by the DNA damage repair gene. Therefore, we tested the expression of the DNA damage repair gene, OGG1. It was found that PB1 can increase the expression of OGG1 and increase the expression of protein. Through the above test, we proved that PB1 can improve the repairability of DNA damage. DNA damage can lead to cell apoptosis; therefore, we also tested the level of apoptosis of blastocysts, and we found that PB1 reduced the level of apoptosis. In summary, our results show that PB1 reduces the accumulation of H_2O_2 by decreasing the level of OS during the in vitro development of SCNT embryos and improves the repairability of DNA damage to reduce cell apoptosis. Our results have important significance for the improvement of the development of SCNT embryos in vitro and provide important reference significance for diseases that can be treated using SCNT technology.

Keywords: procyanidin B1; mouse; SCNT; embryo; reactive oxygen species

Citation: Gao, W.; Yu, T.; Li, G.; Shu, W.; Jin, Y.; Zhang, M.; Yu, X. Antioxidant Activity and Anti-Apoptotic Effect of the Small Molecule Procyanidin B1 in Early Mouse Embryonic Development Produced by Somatic Cell Nuclear Transfer. *Molecules* **2021**, *26*, 6150. https://doi.org/10.3390/molecules26206150

Academic Editors: Stefano Castellani and Massimo Conese

Received: 30 August 2021
Accepted: 10 October 2021
Published: 12 October 2021

Publisher's Note: MDPI stays neutral with regard to jurisdictional claims in published maps and institutional affiliations.

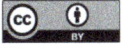

Copyright: © 2021 by the authors. Licensee MDPI, Basel, Switzerland. This article is an open access article distributed under the terms and conditions of the Creative Commons Attribution (CC BY) license (https://creativecommons.org/licenses/by/4.0/).

1. Introduction

Somatic cell nuclear transfer (SCNT) is a technology that transfers the nuclei of non-pluripotent differentiated somatic cells into mature oocytes, so that the transplanted oocytes have pluripotency and can develop into normal individuals. SCNT technology can be used to obtain embryonic stem cells derived from nuclear transfer (ntESCs); ntESCs were first obtained from mice [1], and then, scientists obtained ntESCs from rhesus monkeys [2]. Then, scientists used their experience in rhesus monkeys to obtain fibroblasts using fetuses or infants [3]. Both normal humans and type 1 diabetes (T1D) patients have produced ntESCs (nuclei of ntESC cell lines as donors and nuclei of adult somatic cells as donors for nuclear transfer) [4,5]. Studies have shown the potential use of ntESCs in cell replacement therapy [5]. Reproductive cloning has great potential to expand the population of important agricultural economic animals and save endangered animals without sacrificing donor animals [6–9]. Another potential application of SCNT technology is the generation of new animal models for human diseases [10,11]. Because of the huge application potential of nuclear transfer, in addition to improving the efficiency of nuclear transfer from the perspective of epigenetic modification, it is also very important to explore other aspects to improve the efficiency of nuclear transfer.

Oxidative stress (OS) is a challenging problem in embryo culture and development in vitro. When the embryos are exposed outside the body for manipulation, such as during in vitro fertilization (IVF) [12], intracytoplasmic sperm injection (ICSI) [13], parthenogenetic activation (PA) [14], and SCNT [15], they are subjected to oxidative stress. Under these conditions, embryos produce higher levels of reactive oxygen species (ROS) and reduce the levels of GSH [16], with disruption of the mitochondrial membrane potential [17]. Due to the increase in oxidative stress, a large number of free radicals (such as the hydroxyl radical (-OH)) and non-radical species (such as hydrogen peroxide (H_2O_2)) are produced in cells [18,19]. Again, free radical and non-radical species cause oxidative stress, among which H_2O_2 is the most typical non-radical species. H_2O_2 can be converted to -OH by Fe^{2+}/Cu^+ [18]. Free radicals can cause DNA damage and induce cell apoptosis. In order to enhance the antioxidant capacity of somatic cell nuclear transfer embryos, improve the in vitro development ability of somatic cell nuclear transfer embryos, and reduce the apoptosis level of somatic cell nuclear transfer embryos, it is very necessary to select antioxidants with strong antioxidant activity to be added to the in vitro culture system of somatic cell nuclear transfer embryos.

Procyanidin B1(PB1) is a small-molecule compound, extracted from a variety of plants [20–23], especially grapes [24–26], and it has strong antioxidant effects [22,24,27–29]. The antioxidant function of PB1 works by reducing the LPS-induced production of ROS and inhibiting extracellular signal-regulated kinase (ERK)1/2 and IkB kinase beta (IKKb) activity [30]. Additionally, the antioxidant function of PB1 also operates via the indirect activation of the nuclear factor E2-related factor 2 (Nrf2) antioxidant response element (ARE) signaling pathway, which reduces the in vitro and in vivo oxidant levels in HepG2 cells [22]. The antioxidant effects of PB1 can also reduce neuronal death via the attenuation of the activation of caspase-3 by inhibiting the activation of caspase-8 and caspase-9 [28]. Additionally, procyanidin B1 also has anti-inflammatory [30,31], and anti-tumor [32] effects. Furthermore, the antioxidant procyanidin B1 contained in grape extracts protects from chronic metabolic diseases such as diabetes and hypertension, and also prevents the development of chronic kidney disease (CKD) and cardiovascular disease [33]. Thus, PB1 has beneficial effects on health and disease due to its antioxidant effects, and PB1 also benefits the in vitro development of PA embryos [29]. So, PB1 may be a potential and beneficial small molecules drug in relation to SCNT embryo development.

2. Results

2.1. Determination of the Concentration of PB1 and the Effect of 50 µM PB1 on the Development of SCNT Embryos

SCNT embryos (Figure 1A) were cultured in KSOM media supplemented with 0, 20, 50, 80, 100, 120, and 150 µM PB1 to determine the blastocyst rate. Supplemented 50 µM PB1 significantly increased the blastocyst rate compared with the control group (38.12% ± 1.55% vs. 34.26% ± 1.60%, Figure 1D).

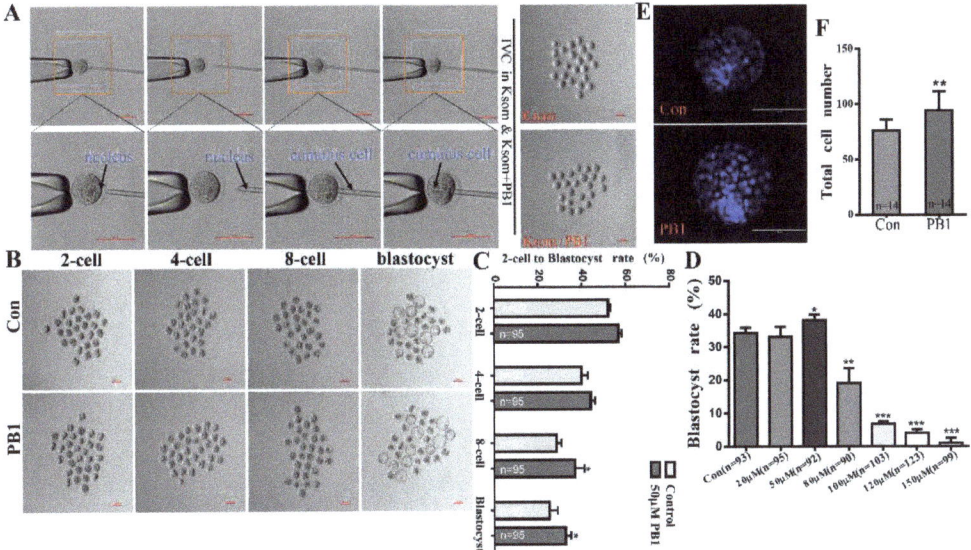

Figure 1. Effects of PB1 on SCNT embryo development. (**A**) Images of SCNT experimental protocol. Scale bar = 100 µm. Below is the display picture of the magnification. Scale bar = 200 µm. (**B**) Picture of 2-cell to blastocyst rates for control and 50 µM PB1 groups. (**C**) Histogram of 2-cell, 4-cell, 8-cell, and blastocyst rate for control and 50 µM PB1 groups. (**D**) Shows the blastocyst rate of control and 20, 50, 80, 100, 120, or 150 µM PB1-exposed groups. (**E**) Picture of blastocyst total cell numbers for control and 50 µM PB1 groups. (**F**) Histogram of blastocyst total cell numbers for control and 50 µM PB1 groups. Values shown are mean ± standard deviation of three independent experiments. * $p < 0.05$, ** $p < 0.01$ and *** $p < 0.001$. $p < 0.05$ indicates a significant difference between the two groups.

Supplemented 50 µM PB1 affected the development of SCNT embryos; at the eight-cell and blastocyst stage, the eight-cell and blastocyst rate were significantly increased compared with the control group (36.90% ± 4.36% vs. 27.34% ± 2.04%, $p < 0.05$; and 32.65% ± 2.46% vs. 25.27% ± 3.78%, $p < 0.05$, Figure 1B,C).

In regard to the total blastocyst cell numbers in SCNT embryos of cultured with KSOM medium supplemented with 0 and 50 µM PB1, the result showed that the group with supplemented 50 µM PB1 total blastocyst cell numbers were significantly increased compared with the control group (93.86 ± 17.52 vs. 76.00 ± 10.18, $p < 0.01$, Figure 1E,F).

2.1.1. ROS, GSH and JC-1 Ratio Levels in Two-Cell, Four-Cell, Eight-Cell and Blastocyst Embryos Cultured in KSOM Medium Supplemented in 50 µM PB1

At the two-cell stage, the GSH levels were significantly higher than those in the control group (37.03 ± 3.10 vs. 33.70 ± 3.65, $p < 0.01$, Figure 2D–F). At the four-cell stage, there were no significant results. At the eight-cell stage, the GSH levels significantly increased compared with the control group (41.99 ± 4.80 vs. 38.03 ± 3.52 pixels per embryo, $p < 0.05$, Figure 2D–F) and the ROS levels significantly decreased compared with the control group (4.74 ± 1.12 vs. 6.04 ± 2.12 pixels per embryo, $p < 0.05$, Figure 2A–C). JC-1 red represents the JC-1 polymer in the mitochondrial membrane, JC-1 green represents the JC-1 monomer outside the mitochondrial membrane, and JC-1 ratio is the ratio of JC-1 red to JC-1 green, representing the level of mitochondrial membrane potential (MMP). The decrease in MMP level is a landmark event in the early stage of apoptosis. At the blastocyst stage, the JC-1 ratio levels significantly increased compared with the control group (2.86 ± 0.91 vs. 2.32 ± 0.33 pixels per embryo, $p < 0.05$, Figure 2G–I) and the ROS levels significantly decreased compared with the control group (5.59 ± 1.40 vs. 7.25 ± 2.05 pixels per embryo, $p < 0.05$, Figure 2A–C).

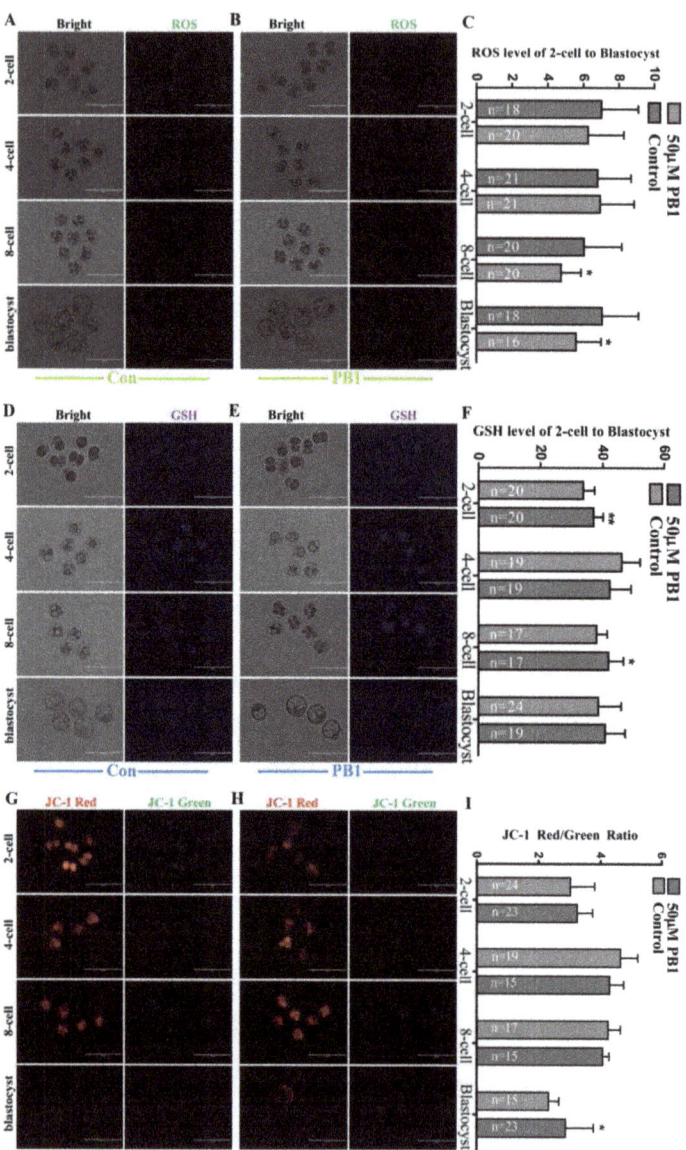

Figure 2. ROS, GSH and MMP levels in 2-cell, 4-cell, 8-cell, and blastocyst embryos. (**A**) Intracellular H2DCFDA-stained (ROS) in 2-cell, 4-cell, 8-cell, and blastocyst embryos of control group. (Scale bar = 200 μm). (**B**) Intracellular H2DCFDA-stained (ROS) in 2-cell, 4-cell, 8-cell, and blastocyst embryos of 50 μM PB1 group. (Scale bar = 200 μm). (**C**) The ROS signal intensity of control group and 50 μM PB1 group. (**D**) Intracellular CMF2HC-stained (GSH) in 2-cell, 4-cell, 8-cell, and blastocyst embryos of control group. (**E**) Intracellular CMF2HC-stained (GSH) in 2-cell, 4-cell, 8-cell, and blastocyst embryos of 50 μM PB1 group. (Scale bar = 200 μm). (**F**) The GSH signal intensity of control group and 50 μM PB1 group. (**G**) JC-red and JC-green in 2-cell, 4-cell, 8-cell, and blastocyst embryos of control group. (Scale bar = 200 μm). (**H**) JC-red and JC-green in 2-cell, 4-cell, 8-cell, and blastocyst embryos of 50 μM PB1 group. (Scale bar = 200 μm). (**I**) The JC-1 ratio (JC-red signal intensity to JC-green signal intensity) of control group and 50 μM PB1 group. The experiment was repeated three times, and values shown are mean ± standard deviation. * $p < 0.05$, ** $p < 0.01$.

2.1.2. The Levels of Catalase (CAT) in Two-Cell, Four-Cell, Eight-Cell and Blastocyst Embryos and the DNA Damage Repairability of PB1

At the two-cell and eight-cell stage, the CAT levels of the group cultured in KSOM medium supplemented in 50 µM PB1 were significantly higher than the control group (39.20 ± 3.07 vs. 36.92 ± 2.06 pixels per embryo, $p < 0.01$; 38.71 ± 2.94 vs. 35.13 ± 1.96 pixels per embryo, $p < 0.01$, Figure 3A–C).

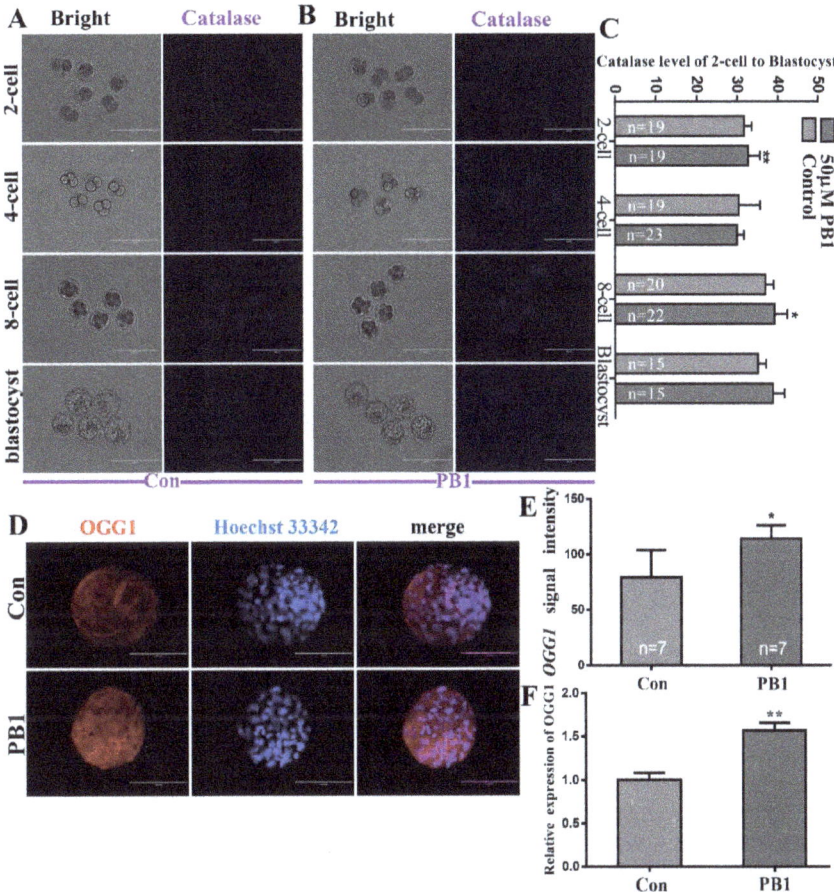

Figure 3. The levels of CAT in 2-cell, 4-cell, 8-cell, and blastocyst embryos and the DNA damage repairability of PB1. (**A**) The CAT levels in 2-cell, 4-cell, 8-cell, and blastocyst embryos of control group. (Scale bar = 200 µm). (**B**) The CAT levels in 2-cell, 4-cell, 8-cell, and blastocyst embryos of 50 µM PB1 group. (Scale bar = 200 µm). (**C**) The CAT signal intensity of control group and 50 µM PB1 group. (**D**) OGG1 levels in blastocyst, with proteins labeled with red fluorescence and blue indicating nuclei. (Scale bar = 100 µm) (**E**) Signal strength of OGG1 protein expression. (**F**) Relative expression levels of OGG1 mRNA in blastocyst. The experiment was repeated three times, and values shown are mean ± standard deviation. * $p < 0.05$, ** $p < 0.01$.

To determine the DNA damage repairability of PB1, we detected the OGG1 mRNA and protein expression in blastocysts; the results showed that the OGG1 mRNA expression was significantly increased and protein expression was increased in the 50 µM PB1 group compared with the control group (114.27 ± 11.86 vs. 79.12 ± 24.82 pixels per embryo, $p < 0.05$, Figure 3D,E, respectively).

2.1.3. Apoptosis of Blastocysts Cultured in KSOM Medium Supplemented in 50 µM PB1

To determine their ability to inhibit apoptosis of PB1, we evaluated P53 and caspase-3 mRNA and protein expression through immunofluorescence staining. There were no significant differences in the caspase-3 protein expression. However, the caspase-3 mRNA expression significantly decreased. Additionally, the P53 mRNA expression also significantly decreased. The expression of P53 protein in blastocysts decreased in the 50 µM PB1 group compared with the control group (73.47 ± 29.36 vs. 113.33 ± 50.85 pixels per embryo, $p < 0.05$, Figure 4A,B,D, respectively). The TUNEL results show that the 50 µM PB1 group showed a significant decrease in apoptosis level compared with the control group (7.67 ± 0.50 vs. 8.43 ± 1.15 pixels per blastocyst, $p < 0.05$, Figure 4C,F, respectively).

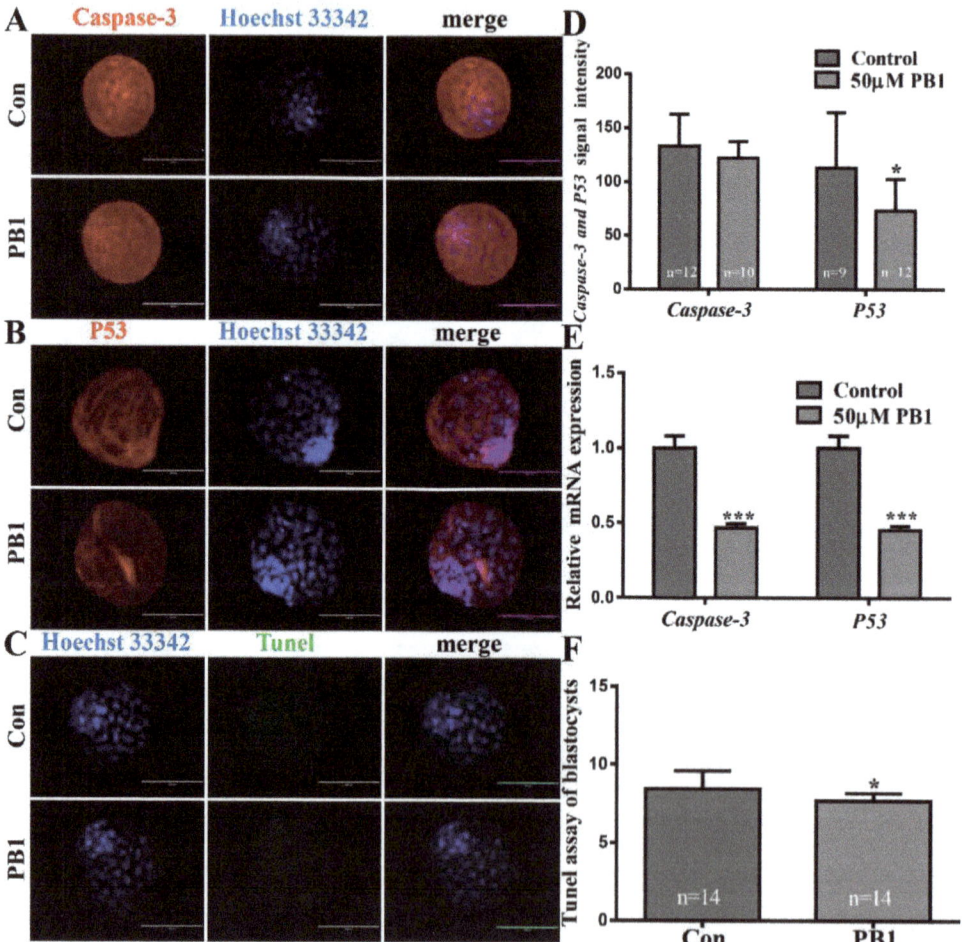

Figure 4. Apoptosis levels of blastocyst. (**A**) Caspase-3 and P53 levels in blastocyst, with proteins labeled with red fluorescence and blue indicating nuclei. Scale bar = 200 µm. (**B**) P53 levels in blastocyst, with proteins labeled with red fluorescence and blue indicating nuclei. Scale bar = 200 µm. (**C**) dUTPs labeled with green fluorescence and blue, indicating nuclei, in blastocysts. Scale bar = 100 µm. (**D**) Signal strength of caspase-3 and P53 protein. (**E**) Relative caspase-3 and P53 mRNA expression levels in blastocysts. (**F**) Percentage of apoptotic blastocysts. Values indicate mean ± standard deviation of three independent experiments. * $p < 0.05$, *** $p < 0.001$.

3. Discussion

Based on the results of previous studies [22,25,29], we can determine that PB1 is a small-molecule drug with antioxidant effects. In addition, we can confirm that it can improve the developmental ability of embryos during early development [29]. The in vitro development of embryos is inefficient compared to embryos derived in vivo [34]; embryos cultured in vitro exhibit increased ROS levels, especially SCNT embryos during the process of micromanipulation in vitro [35]. SCNT technology in embryos can also cause damage to mitochondrial membrane potential, DNA, and gene and protein expression [35,36]. This experiment focuses on the effect of PB1 on the early development of SCNT embryos to reduce the level of OS in SCNT embryos development. Firstly, the optimal concentration of PB1 during SCNT embryos development was selected. In view of the poor treatment effect of 100 µM (the concentration used in the in vitro maturation of pig embryos) [29] and the lower rate of blastocysts, we believe that the processing time for SCNT embryos in mice is longer; it takes 3.5 days. We finally determined the best concentration to be 50 µM. In the SCNT embryos treated at this concentration, the eight-cell rate and the blastocyst rate were significantly improved, and the number of blastocyst cells was more than that of the control group without PB1. The above results can show that PB1 at a concentration of 50 µM promotes the development of mouse embryos in vitro.

Scientists engaged in embryo development research have been committed to finding ways to reduce the oxidative stress of embryo development in vitro. The most common method is the addition of antioxidants to in vitro embryo culture medium, and the most representative one is vitamin C (VC); VC can reduce excessive ROS levels and reduce DNA damage and apoptosis [37]. With the progress of chemical extraction methods and the continuous discovery of new chemical molecules, increasing numbers of antioxidants have been discovered and used to improve oxidative stress in biological research, especially in the field of embryonic development, such as asiatic acid [38] and melatonin [39]. Using PB1 as an antioxidant, we analyzed the effect of PB1 on the level of ROS in SCNT embryos and found that in the late stage of embryonic development (eight-cell and blastocyst stage), the level of ROS showed a significant decrease, indicating that PB1 can play a role in scavenging ROS during development, and that it takes time to accumulate so that it can play a role. The finding that PB1 can reduce the level of active oxygen is consistent with the results of previous studies [29,30].

As an important regulatory metabolite in cells, GSH has an antioxidant effect which plays an important reducing role and is significantly increased during the two-cell and eight-cell stage of SCNT embryo development during PB1 processing, which is consistent with the previous results found in the maturation of pig oocytes [29], and the results are consistent with those found in intestinal normal-like cells [40]. The improvement of GSH level occurred earlier, in the two-cell stage. From this, we guessed that PB1 first increased the GSH level, and GSH then played a role to reduce the ROS level in the eight-cell and blastocyst stages. In addition, the endogenous source of ROS is mainly mitochondria. MMP plays a key role in mitochondrial respiration. When MMP is depolarized, a large amount of ROS is produced [29]. Additionally, GSH can also attenuate the depolarization of MMP [41]. Our results show that when the MMP in the blastocyst increases, there is a corresponding decrease in ROS in the blastocysts. In addition, in the process of redox in the cell, GSH and GSSG (L-Glutathione Oxidized) are continuously circulated under the action of the glutathione cycle. H_2O_2 can be degraded into H_2O through the process of converting GSH to GSSG, thereby reducing oxidative stress. Therefore, we believe that this process may be due to PB1 increasing the conversion rate of GSSG to GSH, and the underlying mechanism may be that PB1 promotes the activity of glutathione-related invertase, and decreases glutathione reductase level.

In the process of oxidative stress, some metabolic by-products, such as H_2O_2, can be produced [42]. These metabolic by-products of oxidative stress can cause serious damage to cells. H_2O_2 can cause cell DNA damage and cell apoptosis [43]. The decrease in CAT levels causes an increase in H_2O_2 levels [44]. We analyzed the level of CAT that can decompose

H_2O_2, and after PB1 treatment, the level of CAT in SCNT embryos (two-cell and eight-cell stage) showed a significant increase. The above results can show that PB1 increases the expression level of CAT, which in turn can reduce the production of H_2O_2. The possible mechanism is that PB1 activates the expression of the CAT gene, and the activated CAT gene promotes the level of CAT. CAT can reduce the H_2O_2 level, so the H_2O_2 harm is reduced, which reduces DNA damage and cell apoptosis, thereby reducing DNA damage and cell apoptosis. The blastocyst stage is the final stage of early embryo development and the longest PB1 treatment stage. Therefore, we tested the blastocyst DNA damage repairability and the level of blastocyst apoptosis in the blastocyst stage. Since the protein encoded by OGG1 (DNA damage repair gene) can protect DNA from ROS damage [45], we detected the expression of the OGG1 gene in blastocysts. We found that the expression of the OGG1 gene in blastocysts treated with PB1 was significantly increased compared with the group without PB1, and protein expression was also significantly increased compared with the group without PB1. We also carried out a correlation analysis on the level of apoptosis of blastocyst stage cells. Although immunofluorescence staining showed that the protein level of caspase-3 did not decrease significantly, the level of mRNA showed a significant decrease in the expression of caspase-3. Another representative apoptotic protein, P53, showed a significant reduction in protein and mRNA levels. TUNEL analysis also showed a significant reduction in apoptosis. The above results can prove that PB1 can enhance the embryo's DNA repairability and reduce cell apoptosis.

In summary, our results show that PB1 can reduce the level of oxidative stress during the early development of SCNT embryos, improve the embryo's ability to remove oxidative stress metabolites, and enhance the embryo's DNA damage repairability, thereby reducing the level of apoptosis and promoting the development ability of SCNT embryos.

4. Materials and Methods

4.1. Ethics Statement

The mice used for our experiments were kept in a comfortable environment (12 h of light, 12 h of darkness, 20 °C, moderate humidity). Our experiments complied with the Animal Care and Use Committee of Jilin University, Changchun, China (Grant No. SY202009068).

4.2. Reagents and Animals

We purchased all chemicals and reagents from Sigma-Aldrich (St. Louis, MO, USA), unless stated otherwise.

We used 8-week-old female offspring (B6D2F1) produced after mating of C57 BL/6J (female) and DBA/2 (male) as experimental animals for SCNT.

4.3. Drug Treatment and Experimental Design

Based on our and others' previous research on porcine [30] and on mouse embryos, we analyzed the concentration of PB1 by treating the embryos with 0, 20, 50, 80, 100, 120, and 150 µM. We found 50 µM to be the most suitable concentration. We dissolved PB1 in KSOM solution to make a storage solution with a concentration of 500 mM and stored it at −20 °C. When we came to use the working solution, we first diluted it to 500 µM with KSOM solution, and then diluted it to the required concentration.

Regarding MII oocytes after SCNT, we chose good SCNT embryos and transferred them to the new in vitro culture (IVC) KSOM medium (NaCl 555 mg/100 mL, KCl 18.5 mg/100 mL, KH_2PO_4 4.75 mg/100 mL, $MgSO_4$ $7H_2O$ 4.95 mg/100 mL, $CaCl_2$ $2H_2O$ 25 mg/100 mL, $NaHCO_3$ 210 mg/100 mL, Glucose 3.6 mg/100 mL, Na-Pyruvate 2.2 mg/100 mL, DL-Lactic Acid, sodium salt 0.174 mL/100 mL, 10 mM EDTA 100 µL/100 mL, Streptomycin 5 Penicillin 6.3 mg/100 mL, 0.5% phenol red 0.1 mL/100 mL, L-Glutamine 14.6 mg/100 mL, MEM Essential Amino Acids 1 mL/100 mL, MEM Non-essential AA 0.5 mL/100 mL, BSA 100 mg/100 mL) and KSOM medium supplemented with 50 µM of PB1. During the

IVC process, we counted the 2-cell, 4-cell, 8-cell, and blastocyst embryos at 24, 48, 48–60, 72–84 h after SCNT.

4.4. SCNT Protocol and Embryonic IVC

Each female B6D2F1 mouse was injected with 7.5 IU PMSG (pregnant mare serum gonadotropin; Merck Millipore, San Francisco, CA, USA) at 6:30 p.m. Forty-eight hours later, the mice were injected with 7.5 IU hCG (human chorionic gonadotropin; Sigma, St. Louis, MO, USA). After 13–15 h, we killed the mice by cervical dislocation, and the oviducts were removed and put into HCZB [CZB stock medium 94 mL (500 mL of CZB stock medium: special media ultra-pure water (470 mL), NaCl (2380 mg), KCl (180 mg), $MgSO_4 \cdot 7H_2O$ (145 mg), $EDTA \cdot 2Na$ (20 mg), D-Glucose (500 mg), KH_2PO_4 (80 mg), Na-Lactate (2.65 mL)), PVA (10 mg), Hepes (476 mg), $NaHCO_3$ (42 mg), $CaCl_2 \cdot 2H_2O$ 100× stock (42 mg), $CaCl_2 \cdot 2H_2O$ 100× stock (1 mL), Na-Pyruvate (3.7 mL), Glutamax (1mL)]. Next, the cumulus–oocyte complexes (COCs) were picked from the magnum tubae uterinae of the oviducts; we detached cumulus cells from B6D2F1 COCs with 2% hyaluronidase melted in HCZB, and washed them 3 times using HCZB. B6D2F1 MII oocytes were prepared for SCNT. The restoration, activation, and culture of embryos were carried out at 37 °C with 5% CO_2/95% air conditions, and all media overlaid with mineral oil were prepared for use in an incubator.

SCNT protocol: We removed the B6D2F1 MII oocytes nucleus using a micromanipulator in HCZB containing 0.5 μg/mL CB [HCZB + CB(Cytochalasin B)], and we used cumulus cells of B6D2F1 mice as donor cells. After that, we injected cumulus cells into B6D2F1 MII oocytes without nuclei. All manipulations were completed within 18 h after the HCG injection. Next, we put the SCNT embryos in KSOM medium to recover for 1 h, and then we put the SCNT embryos into Ca^{2+}-free CZB containing 10 μM of Sr^{2+} and 0.5 μg/mL of CB for 6 h. After that, we transferred SCNT embryos to a KSOM medium containing 0.5 nM of TSA(trichostatin A) for 4 h. Finally, we transferred SCNT embryos into fresh KSOM medium. The KSOM culture medium supplemented with 50 μM of PB1 was used as the experimental group, and the KSOM culture medium without any addition was used as the control group.

4.5. Assay of Total Blastocyst Cell Numbers

SCNT blastocysts were collected in order to count the total cell numbers. All blastocysts were washed three times using PBS-PVA (phosphate-buffered saline mixed with 1 g/L of PVA) and fixed with 4% (w/v) paraformaldehyde; fixed blastocysts were washed three times again and incubated in 5 μg/mL of Hoechst 33342 for 10 min at 37 °C. After that, blastocysts were washed three times again; washed blastocysts were mounted on a glass slide under a glass coverslip, and photographed using EVOS FL.

4.6. Immunofluorescence Staining and Quantitative Real-Time Polymerase Chain Reaction (Q-PCR) Protocol

Blastocysts (the control group and 50 μM PB1-treated group) were fixed with 4% (w/v) paraformaldehyde solution after being washed three times with PBS-PVA, and incubated with 0.2% (v/v) Triton X-100 for 15 min. Then, after being washed 3 times, all fixed blastocysts were incubated with 1% (w/v) BSA for 1 h. After they were fixed, blastocysts were incubated with anti-P53 (1:100; Abcam, Cambridge, UK), anti-caspase-3 (1:100; Abcam) and anti-OGG1 (1:100; GeneTex, Irvine, CA USA) antibodies at 4 °C overnight. The next day, they were washed 3 times and incubated with a secondary antibody (1:100; CY3-goat anti-rabbit; Boster Biological Technology, Wuhan, China) at 37 °C for 2 h. After being incubated with a secondary antibody and washed three times, we placed the blastocysts in Hoechst 33342 for 10 min at room temperature. Blastocysts were washed three times again; washed blastocysts were mounted on a glass slide under a glass coverslip, and photographed using EVOS FL (Waltham, MA, USA).

Total mRNA was extracted from about 20–30 blastocysts using a microRNA extraction kit (cat. 74181, Qiagen, Dusseldorf, Germany) and reverse transcribed into cDNA using a reverse transcription kit (Tiangen Biotech, Beijing, China). We added SYBR green fluorescent dye (Tiangen Biotech), cDNA, ddH$_2$O, and primers (Table 1) to a 96-well PCR Cell PCR-plate using an RT-PCR instrument (Eppendorf, Hamburg, Germany). The RT-PCR cycles were as follows: pre-denaturation at 95 °C for 15 min, 95 °C for 10 s (denaturation), 60 °C for 20 s (annealing), and 72 °C for 30 s (extension) for 45 cycles. The β-actin gene was used for standardization. Three independent experiments were performed; we used the 2 − ΔΔCt (ΔΔCt = ΔCt (case) − ΔCt (control)) method to calculate relative mRNA expression. The primer sequences used for real-time PCR are shown in Table 1.

Table 1. Primer sequences used for real-time PCR.

Gene		Primer	Sequence	Annealing
OGG1	[45]	Forward	CTGCCTAGCAGCATGAGACAT	61 °C
		Reverse	CAGTGTCCATACTTGATCTGCC	
P53	[46]	Forward	CAGCCAAGTCTGTGACTTGCACGTAC	61 °C
		Reverse	CTATGTCGAAAAGTGTTTCTGTCATC	
Caspase3	[47]	Forward	CCAACCTCAGAGAGACATTC	61 °C
		Reverse	TTTCGGCTTTCCAGTCAGAC	
β-actin	[48]	Forward	GGGAAATCGTGCGTGACATT	61 °C
		Reverse	GCGGCAGTGGCCATCTC	

4.7. TUNEL Method

Blastocysts (control group and 50 μM PB1 treated group) were removed from the KSOM medium, washed with PBS-PVA three times, and fixed with 4% (w/v) paraformaldehyde solution for 10 min, then washed 3 times, and transferred to 0.2% (v/v) Triton X-100 for 15 min. Then, we washed the blastocysts 3 times, and we incubated the blastocysts with TdT and fluorescein-conjugated dUTPs (In Situ Cell Death Detection Kit; Roche, Mannheim, Germany) in the dark for 30 min at 37 °C. After that, we washed the embryos 3 times and transferred the blastocysts to Hoechst 33342 for 5 min at 37 °C, and they were washed again three times with PBS-PVA. The processed blastocysts were fixed on a glass slide, and observed and photographed using EVOS FL.

4.8. ROS, GSH and MMP Level Assay

Two-cell, four-cell, eight-cell, and blastocyst embryos were collected to measure ROS, GSH and MMP levels. All the embryos (2-cell, 4-cell, 8-cell, and blastocyst) were washed 3 times to examine ROS levels, embryos were incubated with PBS-PVA containing 10 μM 2,7-dichlorodihydrofluorescein diacetate (H2DCFDA; Solarbio Life Sciences, Beijing, China) for 5 min, and after being washed three times, they were photographed using EVOS FL (green fluorescence, UV filters, 490 nm, Waltham, MA, USA). To detect GSH levels, 2-cell, 4-cell, 8-cell, and blastocyst embryos were incubated with PBS-PVA containing 10 μM 4-chloromethyl-6,8-difluoro-7-hydroxycoumarin (CMF2HC, Solarbio Life Sciences, Beijing, China) for 5 min, then washed three times, and photographed using EVOS FL (blue fluorescence, UV filter, 370 nm, Waltham, MA, USA). To detect MMP levels, we incubated all cells with PBS-PVA containing JC-1 fluorescent probe (Solarbio Life Sciences, Beijing, China) at 37 °C for 30 min. Cells were photographed using a fluorescence microscope (EVOS FL, Waltham, MA, USA) with 490 nm (green fluorescence) and 530 nm (red fluorescence) excitation, and the MMP was calculated as the ratio of red fluorescence (corresponding to activated mitochondria) to green fluorescence (corresponding to less activated mitochondria, J-monomer).

4.9. CAT Levels Method

Two-cell, four-cell, eight-cell and blastocyst embryos were collected to measure CAT levels; all embryos were washed 3 times, then incubated with 200 μL of solution 1 mixed with 1 μL of solution 2 (cat. BC0205, Solarbio Life Sciences, Beijing, China) for 5 min; after that, we placed the embryos in KSOM medium to recover for 5 min, and photographed them using fluorescence microscope (EVOS FL, Waltham, MA, USA) (blue fluorescence, UV filter) excitation.

4.10. Statistical Analysis

We repeated each experiment at least three times and analyzed the data using SPSS 20.0 software (IBM, Armonk, NY, USA). We used the Student's t-test to analyze comparisons of the two groups (treatment and control groups) and the ANOVA test to analyze comparisons of more than two groups and Dunnett's test to analyze Figure 1D. $p < 0.05$ was considered statistically significant.

5. Conclusions

The above research results indicate that as an antioxidant small molecule, PB1 can reduce the oxidative stress level during the early development of SCNT embryos by reducing the level of ROS and increasing the level of GSH. Additionally, it can improve the ability of embryos to scavenge free radicals such as H_2O_2, improve DNA damage repairability, and reduce the expression level of embryonic apoptosis markers, as well as reduce the level of apoptosis of SCNT embryonic blastocysts, thereby reducing the level of apoptosis. All the results support the idea that PB1 can be used as a supplement to promotes the development of SCNT embryos.

Author Contributions: Conceptualization, W.G. and X.Y.; validation, T.Y. and G.L.; formal analysis, W.S.; investigation, Y.J.; resources, M.Z. and X.Y.; data curation, W.G.; writing—original draft preparation, W.G.; writing—review and editing, X.Y.; visualization, W.G.; supervision, X.Y.; project administration, X.Y.; funding acquisition, X.Y. All authors have read and agreed to the published version of the manuscript.

Funding: This research was funded by the Jilin Province Science and Technology Development Project (No. 20180623023TC), Fundamental Research Funds for the Central Universities (No. 45119031C101).

Institutional Review Board Statement: The study was conducted according to the guidelines of the Declaration of Helsinki and approved by the Institutional Animal Care and Use Committee of Jilin University (SY202009068, 1 September 2020).

Informed Consent Statement: Not applicable.

Data Availability Statement: The data presented in this study are available on request from the corresponding author.

Acknowledgments: We thank Lin Jiangwei, Principal Investigator (Group of Non-Human Primates of Reproductive and Stem Cell, Kunming Institute of Zoology, CAS), for assisting with the experimental protocol.

Conflicts of Interest: The authors declare no conflict of interest.

Sample Availability: Samples are available from the authors.

References

1. Rideout, W.M., 3rd; Hochedlinger, K.; Kyba, M.; Daley, G.Q.; Jaenisch, R. Correction of a genetic defect by nuclear transplantation and combined cell and gene therapy. *Cell* **2002**, *109*, 17–27. [CrossRef]
2. Byrne, J.A.; Pedersen, D.A.; Clepper, L.L.; Nelson, M.; Sanger, W.G.; Gokhale, S.; Wolf, D.P.; Mitalipov, S.M. Producing primate embryonic stem cells by somatic cell nuclear transfer. *Nature* **2007**, *450*, 497–502. [CrossRef] [PubMed]
3. Tachibana, M.; Amato, P.; Sparman, M.; Gutierrez, N.M.; Tippner-Hedges, R.; Ma, H.; Kang, E.; Fulati, A.; Lee, H.S.; Sritanaudomchai, H.; et al. Human embryonic stem cells derived by somatic cell nuclear transfer. *Cell* **2013**, *153*, 1228–1238. [CrossRef]

4. Chung, Y.G.; Eum, J.H.; Lee, J.E.; Shim, S.H.; Sepilian, V.; Hong, S.W.; Lee, Y.; Treff, N.R.; Choi, Y.H.; Kimbrel, E.A.; et al. Human somatic cell nuclear transfer using adult cells. *Cell Stem Cell* **2014**, *14*, 777–780. [CrossRef] [PubMed]
5. Yamada, M.; Johannesson, B.; Sagi, I.; Burnett, L.C.; Kort, D.H.; Prosser, R.W.; Paull, D.; Nestor, M.W.; Freeby, M.; Greenberg, E.; et al. Human oocytes reprogram adult somatic nuclei of a type 1 diabetic to diploid pluripotent stem cells. *Nature* **2014**, *510*, 533–536. [CrossRef] [PubMed]
6. Beyhan, Z.; Iager, A.E.; Cibelli, J.B. Interspecies nuclear transfer: Implications for embryonic stem cell biology. *Cell Stem Cell* **2007**, *1*, 502–512. [CrossRef] [PubMed]
7. Loi, P.; Ptak, G.; Barboni, B.; Fulka, J.; Cappai, P., Jr.; Clinton, M. Genetic rescue of an endangered mammal by cross-species nuclear transfer using post-mortem somatic cells. *Nat. Biotechnol.* **2001**, *19*, 962–964. [CrossRef]
8. Kamimura, S.; Inoue, K.; Ogonuki, N.; Hirose, M.; Oikawa, M.; Yo, M.; Ohara, O.; Miyoshi, H.; Ogura, A. Mouse cloning using a drop of peripheral blood. *Biol. Reprod.* **2013**, *89*, 24. [CrossRef]
9. Wakayama, S.; Ohta, H.; Hikichi, T.; Mizutani, E.; Iwaki, T.; Kanagawa, O.; Wakayama, T. Production of healthy cloned mice from bodies frozen at −20 degrees C for 16 years. *Proc. Natl. Acad. Sci. USA* **2008**, *105*, 17318–17322. [CrossRef]
10. Doudna, J.A.; Charpentier, E. Genome editing. The new frontier of genome engineering with CRISPR-Cas9. *Science* **2014**, *346*, 1258096. [CrossRef]
11. Hsu, P.D.; Lander, E.S.; Zhang, F. Development and applications of CRISPR-Cas9 for genome engineering. *Cell* **2014**, *157*, 1262–1278. [CrossRef]
12. Kumar, S.; Mishra, V.; Thaker, R.; Gor, M.; Perumal, S.; Joshi, P.; Sheth, H.; Shaikh, I.; Gautam, A.K.; Verma, Y. Role of environmental factors & oxidative stress with respect to in vitro fertilization outcome. *Indian J. Med. Res.* **2018**, *148*, S125–S133. [PubMed]
13. Ashibe, S.; Miyamoto, R.; Kato, Y.; Nagao, Y. Detrimental effects of oxidative stress in bovine oocytes during intracytoplasmic sperm injection (ICSI). *Theriogenology* **2019**, *133*, 71–78. [CrossRef] [PubMed]
14. Luo, D.; Zhang, J.-B.; Li, S.-P.; Liu, W.; Yao, X.-R.; Guo, H.; Jin, Z.-L.; Jin, Y.-X.; Yuan, B.; Jiang, H.; et al. Imperatorin Ameliorates the Aging-Associated Porcine Oocyte Meiotic Spindle Defects by Reducing Oxidative Stress and Protecting Mitochondrial Function. *Front. Cell. Dev. Biol.* **2020**, *8*, 592433. [CrossRef] [PubMed]
15. An, Q.; Peng, W.; Cheng, Y.; Lu, Z.; Zhou, C.; Zhang, Y.; Su, J. Melatonin supplementation during in vitro maturation of oocyte enhances subsequent development of bovine cloned embryos. *J. Cell. Physiol.* **2019**, *234*, 17370–17381. [CrossRef] [PubMed]
16. Takahashi, M. Oxidative stress and redox regulation on in vitro development of mammalian embryos. *J. Reprod. Dev.* **2012**, *58*, 1–9. [CrossRef]
17. Al-Zubaidi, U.; Liu, J.; Cinar, O.; Robker, R.L.; Adhikari, D.; Carroll, J. The spatio-temporal dynamics of mitochondrial membrane potential during oocyte maturation. *Mol. Hum. Reprod.* **2019**, *25*, 695–705. [CrossRef]
18. Poprac, P.; Jomova, K.; Simunkova, M.; Kollar, V.; Rhodes, C.J.; Valko, M. Targeting Free Radicals in Oxidative Stress-Related Human Diseases. *Trends Pharmacol. Sci.* **2017**, *38*, 592–607. [CrossRef] [PubMed]
19. Firuzi, O.; Miri, R.; Tavakkoli, M.; Saso, L. Antioxidant therapy: Current status and future prospects. *Curr. Med. Chem.* **2011**, *18*, 3871–3888. [CrossRef]
20. Matta, F.V.; Xiong, J.; Lila, M.A.; Ward, N.I.; Felipe-Sotelo, M.; Esposito, D. Chemical Composition and Bioactive Properties of Commercial and Non-Commercial Purple and White Acai Berries. *Foods* **2020**, *9*, 1481. [CrossRef]
21. Zhang, X.; Li, X.; Su, M.; Du, J.; Zhou, H.; Li, X.; Ye, Z. A comparative UPLC-Q-TOF/MS-based metabolomics approach for distinguishing peach (Prunus persica (L.) Batsch) fruit cultivars with varying antioxidant activity. *Food Res. Int.* **2020**, *137*, 109531. [CrossRef] [PubMed]
22. Li, T.; Li, Q.; Wu, W.; Li, Y.; Hou, D.-X.; Xu, H.; Zheng, B.; Zeng, S.; Shan, Y.; Lu, X.; et al. Lotus seed skin proanthocyanidin extract exhibits potent antioxidant property via activation of the Nrf2-ARE pathway. *Acta Biochim. Biophys. Sin.* **2019**, *51*, 31–40. [CrossRef] [PubMed]
23. Gillmeister, M.; Ballert, S.; Raschke, A.; Geistlinger, J.; Kabrodt, K.; Baltruschat, H.; Deising, H.B.; Schellenberg, I. Polyphenols from Rheum Roots Inhibit Growth of Fungal and Oomycete Phytopathogens and Induce Plant Disease Resistance. *Plant Dis.* **2019**, *103*, 1674–1684. [CrossRef] [PubMed]
24. Fia, G.; Bucalossi, G.; Gori, C.; Borghini, F.; Zanoni, B. Recovery of Bioactive Compounds from Unripe Red Grapes (cv. Sangiovese) through a Green Extraction. *Foods* **2020**, *9*, 566. [CrossRef] [PubMed]
25. Sano, A.; Yamakoshi, J.; Tokutake, S.; Tobe, K.; Kubota, Y.; Kikuchi, M. Procyanidin B1 is detected in human serum after intake of proanthocyanidin-rich grape seed extract. *Biosci. Biotechnol. Biochem.* **2003**, *67*, 1140–1143. [CrossRef] [PubMed]
26. Mao, J.T.; Xue, B.; Smoake, J.; Lu, Q.Y.; Park, H.; Henning, S.M.; Burns, W.; Bernabei, A.; Elashoff, D.; Serio, K.J.; et al. MicroRNA-19a/b mediates grape seed procyanidin extract-induced anti-neoplastic effects against lung cancer. *J. Nutr. Biochem.* **2016**, *34*, 118–125. [CrossRef]
27. Zuriarrain, A.; Zuriarrain, J.; Puertas, A.I.; Duenas, M.T.; Ostra, M.; Berregi, I. Polyphenolic profile in cider and antioxidant power. *J. Sci. Food Agric.* **2015**, *95*, 2931–2943. [CrossRef]
28. Kanno, H.; Kawakami, Z.; Tabuchi, M.; Mizoguchi, K.; Ikarashi, Y.; Kase, Y. Protective effects of glycycoumarin and procyanidin B1, active components of traditional Japanese medicine yokukansan, on amyloid beta oligomer-induced neuronal death. *J. Ethnopharmacol.* **2015**, *159*, 122–128. [CrossRef]

29. Gao, W.; Jin, Y.; Hao, J.; Huang, S.; Wang, D.; Quan, F.; Ren, W.; Zhang, J.; Zhang, M.; Yu, X. Procyanidin B1 promotes in vitro maturation of pig oocytes by reducing oxidative stress. *Mol. Reprod. Dev.* **2021**, *88*, 55–66. [CrossRef]
30. Terra, X.; Palozza, P.; Fernandez-Larrea, J.; Ardévol, A.; Bladé, C.; Pujadas, G.; Salvado, J.; Arola, L.; Blay, M.T. Procyanidin dimer B1 and trimer C1 impair inflammatory response signalling in human monocytes. *Free Radic. Res.* **2011**, *45*, 611–619. [CrossRef]
31. Xing, J.; Li, R.; Li, N.; Zhang, J.; Li, Y.; Gong, P.; Gao, D.; Liu, H.; Zhang, Y. Anti-inflammatory effect of procyanidin B1 on LPS-treated THP1 cells via interaction with the TLR4-MD-2 heterodimer and p38 MAPK and NF-kappaB signaling. *Mol. Cell. Biochem.* **2015**, *407*, 89–95. [CrossRef] [PubMed]
32. Na, W.; Ma, B.; Shi, S.; Chen, Y.; Zhang, H.; Zhan, Y.; An, H. Procyanidin B1, a novel and specific inhibitor of Kv10.1 channel, suppresses the evolution of hepatoma. *Biochem. Pharmacol.* **2020**, *178*, 114089. [CrossRef]
33. Zhu, J.; Du, C. Could grape-based food supplements prevent the development of chronic kidney disease? *Crit. Rev. Food Sci. Nutr.* **2020**, *60*, 3054–3062. [CrossRef]
34. Ma, Y.; Gu, M.; Chen, L.; Shen, H.; Pan, Y.; Pang, Y.; Miao, S.; Tong, R.; Huang, Y.; Zhu, Y.; et al. Recent advances in critical nodes of embryo engineering technology. *Theranostics* **2021**, *11*, 7391–7424. [CrossRef] [PubMed]
35. Su, J.; Wang, Y.; Xing, X.; Zhang, L.; Sun, H.; Zhang, Y. Melatonin significantly improves the developmental competence of bovine somatic cell nuclear transfer embryos. *J. Pineal Res.* **2015**, *59*, 455–468. [CrossRef] [PubMed]
36. Hwang, I.S.; Bae, H.K.; Cheong, H.T. Mitochondrial and DNA damage in bovine somatic cell nuclear transfer embryos. *J. Vet. Sci.* **2013**, *14*, 235–240. [CrossRef]
37. Zhang, X.; Zhou, C.; Cheng, W.; Tao, R.; Xu, H.; Liu, H. Vitamin C protects early mouse embryos against juglone toxicity. *Reprod. Toxicol.* **2020**, *98*, 200–208. [CrossRef] [PubMed]
38. Qi, J.J.; Li, X.X.; Diao, Y.F.; Liu, P.L.; Wang, D.L.; Bai, C.Y.; Yuan, B.; Liang, S.; Sun, B.X. Asiatic acid supplementation during the in vitro culture period improves early embryonic development of porcine embryos produced by parthenogenetic activation, somatic cell nuclear transfer and in vitro fertilization. *Theriogenology* **2020**, *142*, 26–33. [CrossRef]
39. Qu, P.; Shen, C.; Du, Y.; Qin, H.; Luo, S.; Fu, S.; Dong, Y.; Guo, S.; Hu, F.; Xue, Y.; et al. Melatonin Protects Rabbit Somatic Cell Nuclear Transfer (SCNT) Embryos from Electrofusion Damage. *Sci. Rep.* **2020**, *10*, 2186. [CrossRef]
40. Attanzio, A.; D'Anneo, A.; Pappalardo, F.; Bonina, F.P.; Livrea, M.A.; Allegra, M.; Tesoriere, L. Phenolic Composition of Hydrophilic Extract of Manna from Sicilian Fraxinus angustifolia Vahl and its Reducing, Antioxidant and Anti-Inflammatory Activity in Vitro. *Antioxidants* **2019**, *8*, 494. [CrossRef] [PubMed]
41. Kelly-Aubert, M.; Trudel, S.; Fritsch, J.; Nguyen-Khoa, T.; Baudouin-Legros, M.; Moriceau, S.; Jeanson, L.; Djouadi, F.; Matar, C.; Conti, M.; et al. GSH monoethyl ester rescues mitochondrial defects in cystic fibrosis models. *Hum. Mol. Genet.* **2011**, *20*, 2745–2759. [CrossRef] [PubMed]
42. Del Rio, L.A.; Lopez-Huertas, E. ROS Generation in Peroxisomes and its Role in Cell Signaling. *Plant Cell Physiol.* **2016**, *57*, 1364–1376. [CrossRef]
43. Mizutani, H.; Hayashi, Y.; Hashimoto, M.; Imai, M.; Ichimaru, Y.; Kitamura, Y.; Ikemura, K.; Miyazawa, D.; Ohta, K.; Ikeda, Y.; et al. Oxidative DNA Damage and Apoptosis Induced by Aclarubicin, an Anthracycline: Role of Hydrogen Peroxide and Copper. *Anticancer Res.* **2019**, *39*, 3443–3451. [CrossRef] [PubMed]
44. Cheng, C.H.; Ma, H.L.; Deng, Y.Q.; Feng, J.; Jie, Y.K.; Guo, Z.X. Oxidative stress, cell cycle arrest, DNA damage and apoptosis in the mud crab (Scylla paramamosain) induced by cadmium exposure. *Chemosphere* **2021**, *263*, 128277. [CrossRef] [PubMed]
45. Mori, Y.; Ogonuki, N.; Hasegawa, A.; Kanatsu-Shinohara, M.; Ogura, A.; Wang, Y.; McCarrey, J.R.; Shinohara, T. OGG1 protects mouse spermatogonial stem cells from reactive oxygen species in culturedagger. *Biol. Reprod.* **2021**, *104*, 706–716. [CrossRef] [PubMed]
46. Kunimura, N.; Kitagawa, K.; Sako, R.; Narikiyo, K.; Tominaga, S.; Bautista, D.S.; Xu, W.; Fujisawa, M.; Shirakawa, T. Combination of rAd-p53 in situ gene therapy and anti-PD-1 antibody immunotherapy induced anti-tumor activity in mouse syngeneic urogenital cancer models. *Sci. Rep.* **2020**, *10*, 17464. [CrossRef]
47. De Santis, R.; Liepelt, A.; Mossanen, J.C.; Dueck, A.; Simons, N.; Mohs, A.; Trautwein, C.; Meister, G.; Marx, G.; Ostareck-Lederer, A.; et al. miR-155 targets Caspase-3 mRNA in activated miR-155 targets Caspase-3 mRNA in activated macrophages. *RNA Biol.* **2016**, *13*, 43–58. [CrossRef]
48. Kong, D.; Yan, Y.; He, X.Y.; Yang, H.; Liang, B.; Wang, J.; He, Y.; Ding, Y.; Yu, H. Effects of Resveratrol on the Mechanisms of Antioxidants and Estrogen in Alzheimer's Disease. *BioMed Res. Int.* **2019**, *2019*, 8983752. [CrossRef]

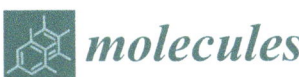

Review

Polyphenolic Flavonoid Compound Quercetin Effects in the Treatment of Acute Myeloid Leukemia and Myelodysplastic Syndromes

Cristiane Okuda Torello *, Marisa Claudia Alvarez and Sara T. Olalla Saad *

Hematology and Transfusion Medicine Center—Hemocentro, University of Campinas, Campinas 13083-878, Brazil; marisacalvarez@yahoo.com
* Correspondence: cris.okuda@gmail.com (C.O.T.); sara@unicamp.br (S.T.O.S.);
Tel.: +55-(19)-35218734 (C.O.T.); +55-(19)-35218733 (S.T.O.S.)

Abstract: Flavonoids are ubiquitous groups of polyphenolic compounds present in most natural products and plants. These substances have been shown to have promising chemopreventive and chemotherapeutic properties with multiple target interactions and multiple pathway regulations against various human cancers. Polyphenolic flavonoid compounds can block the initiation or reverse the promotion stage of multistep carcinogenesis. Quercetin is one of the most abundant flavonoids found in fruits and vegetables and has been shown to have multiple properties capable of reducing cell growth in cancer cells. Acute myeloid leukemia (AML) and myelodysplastic syndromes (MDS) therapy remains a challenge for hematologists worldwide, and the outcomes for patients with both disorders continue to be poor. This scenario indicates the increasing demand for innovative drugs and rational combinative therapies. Herein, we discuss the multitarget effects of the flavonoid quercetin, a naturally occurring flavonol, on AML and MDS.

Keywords: polyphenolic compounds; quercetin; hematological disorders; anti-proliferative effect; apoptosis; autophagy; epigenetic modifications

Citation: Torello, C.O.; Alvarez, M.C.; Olalla Saad, S.T. Polyphenolic Flavonoid Compound Quercetin Effects in the Treatment of Acute Myeloid Leukemia and Myelodysplastic Syndromes. *Molecules* 2021, 26, 5781. https://doi.org/10.3390/molecules26195781

Academic Editors: Stefano Castellani and Massimo Conese

Received: 26 August 2021
Accepted: 20 September 2021
Published: 24 September 2021

Publisher's Note: MDPI stays neutral with regard to jurisdictional claims in published maps and institutional affiliations.

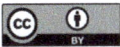

Copyright: © 2021 by the authors. Licensee MDPI, Basel, Switzerland. This article is an open access article distributed under the terms and conditions of the Creative Commons Attribution (CC BY) license (https://creativecommons.org/licenses/by/4.0/).

1. Introduction

Flavonoids are ubiquitous groups of polyphenolic compounds present in natural products and plants such as fruits, vegetables, grains, bark, roots, stems, flowers, tea, and wine [1]. These natural substances have been shown to present promising chemopreventive and chemotherapeutic properties with multiple target interactions and multiple pathway regulation against various human cancers. Polyphenolic flavonoid compounds can block the initiation or reverse the promotion stage of multistep carcinogenesis [2]. Flavonoids are usually classified into six main subgroups: flavone (baicalein, apigenin), flavonol (fisetin, quercetin), flavanone (eriodyctiol, hesperidin), flavanol (catechin, epicatechin), anthocyanidin (cyaniding, apigeninidin), and isoflavone (daidzein, prunetin) (Figure 1).

Quercetin (3,3′,4′,5,7-pentahidroxiflavonol) is one of the most abundant flavonoids (Figure 2) belonging to the flavonol subgroup, found in fruits, vegetables, tea, and red wine [3,4]. Quercetin is also found in medicinal plants including *Allium cepa* (Liliaceae), *Allium fistulosum* (Amaryllidaceae), *Apium graveolens* (Apiaceae), *Asopargus officinalis* (Aspargaceae), *Camellia sinensis* (Theaceae), *Capparis spinosa* (Capparaceae), *Calamus scipionum* (Calamoidaceae), *Centella asiatica* (Apiaceae), *Coriandrum sativum* (Apiaceae), *Ginkgo biloba* (Ginkgoaceae), *Hypericum perforatum* (Hyperiaceae), *Hypericum hiricinum* (Clusiaceae), *Lactuca sativa* (Asteraceae), *Moringa oleifera* (Moringa), *Morus alba* (Moraceae), *Nasturtium officinale* (Brassicaceae), *Solanum lycopersicum* (Solanaceae), *Vitis vinifera* (Vitaceae), and *Sambucus canadensis* (Adoxaceae) [5–7]. Quercetin has anti-inflammatory, anticancer, cardiovascular protection, antiviral, antidiabetic, immunomodulatory, antiallergy, and antihypertensive therapeutic properties, in addition to gastroprotective effects. Quercetin is a yellow-colored crystalline insoluble solid substance and has a bitter taste. Quercetin is slightly soluble in alcohol, aqueous alkaline solutions, and glacial acetic acid [5].

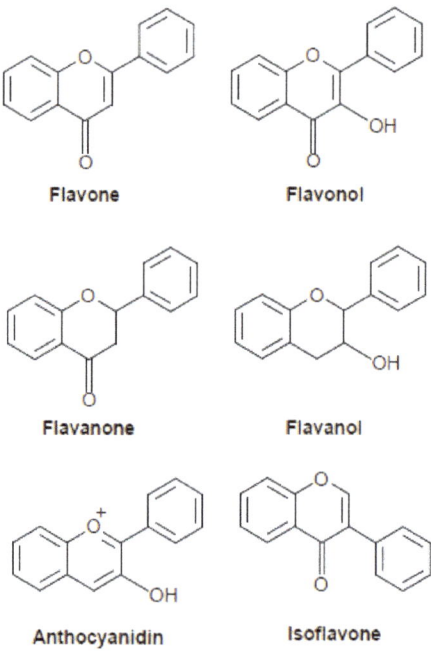

Figure 1. Structure of the major classes of flavonoids.

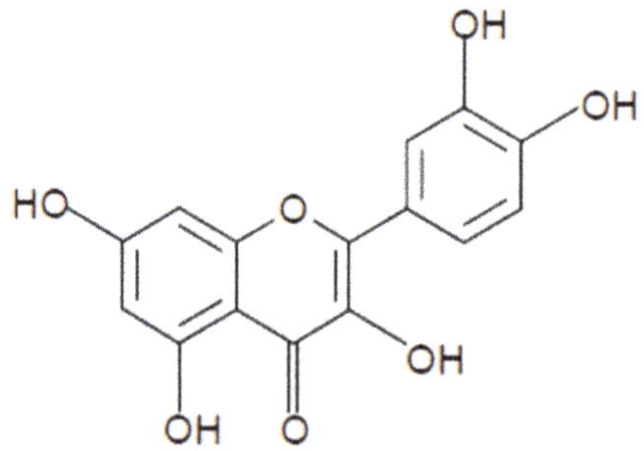

Figure 2. Structure of quercetin. Quercetin contains the basic structure of flavonoids: diphenyl-propane (C6–C3–C6) with hydroxyl groups attached to the rings. The official nomenclature according to IUPAC is 2-(3,4-dihydroxyphenyl)-3,5,7-trihydroxy-4H-chromen-4-one. Other names include 5,7,3′,4′-flavon-3-ol, sophoretin, meletin, quercetine, xanthaurine, quercetol, quercitin, quertine, and flavin meletin. Chemical formula: $C_{15}H_{10}O_7$.

Quercetin biosynthesis occurs though the phenylpropanoid metabolic pathway. Firstly, phenylalanine is converted to cinnamic acid; this reaction is catalyzed by the enzyme phenylalanine ammonialyase (Figure 3). Cinnamic acid undergoes the action of the enzyme cinnamate 4-hydroxylase to produce p-coumaric acid. This carboxylic group of synthesized p-coumaric acid undergoes ligation with CoA and produces 4-coumaroyl-CoA; this reaction is catalyzed by the enzyme p-coumarate:CoA ligase. Naringenin chalcone is produced by the enzyme chalcone synthase from one molecule of 4-coumaroyl-CoA and three molecules of malonyl-CoA to form the essential A and B rings of the flavonoid skeleton (i.e., C6–C3–C6). The chalcone isomerase synthesizes naringenin (a flavanone); this reaction enables the construction of the heterocyclic C ring. Flavanone 3β-hydroxylase undergoes hydroxylation of naringenin and produces dihydrokaempferol. Flavonol 3′-hydroxylase undergoes the hydroxylation reaction on dihydrokaempferol to produce dihydroquercetin. Finally, the activity of the enzyme flavonol synthase on dihydroquercetin catalyzes the biosynthesis of quercetin [8,9].

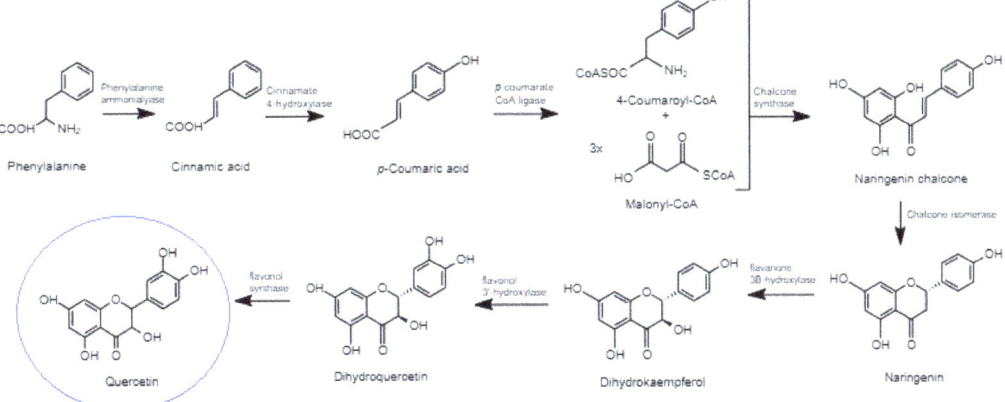

Figure 3. Quercetin biosynthesis.

Quercetin has high bioavailability due to its aglycone structure, i.e., without a sugar group. The daily intake of quercetin in the diet is estimated to be 5–40 mg/day [2]; however, these values may be as high as 200–500 mg/day in individuals who consume large amounts of fruits and vegetables rich in quercetin (apples, onions, and tomatoes) [10]. In food, quercetin is found in a glycosylated pattern with bioavailability, which depends on the type of glycoside present in the molecule. After absorption, quercetin is metabolized in different organs, such as the intestine, colon, liver, and kidneys, where the molecule is conjugated to methyl, sulfate, and glucuronic acid [11]. The total amount of quercetin available in the plasma deriving from the diet is usually in the nanomolar concentration range (<100 nM); however, upon quercetin supplementation, this availability may increase to the high nanomolar or low micromolar range. For example, after 28 days of supplementation with 1 g/day of quercetin, concentrations of up to 1.5 µM have been observed [12,13].

In vivo studies reported that low doses of 50–500 mg/kg per day of quercetin do not cause relevant adverse effects or carcinogenic effects in animals [13]. In humans, a phase I clinical study recommended a dose of 1400 mg/m^2, i.e., 2.5 g for subjects weighing 70 kg, administered via intravenous infusions for 3 weeks at weekly intervals. High doses exceeding 50 mg/kg (i.e., 3.5 g/70 kg) produced renal toxicity without signs of nephritis or obstructive uropathy [14]. Other studies found no adverse effects associated with oral administration of quercetin in a single dose of up to 4 g or after one month with 500 mg twice daily [15]. In 1999, the International Agency for Research on Cancer concluded that quercetin is not classified as carcinogenic to humans. In the United States and Europe, supplements of quercetin are commercially available, and the beneficial effects of quercetin supplements were reported from clinical trials [16].

Quercetin has been shown to have multiple properties capable of reducing cell growth in cancer cells due to a variety of biological activities including antioxidant, antiproliferative, apoptotic, and autophagic capacities.

Acute myeloid leukemia (AML) is an aggressive and malignant disorder of hematopoietic stem cells characterized by the clonal expansion of abnormally differentiated blasts of myeloid lineages, having unfavorable prognosis and short life expectancy [17]. Myelodysplastic syndromes (MDS) comprise a heterogeneous group of clonal hematopoietic neoplasms characterized by aberrant myeloid differentiation, ineffective hematopoiesis, refractory cytopenia, and increased rates of AML progression [18].

AML and MDS therapy remains a challenge for hematologists worldwide, and the outcomes of patients with both disorders remain poor. In MDS, the approval of azacitidine, decitabine, and lenalidomide over the last decade represented a major advance for this disease, despite the limited efficacy of these agents and most patients progressing within 2 years. Stem cell transplantation remains the only curative therapy; however, this option is associated with restricted efficacy and toxicity, and the lack or loss of response following standard therapies is related to dismal outcomes [18]. In AML, despite approximately 50% of patients successfully recovering from chemotherapy and bone marrow transplantation, elderly people are not capable of undergoing aggressive therapies, which demonstrates the urgent need for innovative drugs and rational combination therapies [19].

Herein, we discuss the multitarget effects of the flavonoid quercetin, a naturally occurring flavonol, on acute myeloid leukemia and myelodysplastic syndrome (Table 1).

Table 1. Summary of activities for quercetin in AML and SMD.

Activity	Cancer Cell Type	Notes	Reference
Antiproliferative, apoptotic	U937	In vitro	[20]
Antiproliferative, apoptotic, autophagic, antioxidant	P39	In vitro, xenograft	[21]
Antiproliferative, apoptotic, autophagic, antioxidant	HL-60	In vitro	[22]
Antiproliferative, apoptotic, autophagic, antioxidant	HL-60	In vitro, xenograft	[23]
Antiproliferative, apoptotic, autophagic, antioxidant	HL-60	xenograft	[24]
Apoptotic	U937	In vitro	[25]
Apoptotic	HL-60	In vitro	[26]
Apoptotic, antioxidant	HL-60, THP-1, NB4	In vitro	[27]
Apoptotic, antioxidant	HL-60, THP-1, MV4-11, U937	In vitro, xenograft	[28]
Apoptotic	U937	In vitro, xenograft	[29]
Apoptotic	U937	In vitro	[30]
Apoptotic	U937	In vitro	[31]
Antioxidant	THP-1	In vitro	[32]
Antioxidant	NB4	In vitro	[33]
Epigenetic modulation	HL-60, U937	In vitro, xenograft	[34]
Epigenetic modulation	HL-60	In vitro	[35]
Apoptotic	MV4-11, HL-60	In vitro	[36]

2. Multitarget Effects of the Flavonoid Quercetin on Acute Myeloid Leukemia and Myelodysplastic Syndrome

2.1. Antiproliferative Activity

Quercetin inhibits the growth and proliferation of cell lines from different types of cancers (prostate, lung, breast, colon, and neoplasms) [20,37–40], and several mechanisms have been proposed to explain these effects. These studies have identified the ability of this compound to interact with specific regulatory proteins such as cyclins A, B, D and E; cyclin-dependent kinases (CDKs); and CDKs inhibitors (p21 and p27). Depending on the cell type, quercetin is able to block the G2/M or G1/S transition of the cell cycle.

The CDK activity regulator p21 is an important cell growth arrest mediator that inhibits cell entry into the G1 phase in response to DNA damage and hampers the re-entry of G2 cells into the S phase by blocking cyclin E-CDK2 mediated retinoblastoma

(Rb) phosphorylation [41]. Rb is a direct substrate of CDKs and multiple mechanisms are known to potentially inhibit Rb phosphorylation, including proteasomal degradation [42] and inhibition of upstream Ras/RAF/MAPK or PI3K/Akt pathways [43,44].

Quercetin in vitro blocks cell-cycle progression at the G1 phase in P39 cells, a myeloid cell line derived from MDS-chronic myelomonocytic leukemia. Quercetin decreased the levels of CDK2, CDK6, cyclin D, cyclin E, cyclin A, and the phosphorylation of Rb accompanied by induction of p21 and p27 in these cells. In accordance, quercetin induced arrest in the G1 phase of the cell cycle in immunodeficient mice xenografted with P39 cells. The treatment of these mice with quercetin once every four days by intraperitoneal injection at 120 mg/kg body weight decreased the expression of phosphorylated Rb and the cyclin D and cyclin E proteins. Quercetin treatment also resulted in pronounced induction of p21 in xenografts [21]. In addition, pronounced ERK 1/2 and JNK phosphorylation in P39 cells and in P39 xenografts was induced. P39 cells treated with a combination of quercetin and selective inhibitors of ERK 1/2 and/or JNK (PD184352 or SP600125, respectively) decreased cells in the G1 phase, supporting the idea that ERK and JNK activation plays an important role in quercetin-induced G1 phase arrest in P39 cells [21].

Further studies have demonstrated that quercetin suppressed cell proliferation in the HL-60 cell line, derived from a 36-year-old woman with acute promyelocytic leukemia. Quercetin-induced G0/G1-phase arrest occurred [22,23] when expressions of cyclin-dependent kinases CDK2 and CDK4 were inhibited, and the CDK inhibitors, p16 and p21, were induced [23]. Quercetin also displayed antiproliferative activity against the HL-60 xenografts. After 3 weeks of quercetin treatment, a pronounced decrease in the protein levels of CDK2, CDK6, cyclin D, cyclin E and cyclin A were found. Quercetin treatment also resulted in Rb-phosphorylation loss [24].

The antiproliferative effect of quercetin was also demonstrated in the human promonocytic U937 cell line [20]. Quercetin induced antiproliferation and arrest of G2/M phase in these cells. An increase in the level of cyclin B in contrast to decreased levels of cyclin D, cyclin E, E2F1, and E2F2 was found in quercetin-treated U937 cells. Removal of quercetin from the cultures stimulated U937 cells to synchronously re-enter the cell cycle decreased the expression level of cyclin B, and increased the expression level of cyclin D and cyclin E, demonstrating that quercetin promotes reversible G2/M phase arrest. Quercetin further caused DNA fragmentation and increased the sub-G1 population in U937 cells [20].

2.2. Apoptotic Activity

The apoptotic effect of quercetin may result in the activation of multiple pathways in different types of cancer cell lines [25]. In vitro, quercetin led to pronounced apoptosis in the MDS-chronic myelomonocytic leukemia P39 cell line by modulating apoptotic cell death and stimulating the intrinsic and extrinsic apoptosis pathway [21]. Quercetin induced upregulation of the pro-apoptotic protein Bax and suppression of antiapoptotic proteins BcL-2, BcL-xL, and McL-1 in P39 cells. Furthermore, a decline in Rho123 fluorescence intensity and a release of cytochrome c from the mitochondria to the cytoplasm suggested that intracellular events related to P39 cell death caused by quercetin treatment are related to mitochondrial dysfunction and changes in the mitochondrial membrane potential ($\Delta\psi m$). In addition, significant enhancements in cleaved caspase-9, caspase-8, and caspase-3 were observed after quercetin treatment in P39 cells. Improvement in active caspase-8 and increased expression of FasL indicate that the extrinsic or death receptor pathway of apoptosis is activated by quercetin in P39 cells. The results obtained in vivo confirm these findings, since quercetin treatment resulted in the reduction in P39 cell viability and decreased tumor volume of P39 subcutaneously xenografted in immunodeficient mice. Quercetin caused apoptosis activation and decreased the expression of BcL2, BcL-xL, and McL-1 followed by increased Bax expression in P39 xenografts, as well as enhanced cleaved caspase-3 in P39 xenografts [21].

The apoptotic effect of quercetin was also studied in NOD/SCID mice xenografted with HL-60 AML cells. Quercetin reduced the expression of antiapoptotic proteins BcL-

2, BcL-xL, and McL-1, but increased the expression of the proapoptotic protein BAX in xenografts. Induction of caspase-3 activation was further observed after quercetin treatment [24]. Yuan et al. [22] showed that quercetin caused apoptosis in HL-60 cells by decreasing the protein expression of PI3K and Bax, inhibiting Akt phosphorylation, decreasing the levels of BcL-2, and increasing the activation of caspase-2 and caspase-3 [22]. Quercetin induced apoptosis in HL-60 AML cells by increasing the activation of caspase-9, caspase-3, and cleaved poly ADP-ribose polymerase (PARP). Cleaved PARP protein levels were also increased in tumors obtained from HL-60 xenografts [23]. Niu et al. [26] demonstrated that quercetin induced apoptosis in HL-60 cells in a caspase-3-dependent manner by regulating the expression of downstream apoptotic proteins Bcl-2 and Bax [26]. Quercetin further potentiated the apoptosis induced by the glycolytic inhibitor 2-deoxy-d-glucose (2-DG) in HL-60 cells. Cotreatment with quercetin and 2-DG elicited the opening of mitochondria pore transition, which preceded the triggering of apoptosis [27]. Quercetin induced the activation of ERK, and the inhibition of ERK by an ERK inhibitor abolished the quercetin-induced cell apoptosis in HL-60 cells, as confirmed by the activation of caspase-8, caspase-9, caspase-3, PARP cleavage, and mitochondrial membrane depolarization in these AML cells. In vivo experiments corroborated these findings by demonstrating that quercetin reduced tumor growth through activating the ERK pathway and the subsequent cell apoptosis in HL-60 xenografts [28].

The ability of quercetin to induce apoptosis via the mitochondrial pathway was also demonstrated in human promonocytic U937 cells: loss of mitochondrial membrane potential prompted the release of cytochrome c in the cytoplasm with the activation of caspase-3 [20]. Cheng et al. [29] reported that the administration of quercetin led to pronounced apoptosis in the human leukemia cell line U937 by Mcl-1 downregulation, Bax conformational change, and mitochondrial translocation that triggered cytochrome c release. To prove quercetin's effects, knockdown of Bax by siRNA was found to reverse quercetin-induced apoptosis and abolish the apoptosis and activation of caspase. Knockdown of Mcl-1 by siRNA improved Bax activation and translocation, and cell death induced by quercetin. Furthermore, in vivo administration of quercetin mitigated tumor growth and increased TUNEL-positive apoptotic cells in tumor sections of U937 xenografts. Quercetin also increased the expression of the pro-apoptotic protein Bax and inhibited the antiapoptotic McL-1 protein in xenografts [29]. Quercetin in combination with shHSP27 synergistically induced apoptosis by decreasing the Bcl2-to-Bax ratio in U937 cells [30]. The apoptosis induced in U937 cells occurred by downregulation of Mcl-1 acting directly or indirectly on mRNA stability and protein degradation [31]. Quercetin was also reported to cause the induction of PARP cleavage in the three AML cell lines: THP-1, MV4-11, and U937 [28]. Quercetin induced cell death by downregulating VEGRF2 and PI3K/Akt signaling; these pathways were related to quercetin's action on mitochondria and BCL2 proteins [36]. Increased VEGRF2 is related to chemotherapy resistance in human leukemia cells, and VEGRF2 reduction sensitizes AML cells to chemotherapy treatment, leading to an increase in mitochondrial mass and oxidative stress [45]. These findings reveal quercetin as a promising compound targeting VEGRF2. These data suggest that the ability of quercetin to induce apoptosis (both intrinsically and extrinsically) into cancer cells establishes quercetin, without a doubt, as a promising molecule in the field of oncology.

2.3. Autophagic Activity

Quercetin demonstrated autophagic activity on both acute myeloid leukemia and myelodysplastic syndrome cell lines. Quercetin was found to induce autophagy and cell death [46] and, apparently, autophagy activation is an attempt to rescue cells from induced apoptosis [47]. This flavonol may induce sirtuins [48], reactive oxygen species (ROS) production [49], and JNK 1/2; Mek/ERK [50], all of which are capable of influencing the regulation of the autophagic process. Another target is represented by PI3K pathway proteins, which may positively or negatively affect autophagic regulation. In addition, quercetin assists in the accumulation of hypoxia-induced factor (HIF)-1 alpha, which represses mTOR signaling and induces the expression of BNIP3/BNIP3 ligand, supporting the rupture of the Beclin-1/BcL-2 (BcL-xL) complex for activation of Atg7 and Atg12-Atg5 and the cleavage of LC3 [47]. Conversely, quercetin may further inhibit autophagic flow. This result was obtained by the inhibition of PI3K class III and the NF-κB pathway (which may inhibit or induce autophagy depending on the context) [51]. Another interesting property of quercetin is that, when in combination with other substances, it may potentiate autophagic and apoptotic effects [52].

Quercetin triggered autophagy both in vitro and in vivo in P39 cells in the MDS-derived leukemia cell line [21]. High acidic vesicular organelle formation was detected in quercetin-treated P39 cells. Quercetin increased the expressions of light chain 3 (LC3)-II, PI3K, Beclin-1, Atg5-Atg12, and Atg7 in P39 cells. The inhibition of autophagy in P39 cells using chloroquine (endossomal acidification inhibitor) triggered apoptosis but did not alter the modulation in the G1 phase, suggesting that quercetin-induced autophagy plays a protective role against apoptotic cell death in P39 cells but is not associated with the cell cycle [21]. In accordance with the in vitro results, quercetin increased the expressions of PI3K, Beclin-1, Atg5- Atg-12, and Atg7 in P39 xenografts. Increased cleaved LC3 was further detected in the tumor sections of xenografts by immunohistochemistry. Quercetin additionally dephosphorylated Akt and mTOR in P39 cells and P39 xenografts, underlining the functional importance of Akt–mTOR signaling in quercetin-mediated protective autophagy in P39 cells [21]. Quercetin was described to affect both mTOR activity and activation of PI3K/Akt signaling pathway, giving quercetin the advantage of functioning as a dual-specific mTOR/PI3K inhibitor. Akt-mTOR signaling is a frequently hyperactivated pathway in cancers and, as a key regulator of homeostasis, controls the essential pathways leading to cell growth, protein synthesis, and the autophagic process [53].

The induction of autophagy by quercetin on HL-60 AML xenografts was additionally described [24]. Quercetin increased the expressions of PI3K, Beclin-1, ATG7, and ATG12-ATG5 in HL-60 xenografts, and caused the pronounced induction of the LC3-I to LC3-II switch [24]. Chang et al. [23] reported the effect of quercetin on autophagy both in vitro and in vivo in the HL-60 AML cell line. Increased expression of LC3-II, decreased expression of p62, and formation of acidic vesicular organelles were found after quercetin treatment [23]. Decreased protein expression of PI3K and phosphorylated Akt were reported in the HL-60 cell line after quercetin treatment [22].

2.4. Antioxidant Activity

Quercetin is considered one of the most prominent dietary antioxidants [11]. The antioxidant effect of quercetin has been extensively described [54]. Quercetin is a potent scavenger of ROS, including superoxide (O^{2-}), and reactive nitrogen species (RNS) such as nitric oxide (NO) and peroxynitrite (ONOO–). These antioxidative capacities of quercetin are attributed to the presence of two pharmacophores within the molecule that have the optimal configuration for free radical scavenging: the catechol group in the B ring and the OH group at position 3 of the AC ring [11].

During antioxidative activities, quercetin becomes oxidized into oxidation products (QQ: ortho-quinone) and reacts with glutathione (GSH) to form 6-glutathionyl quercetin (6-GSQ) and 8-GSQ (Figure 4). Oxidation products such as semiquinone radicals and quinones have been well-described to display various toxic effects in vitro only due to their ability to arylate protein thiols [11]. The antioxidative mechanism of quercetin occurs primarily with the O_2 bond yielding the ortho-quinone and H_2O_2 radicals. Quercetin further reacts with H_2O_2 in the presence of peroxidase, decreasing H_2O_2 levels. In addition, the antioxidant capacity of quercetin depends on the availability of intracellular glutathione (GSH).

The antioxidative aspect of quercetin was associated with the amelioration of adverse side effects derived from cancer therapy, which is considered a suitable strategy for the prevention and treatment of cancer [55]. This property of quercetin was demonstrated in both acute myeloid leukemia and myelodysplastic syndrome.

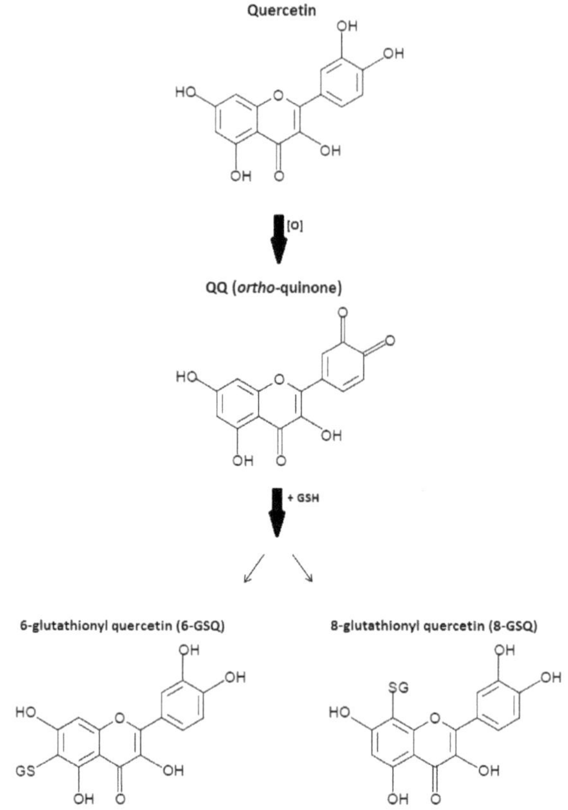

Figure 4. Antioxidative mechanism of quercetin. Quercetin is oxidized into oxidation products (QQ: ortho-quinone) and reacts with glutathione (GSH) to form 6-glutathionyl quercetin (6-GSQ) and 8-GSQ.

Quercetin decreased ROS levels in P39 MDS-derived leukemia cells induced by ter-butylhydroperoxide [21]. The antioxidative activity of quercetin in P39 cells could be explained by its capacity to interact with important antioxidant cellular defense systems, such as the Nrf2/Keap complex. This complex is connected with apoptotic pathways through the regulation of proteins from the Bcl-2 family. Keap1 appears to restrain and destabilize Bcl-2 and decrease Bcl-2:Bax heterodimers, facilitating cancer cells apoptosis [56].

Quercetin further reduced ROS and NO in LPS-stimulated human THP-1 acute monocytic leukemia cells [32]. In contrast, quercetin was shown to induce the cell death of HL-60 AML cells in vitro and in vivo through the induction of intracellular oxidative stress following activation of ERK. The authors demonstrated that mitochondrial superoxide and intracellular peroxide levels in HL-60 AML cells and HL-60 xenografts were higher after quercetin treatment [28]. In another study, quercetin caused disparate effects on ROS generation in HL60 cells, and did not affect GSH levels [27]. In a human acute promyelocytic leukemia NB4 cell line, quercetin increased the levels of Nrf2 in the cytosol, reducing them in the nucleus [33].

2.5. Epigenetic Modulation

An important feature of quercetin was recently reported: the ability to affect epigenetic regulators. Studies evaluating the epigenetic effects of quercetin in MDS are not available.

In AML, quercetin induced cell death in HL-60 and U937 leukemia cell lines by targeting the epigenetic regulators of pro-apoptotic genes [34]. The results showed that quercetin treatment abolishes DNA methyltransferase (DNMT) 1 and DNMT3a expressions partly due to STAT-3 regulation. Downregulation of class I histone deacetylases (HDACs) by quercetin was also detected. Treatment of cells with MG132, a proteasome inhibitor, in combination with quercetin prevented the degradation of class I HDACs compared to cells treated with quercetin alone, indicating increased proteasome degradation of class I HDACs by quercetin. Demethylation of the pro-apoptotic BCL2L11 and DAPK1 genes in a dose- and time-dependent manner was observed after quercetin treatment. Moreover, quercetin caused a global increase in acetylated histone 3 and histone 4, resulting in three- to ten-fold increases in the promoter regions of DAPK1, BCL2L11, BAX, APAF1, BNIP3, and BNIP3L. The increase in the mRNA levels of all these genes induced by quercetin corroborates these findings [34]. Briefly, the induction of apoptosis by quercetin appears to be related to the influence of this flavonoid on DNA demethylation activity, HDAC inhibition, and the enrichment in H3ac and H4ac in the promoter regions of genes involved in the apoptosis pathway, leading to their transcription activation.

Induction of FasL-related apoptosis by quercetin was described by transactivation through activation of c-jun/AP-1 and promotion of histone H3 acetylation in human HL-60 leukemia cells [35].

3. Conclusions

The natural polyphenolic flavonoid compound quercetin has emerged as a molecule possessing multiple properties (Figure 5). Quercetin has been proven to be an excellent antioxidant that also possesses antiproliferative, apoptotic, and autophagy capacities in AML in vitro and in vivo, in addition to exerting effects on epigenetic modulation. The effects on MDS are poorly understood as few studies have been performed. Clinical studies evaluating quercetin's effects on AML and MDS patients are not available. However, we conclude that quercetin has the potential to induce cell death in human AML and MDS-derived leukemia cell lines, both in vitro and in vivo, and that this capacity is related to a mechanism involving multitarget cooperation. The ability of this flavonoid to interfere with different mechanisms involved in cancer development indicates quercetin as an alternative for acute myeloid leukemia and myelodysplastic syndrome.

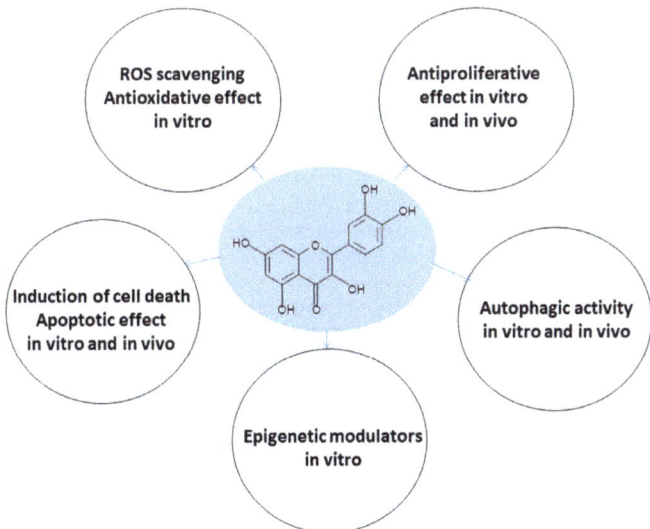

Figure 5. Multitarget effects of quercetin on acute myeloid leukemia and myelodysplastic syndrome.

Author Contributions: Conceptualization, C.O.T. and S.T.O.S.; writing—original draft preparation, C.O.T.; writing—review and editing, C.O.T., M.C.A. and S.T.O.S.; supervision S.T.O.S. All authors have read and agreed to the published version of the manuscript.

Funding: This research was funded by Conselho Nacional de Desenvolvimento Científico e Tecnológico (CNPq), grant number 303405/2018-0; and Fundação de Amparo à Pesquisa do Estado de São Paulo (FAPESP), grant numbers 2017/21801-2 and 14/08939-7.

Institutional Review Board Statement: Not applicable.

Informed Consent Statement: Not applicable.

Data Availability Statement: Not applicable.

Acknowledgments: The authors would like to thank Raquel S. Foglio for the English review. The figures were produced using BKchem 0.13.0 and ChemDraw 19.0.0 software.

Conflicts of Interest: The authors declare no conflict of interest. The funders had no role in the design of the study; in the collection, analyses, or interpretation of data; in the writing of the manuscript; or in the decision to publish the results.

References

1. Panche, A.N.; Diwan, A.D.; Chandra, S.R. Flavonoids: An overview. *J. Nutr. Sci.* **2016**, *5*, e47. [CrossRef] [PubMed]
2. Hertog, M.G.L.; Hollman, P.C.H.; Katan, M.B.; Kromhout, D. Intake of potentially anticarcinogenic flavonoids and their determinants in adults in the Netherlands. *Nutr. Cancer* **1993**, *20*, 21–29. [CrossRef] [PubMed]
3. Formica, J.V.; Regelson, W. Review of the biology of Quercetin and related bioflavonoids. *Food Chem. Toxicol.* **1995**, *33*, 1061–1080. [CrossRef]
4. Park, E.-J.; Pezzuto, J.M. Flavonoids in cancer prevention. *Anticancer. Agents Med. Chem.* **2012**, *12*, 836–851. [CrossRef] [PubMed]
5. Lakhanpal, P.; Rai, D.K. Quercetin: A Versatile Flavonoid. *Internet J. Med. Updat.* **2007**, *2*, 20–35. [CrossRef]
6. Li, Y.; Yao, J.; Han, C.; Yang, J.; Chaudhry, M.T.; Wang, S.; Liu, H.; Yin, Y. Quercetin, Inflammation and Immunity. *Nutrients* **2016**, *8*, 167. [CrossRef]
7. Lwashina, T. The Structure and Distribution of the Flavonoids in Plants. *J. Plant Res.* **2000**, *113*, 287–299. [CrossRef]
8. Singh, P.; Arif, Y.; Bajguz, A.; Hayat, S. The role of quercetin in plants. *Plant Physiol. Biochem.* **2021**, *166*, 10–19. [CrossRef]
9. Nabavi, S.M.; Šamec, D.; Tomczyk, M.; Milella, L.; Russo, D.; Habtemariam, S.; Suntar, I.; Rastrelli, L.; Daglia, M.; Xiao, J.; et al. Flavonoid biosynthetic pathways in plants: Versatile targets for metabolic engineering. *Biotechnol. Adv.* **2020**, *38*, 107316. [CrossRef]
10. Harwood, M.; Danielewska-Nikiel, B.; Borzelleca, J.F.; Flamm, G.W.; Williams, G.M.; Lines, T.C. A critical review of the data related to the safety of quercetin and lack of evidence of in vivo toxicity, including lack of genotoxic/carcinogenic properties. *Food Chem. Toxicol.* **2007**, *45*, 2179–2205. [CrossRef]
11. Boots, A.W.; Haenen, G.R.M.M.; Bast, A. Health effects of quercetin: From antioxidant to nutraceutical. *Eur. J. Pharmacol.* **2008**, *585*, 325–337. [CrossRef]
12. Conquer, J.A.; Maiani, G.; Azzini, E.; Raguzzini, A.; Holub, B.J. Supplementation with Quercetin Markedly Increases Plasma Quercetin Concentration without Effect on Selected Risk Factors for Heart Disease in Healthy Subjects. *J. Nutr.* **1998**, *128*, 593–597. [CrossRef]
13. Manach, C.; Williamson, G.; Morand, C.; Scalbert, A.; Rémésy, C. Bioavailability and bioefficacy of polyphenols in humans. I. Review of 97 bioavailability studies. *Am. J. Clin. Nutr.* **2005**, *81*, 230S–242S. [CrossRef] [PubMed]
14. Ferry, D.R.; Smith, A.; Malkhandi, J.; Fyfe, D.W.; de Takats, P.G.; Anderson, D.; Baker, J.; Kerr, D.J. Phase I clinical trial of the flavonoid quercetin: Pharmacokinetics and evidence for in vivo tyrosine kinase inhibition. *Clin. Cancer Res.* **1996**, *2*, 659–668.
15. Lamson, D.W.; Brignall, M.S. Antioxidants and cancer, part 3: Quercetin. *Altern. Med. Rev.* **2000**, *5*, 196–208. [PubMed]
16. Okamoto, T. Safety of quercetin for clinical application (Review). *Int. J. Mol. Med.* **2005**, *16*, 275–278. [CrossRef]
17. Short, N.J.; Rytting, M.E.; Cortes, J.E. Acute myeloid leukaemia. *Lancet* **2018**, *392*, 593–606. [CrossRef]
18. Zeidan, A.M.; Linhares, Y.; Gore, S.D. Current therapy of myelodysplastic syndromes. *Blood Rev.* **2013**, *27*, 243–259. [CrossRef]
19. Döhner, H.; Estey, E.; Grimwade, D.; Amadori, S.; Appelbaum, F.R.; Büchner, T.; Dombret, H.; Ebert, B.L.; Fenaux, P.; Larson, R.A.; et al. Diagnosis and management of AML in adults: 2017 ELN recommendations from an international expert panel. *Blood* **2017**, *129*, 424–447. [CrossRef] [PubMed]
20. Lee, T.J.; Kim, O.H.; Kim, Y.H.; Lim, J.H.; Kim, S.; Park, J.-W.; Kwon, T.K. Quercetin arrests G2/M phase and induces caspase-dependent cell death in U937 cells. *Cancer Lett.* **2006**, *240*, 234–242. [CrossRef] [PubMed]
21. Maso, V.; Calgarotto, A.K.; Franchi, G.C.; Nowill, A.E.; Filho, P.L.; Vassallo, J.; Saad, S.T.O. Multitarget Effects of Quercetin in Leukemia. *Cancer Prev. Res.* **2014**, *7*, 1240–1250. [CrossRef] [PubMed]
22. Yuan, Z.; Long, C.; Junming, T.; Qihuan, L.; Youshun, Z.; Chan, Z. Quercetin-induced apoptosis of HL-60 cells by reducing PI3K/Akt. *Mol. Biol. Rep.* **2012**, *39*, 7785–7793. [CrossRef] [PubMed]

23. Chang, J.L.; Chow, J.M.; Chang, J.H.; Wen, Y.C.; Lin, Y.W.; Yang, S.F.; Lee, W.J.; Chien, M.H. Quercetin simultaneously induces G_0/G_1-phase arrest and caspase-mediated crosstalk between apoptosis and autophagy in human leukemia HL-60 cells. *Environ. Toxicol.* **2017**, *32*, 1857–1868. [CrossRef] [PubMed]
24. Calgarotto, A.K.; Maso, V.; Junior, G.C.F.; Nowill, A.E.; Filho, P.L.; Vassallo, J.; Saad, S.T.O. Antitumor activities of Quercetin and Green Tea in xenografts of human leukemia HL60 cells. *Sci. Rep.* **2018**, *8*, 3459. [CrossRef] [PubMed]
25. Hashemzaei, M.; Far, A.D.; Yari, A.; Heravi, R.E.; Tabrizian, K.; Taghdisi, S.M.; Sadegh, S.E.; Tsarouhas, K.; Kouretas, D.; Tzanakakis, G.; et al. Anticancer and apoptosis-inducing effects of quercetin in vitro and in vivo. *Oncol. Rep.* **2017**, *38*, 819–828. [CrossRef]
26. Niu, G.; Yin, S.; Xie, S.; Li, Y.; Nie, D.; Ma, L.; Wang, X.; Wu, Y. Quercetin induces apoptosis by activating caspase-3 and regulating Bcl-2 and cyclooxygenase-2 pathways in human HL-60 cells. *Acta Biochim. Biophys. Sin.* **2011**, *43*, 30–37. [CrossRef]
27. De Blas, E.; Estañ, M.C.; del Carmen Gómez de Frutos, M.; Ramos, J.; del Carmen Boyano-Adánez, M.; Aller, P. Selected polyphenols potentiate the apoptotic efficacy of glycolytic inhibitors in human acute myeloid leukemia cell lines. Regulation by protein kinase activities. *Cancer Cell Int.* **2016**, *16*, 70. [CrossRef]
28. Lee, W.J.; Hsiao, M.; Chang, J.L.; Yang, S.F.; Tseng, T.H.; Cheng, C.W.; Chow, J.M.; Lin, K.H.; Lin, Y.W.; Liu, C.C.; et al. Quercetin induces mitochondrial-derived apoptosis via reactive oxygen species-mediated ERK activation in HL-60 leukemia cells and xenograft. *Arch. Toxicol.* **2015**, *89*, 1103–1117. [CrossRef]
29. Cheng, S.; Gao, N.; Zhang, Z.; Chen, G.; Budhraja, A.; Ke, Z.; Son, Y.O.; Wang, X.; Luo, J.; Shi, X. Quercetin Induces Tumor-Selective Apoptosis through Downregulation of Mcl-1 and Activation of Bax. *Clin. Cancer Res.* **2010**, *16*, 5679–5691. [CrossRef]
30. Chen, X.; Dong, X.S.; Gao, H.Y.; Jing, Y.F.; Jin, Y.L.; Chang, Y.Y.; Chen, L.Y.; Wang, J.H. Suppression of HSP27 increases the anti-tumor effects of quercetin in human leukemia U937 cells. *Mol. Med. Rep.* **2016**, *13*, 689–696. [CrossRef]
31. Spagnuolo, C.; Cerella, C.; Russo, M.; Chateauvieux, S.; Diederich, M.; Russo, G.L. Quercetin downregulates Mcl-1 by acting on mRNA stability and protein degradation. *Br. J. Cancer* **2011**, *105*, 221–230. [CrossRef]
32. Zhang, M.; Swarts, S.G.; Yin, L.; Liu, C.; Tian, Y.; Cao, Y.; Swarts, M.; Yang, S.; Zhang, S.B.; Zhang, K.; et al. Antioxidant Properties of Quercetin. *Adv. Exp. Med. Biol.* **2011**, *701*, 283–289.
33. Rubio, V.; García-Pérez, A.I.; Herráez, A.; Diez, J.C. Different roles of Nrf2 and NFKB in the antioxidant imbalance produced by esculetin or quercetin on NB4 leukemia cells. *Chem. Biol. Interact.* **2018**, *294*, 158–166. [CrossRef]
34. Alvarez, M.C.; Maso, V.; Torello, C.O.; Ferro, K.P.; Saad, S.T.O. The polyphenol quercetin induces cell death in leukemia by targeting epigenetic regulators of pro-apoptotic genes. *Clin. Epigenet.* **2018**, *10*, 1–11. [CrossRef] [PubMed]
35. Tseng, W.-J.; Chen, Y.-R.; Tseng, T.-H. Quercetin induces FasL-related apoptosis, in part, through promotion of histone H3 acetylation in human leukemia HL-60 cells. *Oncol. Rep.* **2011**, *25*, 583–591. [CrossRef] [PubMed]
36. Shi, H.; Li, X.Y.; Chen, Y.; Zhang, X.; Wu, Y.; Wang, Z.X.; Chen, P.H.; Dai, H.Q.; Feng, J.; Chatterjee, S.; et al. Quercetin Induces Apoptosis via Downregulation of Vascular Endothelial Growth Factor/Akt Signaling Pathway in Acute Myeloid Leukemia Cells. *Front. Pharmacol.* **2020**, *11*. [CrossRef] [PubMed]
37. Yang, J.H.; Hsia, T.C.; Kuo, H.M.; Chao, P.D.L.; Chou, C.C.; Wei, Y.H.; Chung, J.G. Inhibition of lung cancer cell growth by quercetin glucuronides via G2/M arrest and induction of apoptosis. *Drug Metab. Dispos.* **2006**, *34*, 296–304. [CrossRef] [PubMed]
38. Choi, J.A.; Kim, J.Y.; Lee, J.Y.; Kang, C.M.; Kwon, H.J.; Yoo, Y.D.; Kim, T.W.; Lee, Y.S.; Lee, S.J. Induction of cell cycle arrest and apoptosis in human breast cancer cells by quercetin. *Int. J. Oncol.* **2001**, *19*, 837–844. [CrossRef]
39. Ong, C.S.; Tran, E.; Nguyen, T.T.T.; Ong, C.K.; Lee, S.K.; Lee, J.J.; Ng, C.P.; Leong, C.; Huynh, H. Quercetin-induced growth inhibition and cell death in nasopharyngeal carcinoma cells are associated with increase in Bad and hypophosphorylated retinoblastoma expressions. *Oncol. Rep.* **2004**, *11*, 727–733. [CrossRef]
40. Beniston, R.G.; Campo, M.S. Quercetin elevates p27Kip1 and arrests both primary and HPV16 E6/E7 transformed human keratinocytes in G1. *Oncogene* **2003**, *22*, 5504–5514. [CrossRef]
41. Mitrea, D.M.; Yoon, M.-K.; Ou, L.; Kriwacki, R.W. Disorder-function relationships for the cell cycle regulatory proteins p21 and p27. *Biol. Chem.* **2012**, *393*, 259–274. [CrossRef]
42. Ying, H.; Xiao, Z.-X.J. Targeting Retinoblastoma Protein for Degradation by Proteasomes. *Cell Cycle* **2006**, *5*, 506–508. [PubMed]
43. Bradham, C.; McClay, D.R. p38 MAPK in Development and cancer. *Cell Cycle* **2006**, *5*, 824–828. [CrossRef] [PubMed]
44. Liang, J.; Slingerland, J.M. Multiple roles of the PI3K/PKB (Akt) pathway in cell cycle progression. *Cell Cycle* **2003**, *2*, 339–345. [CrossRef]
45. Nóbrega-Pereira, S.; Caiado, F.; Carvalho, T.; Matias, I.; Graça, G.; Gonçalves, L.G.; Silva-Santos, B.; Norell, H.; Dias, S. VEGFR2–mediated reprogramming of mitochondrial metabolism regulates the sensitivity of acute myeloid leukemia to chemotherapy. *Cancer Res.* **2018**, *78*, 731–741. [CrossRef] [PubMed]
46. Klappan, A.K.; Hones, S.; Mylonas, I.; Brüning, A. Proteasome inhibition by quercetin triggers macroautophagy and blocks mTOR activity. *Histochem. Cell Biol.* **2012**, *137*, 25–36.
47. Wang, K.; Liu, R.; Li, J.; Mao, J.; Lei, Y.; Wu, J.; Zeng, J.; Zhang, T.; Wu, H.; Chen, L.; et al. Quercetin induces protective autophagy in gastric cancer cells: Involvement of Akt-mTOR- and hypoxia-induced factor 1α-mediated signaling. *Autophagy* **2011**, *7*, 966–978. [CrossRef]
48. Howitz, K.T.; Bitterman, K.J.; Cohen, H.Y.; Lamming, D.W.; Lavu, S.; Wood, J.G.; Zipkin, R.E.; Chung, P.; Kisielewski, A.; Zhang, L.-L.; et al. Small molecule activators of sirtuins extend Saccharomyces cerevisiae lifespan. *Nature* **2003**, *425*, 191–196.

49. Mertens-Talcott, S.U.; Bomser, J.A.; Romero, C.; Talcott, S.T.; Percival, S.S. Ellagic Acid Potentiates the Effect of Quercetin on p21waf1/cip1, p53, and MAP-Kinases without Affecting Intracellular Generation of Reactive Oxygen Species In Vitro. *J. Nutr.* **2005**, *135*, 609–614. [CrossRef]
50. Nguyen, T.T.T.; Tran, E.; Nguyen, T.H.; Do, P.T.; Huynh, T.H.; Huynh, H. The role of activated MEK-ERK pathway in quercetin-induced growth inhibition and apoptosis in A549 lung cancer cells. *Carcinogenesis* **2003**, *25*, 647–659. [CrossRef]
51. Gordon, P.B.; Holen, I.; Seglen, P.O. Protection by naringin and some other flavonoids of hepatocytic autophagy and endocytosis against inhibition by okadaic acid. *J. Biol. Chem.* **1995**, *270*, 5830–5838. [CrossRef] [PubMed]
52. Jakubowicz-Gil, J.; Langner, E.; Wertel, I.; Piersiak, T.; Rzeski, W. Temozolomide, quercetin and cell death in the MOGGCCM astrocytoma cell line. *Chem. Biol. Interact.* **2010**, *188*, 190–203. [CrossRef] [PubMed]
53. Kim, Y.-H.; Lee, Y.J. TRAIL apoptosis is enhanced by quercetin through Akt dephosphorylation. *J. Cell. Biochem.* **2007**, *100*, 998–1009. [CrossRef]
54. Vargas, A.J.; Burd, R. Hormesis and synergy: Pathways and mechanisms of quercetin in cancer prevention and management. *Nutr. Rev.* **2010**, *68*, 418–428. [CrossRef] [PubMed]
55. Robaszkiewicz, A.; Balcerczyk, A.; Bartosz, G. Antioxidative and prooxidative effects of quercetin on A549 cells. *Cell Biol. Int.* **2007**, *31*, 1245–1250. [CrossRef] [PubMed]
56. Tian, H.; Zhang, B.; Di, J.; Jiang, G.; Chen, F.; Li, H.; Li, L.; Pei, D.; Zheng, J. Keap1: One stone kills three birds Nrf2, IKKβ and Bcl-2/Bcl-xL. *Cancer Lett.* **2012**, *325*, 26–34. [CrossRef]

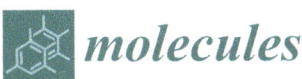

Article

Curcumin and Nano-Curcumin Mitigate Copper Neurotoxicity by Modulating Oxidative Stress, Inflammation, and Akt/GSK-3β Signaling

Wedad S. Sarawi [1], Ahlam M. Alhusaini [1], Laila M. Fadda [1], Hatun A. Alomar [1], Awatif B. Albaker [1], Amjad S. Aljrboa [1], Areej M. Alotaibi [1,2], Iman H. Hasan [1] and Ayman M. Mahmoud [3,*]

[1] Pharmacology and Toxicology Department, Faculty of Pharmacy, King Saud University, Riyadh 11451, Saudi Arabia; wsarawi@ksu.edu.sa (W.S.S.); aelhusaini@ksu.edu.sa (A.M.A.); lfadda@ksu.edu.sa (L.M.F.); hetalomar@ksu.edu.sa (H.A.A.); abaker@ksu.edu.sa (A.B.A.); 441203053@student.ksu.edu.sa (A.S.A.); 442204129@student.ksu.edu.sa (A.M.A.); ihasan@ksu.edu.sa (I.H.H.)
[2] Department of Pharmacology and Toxicology, College of Pharmacy, Umm Al-Qura University, Makkah 21955, Saudi Arabia
[3] Physiology Division, Zoology Department, Faculty of Science, Beni-Suef University, Beni-Suef 62514, Egypt
* Correspondence: ayman.mahmoud@science.bsu.edu.eg

Abstract: Copper (Cu) is essential for multiple biochemical processes, and copper sulphate ($CuSO_4$) is a pesticide used for repelling pests. Accidental or intentional intoxication can induce multiorgan toxicity and could be fatal. Curcumin (CUR) is a potent antioxidant, but its poor systemic bioavailability is the main drawback in its therapeutic uses. This study investigated the protective effect of CUR and N-CUR on $CuSO_4$-induced cerebral oxidative stress, inflammation, and apoptosis in rats, pointing to the possible involvement of Akt/GSK-3β. Rats received 100 mg/kg $CuSO_4$ and were concurrently treated with CUR or N-CUR for 7 days. Cu-administered rats exhibited a remarkable increase in cerebral malondialdehyde (MDA), NF-κB p65, TNF-α, and IL-6 associated with decreased GSH, SOD, and catalase. Cu provoked DNA fragmentation, upregulated BAX, caspase-3, and p53, and decreased BCL-2 in the brain of rats. N-CUR and CUR ameliorated MDA, NF-κB p65, and pro-inflammatory cytokines, downregulated pro-apoptotic genes, upregulated BCL-2, and enhanced antioxidants and DNA integrity. In addition, both N-CUR and CUR increased AKT Ser473 and GSK-3β Ser9 phosphorylation in the brain of Cu-administered rats. In conclusion, N-CUR and CUR prevent Cu neurotoxicity by attenuating oxidative injury, inflammatory response, and apoptosis and upregulating AKT/GSK-3β signaling. The neuroprotective effect of N-CUR was more potent than CUR.

Keywords: curcumin; GSK-3β; inflammation; DNA damage; oxidative stress

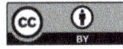

1. Introduction

Copper (Cu) is a redox-active metal found in many organs and tissues. It is essential for a plethora of biochemical processes such as blood clotting, iron absorption, protein homeostasis, energy production, and cellular metabolism [1]. It acts as a cofactor necessary for many redox-regulating proteins [2]. Cu homeostasis is maintained within the normal level by precise regulatory mechanisms that regulate its absorption, excretion, and blood level [3]. Genetic alteration in Cu-regulating ATPases, *ATP7A*, and *ATP7B* can cause Menkes disease (MD) and Wilson disease (WD), respectively [2,4,5]. MD is associated with a defect in Cu absorption and severe Cu deficiency, while WD results in Cu toxicity and affects several organs, including the liver, brain, and eye [2]. Chronic exposure to Cu has been implicated in the pathogenesis of neurodegenerative diseases such as Alzheimer's disease [6], Parkinson's disease [7], and familial amyotrophic lateral sclerosis (ALS) [2,8].

Copper sulphate ($CuSO_4$) is a well-known pesticide used for repelling pests that decreases the crop yield in agriculture. It is commonly used in tissue culture incubators to minimise the contamination risk as it has bactericidal and fungicidal properties. Accidental or intentional CuSO$_4$ intoxication can induce multiorgan dysfunctions that could be fatal. The systemic absorption of Cu occurs through the gastrointestinal tract, lungs, and skin [9]. The clinical manifestations of Cu toxicity are erosive gastropathy, acute liver and kidney injuries, intravascular hemolysis, arrhythmia, rhabdomyolysis, and seizures [10]. Although the mechanisms of CuSO$_4$ toxicity are not fully addressed, they represent a combination of significant oxidative stress and endocrine perturbation in the vulnerable organs of the body [11]. Animal studies showed that the chronic oral administration of CuSO$_4$ causes liver and kidney functional impairment due to increased Cu levels in the respective organs [12]. The toxic effects of Cu on the liver and kidney have been studied extensively, while the toxicities of other vital organs of the body are less documented. Similar to other metals, the management of Cu toxicity includes the use of chelating agents such as D-penicillamine, tetrathiomolybdate, and trientine [13]. Other chelators such as deferoxamine (DFO) have an affinity for Cu binding [14]. Despite the effectiveness of these chelators, they often associated with some serious adverse effects on cardiovascular, gastrointestinal, respiratory, and nervous systems, which necessitates the use of safer alternatives. In addition, the limited or moderate effectiveness of these chelators has been found in some cases.

Curcumin (CUR) is a hydrophobic polyphenolic compound found natively in turmeric [15]. It exhibits antioxidant [16], antimicrobial [17], anti-inflammatory, pulmoprotective [18], anti-diabetic [19], hepatoprotective [20–22], nephroprotective [23], and antitumor actions [24]. In addition to these pharmacological effects, CUR possesses neuroprotective activity where it protected the brain against oxidative injury induced by heavy metals [25]. CUR–cyclodextrin/cellulose nanocrystals (CNCx) exerted more potent antiproliferative effect on prostate and colorectal cancer cell lines than CUR [26]. In addition, CNCx mitigated oxidative stress and improved myelination, and the cellular, electrophysiological, and functional characteristics of Charcot–Marie–Tooth-1A transgenic rats [27]. Recently, Iurciuc-Tincu et al. have immobilized CUR into polysaccharide particles and reported increased stability and bioavailability [28,29]. CUR loading to polysaccharides facilitated overcoming the gastric juice barrier and efficient absorption in the intestine [28,29]. CUR has shown a modulatory effect on glycogen synthase kinase-3 (GSK-3) activity [30], and we have recently reported the involvement of GSK-3β inhibition in mediating its protective efficacy against lead hepatotoxicity [20]. GSK-3β is implicated in neuronal survival; however, the exact mechanism is not clear-cut [31]. Studies have demonstrated increased neuronal death following the overexpression of GSK-3β [32], whereas its knockdown prevents apoptosis [33]. Despite the potent pharmacological effects of CUR, its poor systemic bioavailability and rapid metabolism represent the main drawbacks in its therapeutic uses, which is a problem that was amended by nanoparticle encapsulation [34]. In comparison to the native form, nano-CUR (N-CUR) has a higher solubility and stability but similar activity [15]. Therefore, this nanoformulation can significantly enhance the cell permeability and show more protective effects in vitro and in vivo. This study was conducted to investigate the involvement of the Akt/GSK-3β pathway in CuSO$_4$-induced cerebral oxidative stress, inflammation, and apoptosis in rats and the ameliorative effect of CUR and N-CUR.

2. Results

2.1. N-CUR and CUR Attenuate Cu-Induced Cerebral Oxidative Stress

The ameliorative effect of CUR and N-CUR on oxidative stress in the brain of Cu-exposed rats was evaluated through the assessment of malondialdehyde (MDA), reduced glutathione (GSH), superoxide dismutase (SOD), and catalase (CAT). Cerebral MDA was significantly elevated in Cu-administered rats when compared with the control group ($p < 0.001$; Figure 1A). In contrast, cerebral GSH content (Figure 1B), SOD activity (Figure 1C), and CAT activity (Figure 1D) were decreased in Cu-administered rats ($p < 0.001$). Treatment with DFO, CUR, and N-CUR decreased MDA and increased GSH, SOD, and CAT in the brain of Cu-administered rats. The effect of both CUR and N-CUR on cerebral MDA was significant compared to DFO ($p < 0.01$).

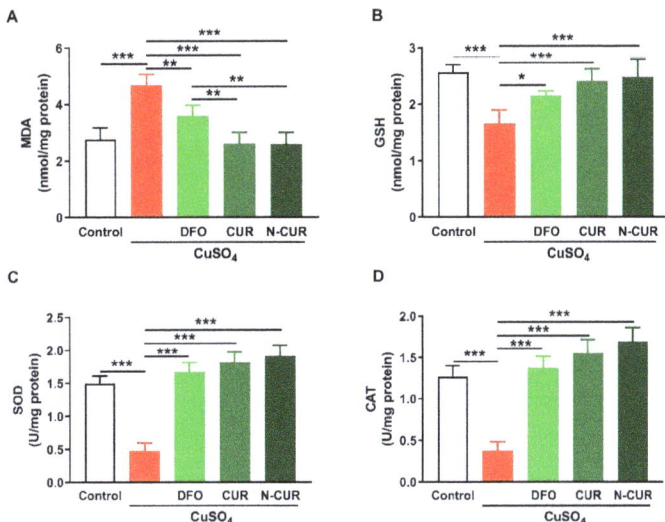

Figure 1. N-CUR and CUR attenuate Cu-induced cerebral oxidative stress. Treatment with N-CUR, CUR, and DFO decreased MDA (**A**) and increased GSH (**B**), SOD (**C**), and CAT (**D**) in the brain of Cu-administered rats. Data are mean ± SEM, (n = 8). * $p < 0.05$, ** $p < 0.01$, and *** $p < 0.001$.

2.2. N-CUR and CUR Suppress Cerebral Inflammation in Cu-Administered Rats

Cerebral levels of NF-κB p65, TNF-α, and IL-6 were assayed to determine the ameliorative effect of CUR and N-CUR on inflammation induced by Cu ingestion (Figure 2). Cu administration increased NF-κB p65 (Figure 2A), TNF-α (Figure 2B), and IL-6 (Figure 2C) in the cerebrum of rats ($p < 0.001$). All treatments (DFO, CUR, and N-CUR) decreased the levels of cerebral NF-κB p65, TNF-α, and IL-6 significantly ($p < 0.001$). N-CUR was more effective in decreasing cerebral NF-κB p65 ($p < 0.05$) than DFO, and TNF-α, and IL-6 as compared to either DFO or CUR.

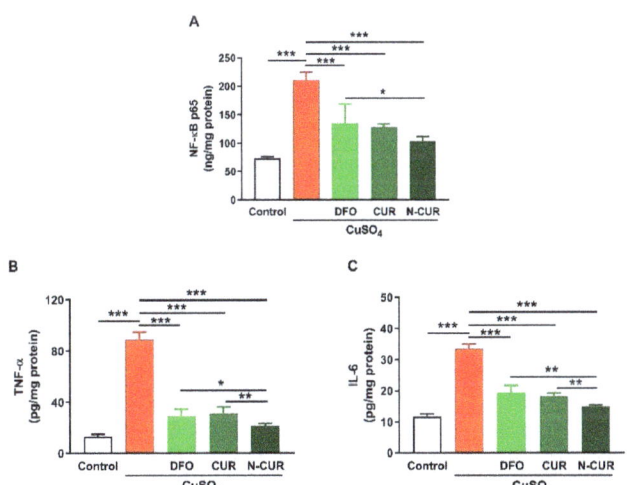

Figure 2. N-CUR and CUR suppress inflammation in Cu-administered rats. Treatment with N-CUR, CUR, and DFO decreased cerebral (**A**) NFκB p65, (**B**) TNF-α, and (**C**) IL-6. Data are mean ± SEM, (n = 8). * $p < 0.05$, ** $p < 0.01$ and *** $p < 0.001$.

2.3. N-CUR and CUR Prevent Apoptosis in Cu-Administered Rats

The expression levels of BAX, caspase-3, and p53 were significantly increased in the cerebrum of rats exposed to Cu as compared to the control group, as depicted in Figure 3. In contrast, rats administered with Cu exhibited a remarkable downregulation of cerebral BCL-2 expression. DFO, CUR, and N-CUR significantly downregulated BAX, p53, and caspase-3 and upregulated BCL-2 in the cerebrum of Cu-administered rats. The effect of N-CUR on BAX and BCL-2 was significant when compared with CUR, whereas its effect was more potent on BAX, caspase-3, and p53 than the effect of DFO.

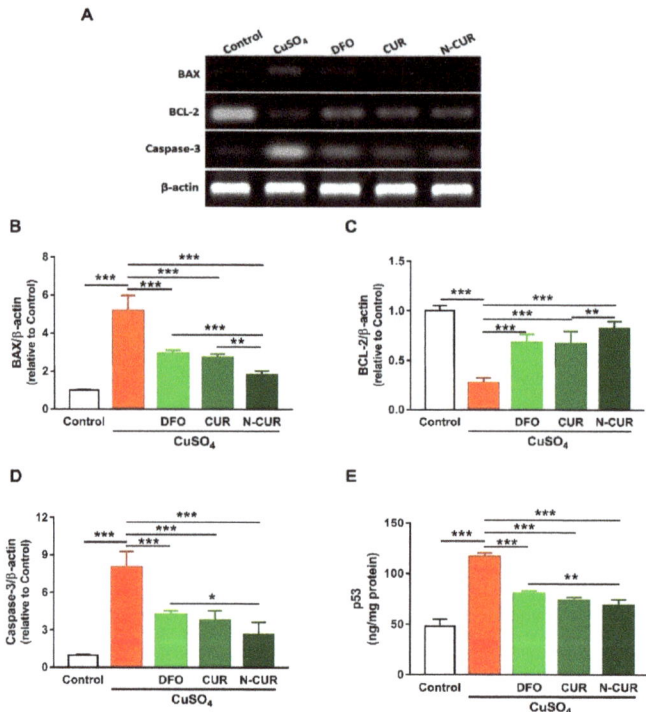

Figure 3. N-CUR and CUR prevent apoptosis in Cu-administered rats. (**A**) Representative blots showing changes in the expression of BAX, BCL-2, and caspase-3. (**B–E**) N-CUR, CUR, and DFO decreased (**B**) BAX, increased (**C**) BCL-2, and downregulated (**D**) caspase-3, and (**E**) p53 expression in the brain of Cu-administered rats. Data are mean ± SEM, (n = 8). * $p < 0.05$, ** $p < 0.01$ and *** $p < 0.001$.

The beneficial effects of CUR and N-CUR against Cu-induced cerebral cell death were further confirmed via assessment of DNA fragmentation (Figure 4). Cu-administered rats showed an increase in DNA fragmentation levels as compared to the control group ($p < 0.001$). All treatments (DFO, CUR and N-CUR) prevented the deleterious effect of Cu on DNA integrity.

2.4. N-CUR and CUR Upregulate AKT/GSK-3β Signaling in Cu-Administered Rats

To investigate the effect of Cu and the ameliorative effect of DFO, CUR, and N-CUR on cerebral AKT/GSK3β signaling, the phosphorylation levels of AKT and GSK3β were determined using Western blotting (Figure 5). Cu-treated rats exhibited a significant decrease in pAKT Ser473 and pGSK-3β Ser9 as compared to the normal rats ($p < 0.001$). Treatment with DFO, CUR, or N-CUR increased cerebral AKT and GSK-3β phosphorylation levels. N-CUR exerted a stronger effect on AKT/GSK-3β signaling than DFO and CUR.

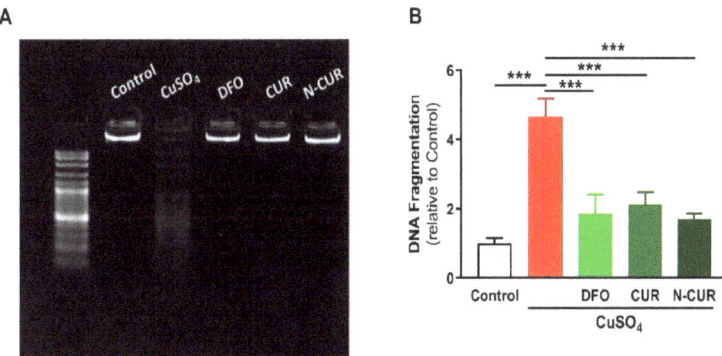

Figure 4. N-CUR, CUR, and DFO prevent DNA fragmentation in the brain of Cu-administered rats. DNA fragmentation was assessed by (**A**) agarose gel electrophoresis and (**B**) colorimetric methods. Data are mean ± SEM, (n = 8). *** $p < 0.001$.

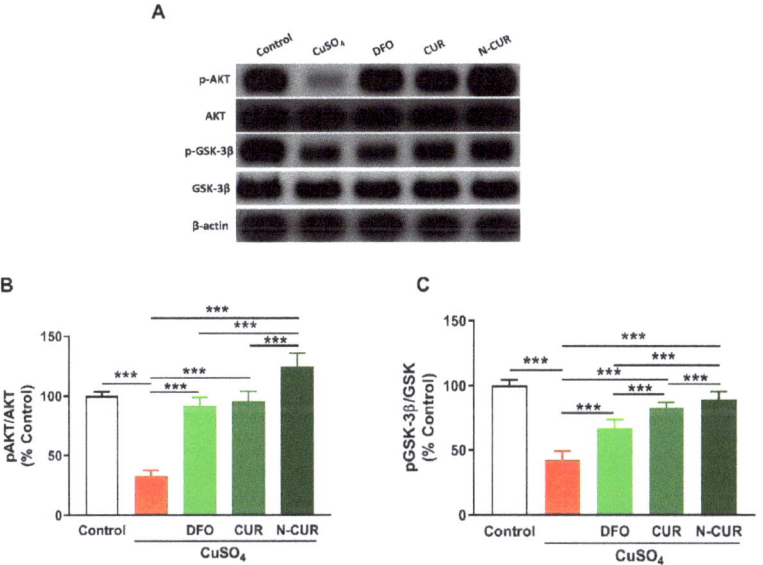

Figure 5. N-CUR and CUR upregulate AKT/GSK-3β signaling in Cu-administered rats. (**A**) Representative blots of pAKT, AKT, pGSK-3β, and GSK-3β. (**B,C**) N-CUR, CUR, and DFO increased AKT Ser473 (**B**) and GSK-3β Ser9 (**C**) phosphorylation in the brain of Cu-administered rats. Data are mean ± SEM, (n = 8). *** $p < 0.001$.

2.5. N-CUR and CUR Upregulate Brain-Derived Neurotrophic Factor (BDNF) in Cu-Administered Rats

The administration of Cu resulted in a significant downregulation of BDNF expression in the cerebrum of rats, as shown in Figure 6. Treatment of the Cu-administered rats with DFO, CUR, or N-CUR increased the levels of cerebral BDNF. While the effect of CUR on BDNF was significant as compared to DFO, the effect of N-CUR was more potent when compared to both treatments.

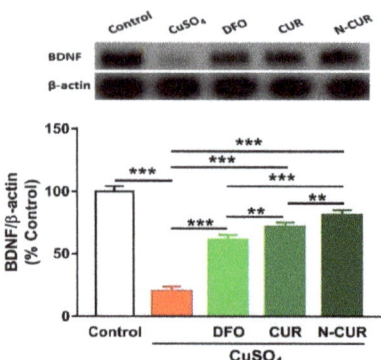

Figure 6. N-CUR and CUR upregulate BDNF in Cu-administered rats. Data are mean ± SEM, (n = 8). ** $p < 0.01$ and *** $p < 0.001$.

3. Discussion

Cu is the third most abundant essential transition metal in humans, and the brain is the second organ containing the highest content after the liver [35]. It is essential for antioxidant defenses, energy homeostasis, and many other physiological processes [1]. However, it may cause neurotoxicity and contribute to the pathogenesis of neurodegenerative diseases [1], where oxidative stress represents the main underlying mechanism [36]. The present results revealed the development of cerebral oxidative stress manifested by elevated MDA and decreased GSH, SOD, and CAT in Cu-administered rats.

Cu cycles easily between stable oxidised and unstable reduced states to coordinate ligands and enzymes and facilitate redox reactions, thereby acting as a cofactor for many enzymes [37]. Although the redox nature makes Cu essential for many biological processes, it renders it toxic because of the generation of highly reactive hydroxyl radicals [36]. In addition, Cu can increase mitochondrial reactive oxygen species (ROS) generation and alter the activity of respiratory chain enzymes [38]. The generated ROS are potent oxidising agents that provoke the oxidative damage of lipids, proteins, and DNA [39], leading to lipid peroxidation (LPO), DNA breaks, and other deleterious effects [40]. Accordingly, LPO was elevated and GSH, SOD, and CAT were declined in the brain of Cu-administered rats in the present study. Given the role of oxidative stress in mediating Cu toxicity, CUR can suppress neurotoxicity via its radical-scavenging and antioxidant properties. Here, rats that received CUR and N-CUR exhibited a remarkable reduction in cerebral MDA levels and enhanced GSH, SOD, and CAT. The antioxidant efficacy of CUR has been reported in numerous studies that employed animal models of neurotoxicity induced by D-galactosamine, fluoride, formaldehyde, rotenone, vincristine, tetrachlorobenzoquinone, pentylenetetrazole, acrylamide, and other agents (reviewed in [41]). In addition, CUR reduced cerebellar LPO in lead-intoxicated rats [25]. These beneficial effects were attributed to the potent radical-scavenging activity of CUR. The activation of nuclear factor erythroid 2-related factor 2 (Nrf2), a redox-sensitive factor that regulates antioxidant genes and suppresses oxidative stress [42], might also have a role in the neuroprotective activity of CUR. In this context, CUR enhanced Nrf2 and antioxidant defenses in rat cerebellar granule neurons challenged with hemin [43] and quinolinic acid-induced neurotoxicity [44].

The upregulation of BDNF in the brain of Cu-administered rats treated with CUR and N-CUR might have a role in boosting the antioxidant defenses through Nrf2 activation. In accordance, a recent study demonstrated that CUR increased BDNF in the brain of quinolinic acid-intoxicated rats, and this activated ERK1/2 and consequently enhanced Nrf2 expression and GSH levels [44]. BDNF belongs to the neurotrophin family and is involved in the maintenance of adult neuronal function [45]. In astrocytes, BDNF has been proposed to play a role in regulating Nrf2 and their metabolic cooperation between neurons [46]. In a model of traumatic brain injury with transplanted neuronal stem cells, BNDF induced Nrf2-mediated antioxidant response [47]. Therefore, this study introduced new information that the upregulation of BDNF plays a role, at least in part, in the protective effect of CUR against Cu neurotoxicity and that N-CUR has a stronger effect on modulating BDNF expression. However, the lack of data showing changes in Nrf2 expression could be considered a limitation of this study.

In addition to the attenuation of oxidative stress, CUR and N-CUR suppressed NF-κB and pro-inflammatory cytokines in the brain of Cu-administered rats. The inflammatory response observed in Cu-administered rats is a direct consequence of excessive ROS generation. The activation of NF-κB and subsequent release of many inflammatory mediators occur as a result of increased cellular ROS [48]. The pro-inflammatory action of Cu is driven by its potential to catalyse ROS generation and decreasing GSH [36], which is an effect reported in the present study. CUR and N-CUR effectively ameliorated cerebral inflammation in Cu-administered rats. N-CUR decreased the levels of TNF-α and IL-6 significantly when compared with CUR, demonstrating enhanced anti-inflammatory activity of the nano form. The ability of CUR to suppress inflammation has been reported in several studies. In a rat model of acrylamide neurotoxicity, Guo et al. [49] showed that CUR attenuated neuroinflammation by decreasing TNF-α and IL-1β levels. In addition, CUR decreased circulating TNF-α in an animal model of lead neurotoxicity [50].

Apoptotic cell death was observed in the brain of Cu-administered rats in the present study. BAX, caspase-3, and p53 were upregulated, whereas the anti-apoptotic BCL-2 was declined in the brain of rats as a result of Cu ingestion. Cu-mediated ROS generation induces mitochondrial permeability transition in astrocytes [51] and hepatocytes [52], leading to cell death via apoptosis. Excess ROS can activate the pro-apoptotic protein BAX, which increases cytochrome c release by promoting the loss of membrane potential via mitochondrial voltage-dependent anion channel [53]. Oxidative stress can also provoke p53 nuclear accumulation and its binding to specific DNA sequences, leading to the transcription of genes involved in cell death [54] and the release of mitochondrial cytochrome c and the activation of caspases [55]. In contrast, BCL-2 suppresses the release of cytochrome c and prevents apoptosis [56]. CUR downregulated the pro-apoptotic factors and increased BCL-2 expression, demonstrating an anti-apoptotic effect that is a direct consequence of its antioxidant and anti-inflammatory properties. The effect of N-CUR on BAX and BCL-2 expression was more potent than CUR. The cytoprotective efficacy of CUR has been reported in a *Drosophila* model of Huntington's disease [57]. In this model, CUR competently ameliorated neurodegeneration, cytotoxicity, and the compromised neuronal function [57].

To further explore the mechanism underlying the neuroprotective effect of CUR in Cu-administered rats and whether N-CUR is more potent, we determined their effect on AKT/GSK-3β signaling. The phosphorylation of AKT Ser473 and GSK-3β Ser9 was decreased in the brain of Cu-administered rats. While CUR ameliorated the altered phosphorylation levels of these proteins, N-CUR remarkably activated AKT/GSK-3β signaling. Activated AKT mediates the regulation of different processes, including cell growth and proliferation through the phosphorylation of GSK-3, mTOR, NF-κB, and other proteins [58]. AKT controls the activity of GSK-3β, which is active in resting cells, through phosphorylation at Ser9 [59]. Increased GSK-3β activity provoked liver injury [60], whereas its inhibition accelerated the generation of hepatocytes and protected against acetaminophen [61] and lead toxicity [62]. In neuronal cells, the overexpression of GSK-3β induced apoptosis [32,63], demonstrating its crucial role in cell death. BAX phosphorylation has been suggested to be stimulated through GSK-3, and the mutation of GSK-3 inhibited BAX mitochondrial translocation [64]. Moreover, GSK-3 can work in concert with JNK to orchestrate neuronal apoptosis [65]. In the current study, Cu ingestion decreased AKT Ser473 and GSK-3β Ser9 phosphorylation. Reduced inhibition of GSK-3β through its phosphorylation at Ser9 due to suppressed AKT coincides with the observed upregulation of BAX and other mediators of apoptosis. Therefore, the neuroprotective effect of CUR could be directly connected to its ability to activate AKT, which then inhibits GSK-3β-mediated apoptosis. Accordingly, activation of the AKT/GSK-3β signaling by CUR conferred protection against liver injury induced by heavy metals [20]. In support of our findings, computational approaches have demonstrated that CUR inhibits GSK-3β by fitting into its binding pocket [66,67]. This inhibitory effect has been confirmed by an in vitro study showing that the IC_{50} of CUR's inhibitory activity was 66.3 nM [66]. Furthermore, studies demonstrating the effect of CUR on GSK-3 activity in several diseases have been reviewed by McCubrey et al. [30].

In addition to the findings of this study, Balasubramanian [68,69] presented important quantum chemical insights into the neuroprotective mechanism of CUR and its efficacy to prevent Alzheimer's disease. The dual property of CUR to be nonpolar in parts and polar in other parts is due to the presence of both phenolic and enolic protons combined with an aliphatic hydrophobic bridge. This property enables CUR to cross the blood–brain barrier (BBB) and bind to and prevent the polymerisation of amyloid-β (Aβ) oligomers [69]. By employing quantum chemical computations, Balasubramanian [68] studied the chelate complexes of CUR with Cu(II) and other transition metal ions that provoke the polymerisation of Aβ and formation of neurotoxic conformations, reporting that the β-diketone bridge, through the loss of an enolic proton of CUR, is the primary site of chelation. CUR can form stable chelate complexes at the β-diketone bridge, thereby scavenging neurotoxic metal ions and inhibiting Aβ polymerisation and the subsequent generation of neurotoxic conformations [68]. Moreover, the ability of piperine, an alkaloid present in black pepper, to enhance the bioavailability and neuroprotective efficacy of CUR is noteworthy of mention. Through the use of quantum chemical and molecular docking, Patil et al. [70] demonstrated that piperine increased the bioavailability of CUR (20-fold) by inhibiting the enzymes mediating CUR glucuronosylation and by intercalating into CUR layers through intermolecular hydrogen bonding [70]. These processes enhance the metabolic transport and consequently the bioavailability of CUR [70]. In support of these findings, Singh et al. [71] reported the protective effect of CUR with piperine, a bioavailability enhancer, against neurotoxicity induced by 3-nitropropionic acid (3-NP) in rats. When supplemented with piperine, CUR improved motor function, attenuated oxidative stress and inflammatory cytokines, and modulated catecholamines and dopamine turnover in the striatum of 3-NP-admninstered rats [71].

4. Materials and Methods

4.1. Chemicals and Reagents

$CuSO_4$, CUR, carboxymethylcellulose (CMC), thiobarbituric acid, agarose, reduced glutathione (GSH), and pyrogallol were obtained from Sigma (St. Louis, MO, USA). Liposomal N-CUR was obtained from Lipolife (Essex, UK), and DFO was purchased from Novartis Pharma AG (Rotkreuz, Switzerland). TNF-α and IL-6 ELISA kits were supplied by R&D Systems (Minneapolis, MN, USA), and the NF-κB p65 ELISA kit was obtained from MyBiosource (San Diego, CA, USA). Antibodies against pAKT Ser473, AKT, pGSK-3β Ser9, GSK-3β, BDNF, and β-actin were supplied by Novus Biologicals (Centennial, CO, USA). Primers were obtained from Sigma (St. Louis, MO, USA). Other chemicals were supplied by standard manufacturers.

4.2. Animals and Treatments

Forty male Wistar rats, weighing 180–200 g, were obtained from the Animals Care Centre at King Saud University. The animals were given free access to food and water and acclimatised for one week under standard conditions and 12 h light/dark cycle and free access to food and water. All experimental procedures were conducted in accordance with the requirements of the research ethics Committee at King Saud University (Ethical reference no. SE-19-129). After acclimatisation, the rats were randomly allocated into five groups ($n = 8$) as follows:

- Group I (Control): received 1% CMC orally for 7 days.
- Group II ($CuSO_4$): received 100 mg/kg $CuSO_4$ dissolved in 1% CMC orally for 7 days [12].

- Group III (DFO): received DFO (23 mg/kg) [72] and 100 mg/kg $CuSO_4$ orally for 7 days.
- Group IV (CUR): received 80 mg/kg CUR suspended in 1% CMC [9,72] and 100 mg/kg $CuSO_4$ orally for 7 days.
- Group V (N-CUR): received 80 mg/kg N-CUR suspended in 1% CMC [9,72] and 100 mg/kg $CuSO_4$ orally for 7 days.

Twenty-four h after the last treatment, the rats were sacrificed under ketamine/xylazine anesthesia. Blood was collected via cardiac puncture and serum was separated by centrifugation. The rats were dissected, and the brain was removed and kept frozen in liquid nitrogen. Other parts from the cerebrum were homogenised in cold PBS (10% w/v), centrifuged at 5000 rpm for 15 min at 4 °C, and the supernatant was used for assessment of MDA, GSH, SOD, CAT, TNF-α, IL-6, and NF-κB p65.

4.3. Determination of MDA and Antioxidants

MDA was determined as previously described [73]. GSH, SOD, and CAT were assayed according to the methods of Ellman [74], Marklund and Marklund [75], and Cohen et al. [76], respectively.

4.4. Determination of NF-κB p65, TNF-α, IL-6, and p53

NF-κB p65 was assayed using a specific ELISA kit (MyBioSource, San Diego, CA, USA), and TNF-α and IL-6 were assayed using R&D Systems (Minneapolis, MN, USA) ELISA kits. p53 was determined using ELISA kit supplied by Novus Biologicals (Centennial, CO, USA).

4.5. Determination of DNA Fragmentation

Agarose electrophoresis and the colorimetric methods [77] were used to assess DNA fragmentation. The results were presented as a fold change of the control.

4.6. Gene Expression

Changes in the expression of BAX, BCL-2, and caspase-3 were determined by RT-PCR as previously described [78]. Briefly, RNA was isolated from the frozen brain samples using TRIzol (ThermoFisher Scientific, Waltham, MA, USA). Following treatment with RNase-free DNase (Qiagen, Hilden, Germany), RNA was quantified using a nanodrop. RNA samples with OD260/OD280 nm ratio of ≥ 1.8 were reverse transcribed into cDNA. The produced cDNA was amplified using PCR master mix (Qiagen, Hilden, Germany) and the primer pairs listed in Table 1. The PCR products were loaded in 1.5% agarose gel, electrophoresed, and the bands were visualised using UV transilluminator. The images were analysed by ImageJ (version 1.32j, NIH, USA), and the values were normalised to β-actin.

Table 1. Primers used for RT-PCR.

Gene	GenBank Accession Number	Primers (5'–3')	Product Size (bp)
BAX	NM_017059.2	F: TGGCGATGAACTGGACAACA R: TGTCCAGCCCATGATGGTTC	223
BCL-2	NM_016993.2	F: GAGGGGCTACGAGTGGGATA R: CAATCCTCCCCCAGTTCACC	359
Caspase-3	NM_012922.2	F: GAGCTTGGAACGCGAAGAAA R: GGCAGTAGTCGCCTCTGAAG	472
β-actin	XM_039089807.1	F: CACTCCAAGTATCCACGGCA R: TGCCTCAACACCTCAAACCA	303

4.7. Western Blotting

The samples were homogenized in RIPA buffer supplemented with proteinase/phosphatase inhibitors, centrifuged, and protein concentration was determined in the supernatant using Bradford protein assay kit (BioBasic, Markham, Canada). Forty µg protein from each sample was subjected to 10% SDS/PAGE and electrotransferred to nitrocellulose membranes. The membranes were subjected to blocking in 5% milk in TBST followed by incubation overnight at 4 °C with primary antibodies against pAKT Ser473, AKT, pGSK-3β Ser9, GSK-3β, BDNF, and β-actin. The probed membranes were washed, and secondary antibodies were added. After washing, the membranes were washed with TBST, developed using Clarity™ Western ECL Substrate from BIO-RAD (Hercules, CA, USA), and then visualised in ImageQuant LAS 4000. The band intensity was quantified using ImageJ (version 1.32j, NIH, USA).

4.8. Statistical Analysis

The obtained data are expressed as mean ± standard error of the mean (SEM). Statistical analysis was performed by one-way ANOVA and Tukey's post hoc test using GraphPad Prism 7 (GraphPad Software, San Diego, CA, USA). A p value < 0.05 was considered significant.

5. Conclusions

These results confer new information on the protective effect of N-CUR on Cu neurotoxicity. N-CUR and CUR attenuated oxidative stress, inflammation, cell death, and oxidative DNA damage in the brain of Cu-administered rats. The modulatory effect of N-CUR and CUR on AKT/GSK-3β signaling was involved, at least in part, in their protective activity against Cu neurotoxicity. The neuroprotective effect of N-CUR was stronger when compared to the native form, which is an effect that could be attributed to the improved properties of CUR.

Author Contributions: Conceptualisation, W.S.S.; A.M.A. (Ahlam M. Alhusaini) and A.M.M.; methodology, W.S.S.; A.M.A. (Ahlam M. Alhusaini); L.M.F.; H.A.A.; A.B.A.; A.S.A.; I.H.H. and A.M.M.; validation, W.S.S.; A.M.A. (Ahlam M. Alhusaini) and A.M.M.; formal analysis, W.S.S.; A.M.A. (Ahlam M. Alhusaini) and A.M.M.; investigation, W.S.S.; A.M.A. (Ahlam M. Alhusaini); L.M.F.; H.A.A.; A.B.A.; I.H.H. and A.M.M.; resources, W.S.S.; A.M.A. (Ahlam M. Alhusaini); A.M.A. (Areej M. Alotaibi) and A.M.M.; data curation, W.S.S. and A.M.M.; writing—original draft preparation, A.M.M.; writing—review and editing, A.M.M.; visualisation, W.S.S.; A.M.A. (Ahlam M. Alhusaini); I.H.H. and A.M.M.; supervision, A.M.A. (Ahlam M. Alhusaini) and A.M.M.; project administration, A.M.A. (Ahlam M. Alhusaini); I.H.H. and W.S.S.; funding acquisition, A.M.A. (Ahlam M. Alhusaini) and W.S.S. All authors have read and agreed to the published version of the manuscript.

Funding: Please add: This research was funded by the Deanship of Scientific Research at King Saud University, grant number RG-1441-546.

Institutional Review Board Statement: The experiment was conducted according to the guidelines of the National Institutes of Health (NIH publication No. 85–23, revised 2011) and was approved by the research ethics Committee at King Saud University (Ethical reference no. SE-19-129).

Informed Consent Statement: Not applicable.

Data Availability Statement: Data analysed or generated during this study are included in this manuscript.

Acknowledgments: The authors extend their appreciation to the Deanship of Scientific Research at King Saud University for funding this work through research group number RG-1441-546.

Conflicts of Interest: The authors declare no conflict of interest.

Sample Availability: Samples of the compounds are not available from the authors.

References

1. Scheiber, I.F.; Mercer, J.F.; Dringen, R. Metabolism and functions of copper in brain. *Prog. Neurobiol.* **2014**, *116*, 33–57. [CrossRef]
2. Uriu-Adams, J.Y.; Keen, C.L. Copper, oxidative stress, and human health. *Mol. Asp. Med.* **2005**, *26*, 268–298. [CrossRef] [PubMed]
3. Denoyer, D.; Masaldan, S.; La Fontaine, S.; Cater, M.A. Targeting copper in cancer therapy: 'Copper that cancer'. *Met. Integr. Biometal Sci.* **2015**, *7*, 1459–1476. [CrossRef] [PubMed]
4. Kim, B.-E.; Nevitt, T.; Thiele, D.J. Mechanisms for copper acquisition, distribution and regulation. *Nat. Chem. Biol.* **2008**, *4*, 176–185. [CrossRef] [PubMed]
5. Kardos, J.; Héja, L.; Simon, Á.; Jablonkai, I.; Kovács, R.; Jemnitz, K. Copper signalling: Causes and consequences. *Cell Commun. Signal* **2018**, *16*, 71. [CrossRef] [PubMed]
6. Brewer, G.J. Alzheimer's disease causation by copper toxicity and treatment with zinc. *Front Aging Neurosci.* **2014**, *6*, 92. [CrossRef]
7. Montes, S.; Rivera-Mancia, S.; Diaz-Ruiz, A.; Tristan-Lopez, L.; Rios, C. Copper and copper proteins in parkinson's disease. *Oxidative Med. Cell. Longev.* **2014**, *2014*, 147251. [CrossRef]
8. Bourassa, M.W.; Brown, H.H.; Borchelt, D.R.; Vogt, S.; Miller, L.M. Metal-deficient aggregates and diminished copper found in cells expressing sod1 mutations that cause als. *Front Aging Neurosci.* **2014**, *6*, 110. [CrossRef]
9. Hashish, E.A.; Elgaml, S.A. Hepatoprotective and nephroprotective effect of curcumin against copper toxicity in rats. *Indian J. Clin. Biochem. IJCB* **2016**, *31*, 270–277. [CrossRef]
10. Gamakaranage, C.S.; Rodrigo, C.; Weerasinghe, S.; Gnanathasan, A.; Puvanaraj, V.; Fernando, H. Complications and management of acute copper sulphate poisoning; a case discussion. *J. Occup. Med. Toxicol.* **2011**, *6*, 34. [CrossRef]
11. Rana, S.V. Perspectives in endocrine toxicity of heavy metals–a review. *Biol. Trace Elem. Res.* **2014**, *160*, 1–14. [CrossRef]
12. Kumar, V.; Kalita, J.; Misra, U.K.; Bora, H.K. A study of dose response and organ susceptibility of copper toxicity in a rat model. *J. Trace Elem. Med. Biol.* **2015**, *29*, 269–274. [CrossRef] [PubMed]
13. Tegoni, M.; Valensin, D.; Toso, L.; Remelli, M. Copper chelators: Chemical properties and bio-medical applications. *Curr. Med. Chem.* **2014**, *21*, 3785–3818. [CrossRef]
14. Lawson, M.K.; Valko, M.; Cronin, M.T.D.; Jomová, K. Chelators in iron and copper toxicity. *Curr. Pharm. Rep.* **2016**, *2*, 271–280. [CrossRef]
15. Gera, M.; Sharma, N.; Ghosh, M.; Huynh, D.L.; Lee, S.J.; Min, T.; Kwon, T.; Jeong, D.K. Nanoformulations of curcumin: An emerging paradigm for improved remedial application. *Oncotarget* **2017**, *8*, 66680–66698. [CrossRef] [PubMed]
16. Pizzo, P.; Scapin, C.; Vitadello, M.; Florean, C.; Gorza, L. Grp94 acts as a mediator of curcumin-induced antioxidant defence in myogenic cells. *J. Cell Mol. Med.* **2010**, *14*, 970–981. [CrossRef]
17. De, R.; Kundu, P.; Swarnakar, S.; Ramamurthy, T.; Chowdhury, A.; Nair, G.B.; Mukhopadhyay, A.K. Antimicrobial activity of curcumin against helicobacter pylori isolates from india and during infections in mice. *Antimicrob. Agents Chemother.* **2009**, *53*, 1592–1597. [CrossRef]
18. Saghir, S.A.M.; Alharbi, S.A.; Al-Garadi, M.A.; Al-Gabri, N.; Rady, H.Y.; Olama, N.K.; Abdulghani, M.A.M.; Al Hroob, A.M.; Almaiman, A.A.; Bin-Jumah, M.; et al. Curcumin prevents cyclophosphamide-induced lung injury in rats by suppressing oxidative stress and apoptosis. *Processes* **2020**, *8*, 127. [CrossRef]
19. Tsuda, T. Curcumin as a functional food-derived factor: Degradation products, metabolites, bioactivity, and future perspectives. *Food Funct.* **2018**, *9*, 705–714. [CrossRef]
20. Alhusaini, A.; Fadda, L.; Hasan, I.H.; Zakaria, E.; Alenazi, A.M.; Mahmoud, A.M. Curcumin ameliorates lead-induced hepatotoxicity by suppressing oxidative stress and inflammation, and modulating akt/gsk-3beta signaling pathway. *Biomolecules* **2019**, *9*, 703. [CrossRef] [PubMed]
21. Al-Dossari, M.H.; Fadda, L.M.; Attia, H.A.; Hasan, I.H.; Mahmoud, A.M. Curcumin and selenium prevent lipopolysaccharide/diclofenac-induced liver injury by suppressing inflammation and oxidative stress. *Biol. Trace Elem. Res.* **2020**, *196*, 173–183. [CrossRef]
22. Galaly, S.R.; Ahmed, O.M.; Mahmoud, A.M. Thymoquinone and curcumin prevent gentamicin-induced liver injury by attenuating oxidative stress, inflammation and apoptosis. *J. Physiol. Pharm.* **2014**, *65*, 823–832.
23. Mahmoud, A.M.; Ahmed, O.M.; Galaly, S.R. Thymoquinone and curcumin attenuate gentamicin-induced renal oxidative stress, inflammation and apoptosis in rats. *Excli J.* **2014**, *13*, 98–110.
24. Aggarwal, B.B.; Harikumar, K.B. Potential therapeutic effects of curcumin, the anti-inflammatory agent, against neurodegenerative, cardiovascular, pulmonary, metabolic, autoimmune and neoplastic diseases. *Int. J. Biochem. Cell Biol.* **2009**, *41*, 40–59. [CrossRef] [PubMed]
25. Abubakar, K.; Muhammad Mailafiya, M.; Danmaigoro, A.; Musa Chiroma, S.; Abdul Rahim, E.B.; Abu Bakar Zakaria, M.Z. Curcumin attenuates lead-induced cerebellar toxicity in rats via chelating activity and inhibition of oxidative stress. *Biomolecules* **2019**, *9*, 453. [CrossRef]
26. Ndong Ntoutoume, G.M.A.; Granet, R.; Mbakidi, J.P.; Brégier, F.; Léger, D.Y.; Fidanzi-Dugas, C.; Lequart, V.; Joly, N.; Liagre, B.; Chaleix, V.; et al. Development of curcumin-cyclodextrin/cellulose nanocrystals complexes: New anticancer drug delivery systems. *Bioorganic Med. Chem. Lett.* **2016**, *26*, 941–945. [CrossRef] [PubMed]
27. Caillaud, M.; Msheik, Z.; Ndong-Ntoutoume, G.M.; Vignaud, L.; Richard, L.; Favreau, F.; Faye, P.A.; Sturtz, F.; Granet, R.; Vallat, J.M.; et al. Curcumin-cyclodextrin/cellulose nanocrystals improve the phenotype of charcot-marie-tooth-1a transgenic rats through the reduction of oxidative stress. *Free Radic. Biol. Med.* **2020**, *161*, 246–262. [CrossRef]

28. Iurciuc-Tincu, C.E.; Atanase, L.I.; Ochiuz, L.; Jérôme, C.; Sol, V.; Martin, P.; Popa, M. Curcumin-loaded polysaccharides-based complex particles obtained by polyelectrolyte complexation and ionic gelation. I-particles obtaining and characterization. *Int. J. Biol. Macromol.* **2020**, *147*, 629–642. [CrossRef]
29. Iurciuc Tincu, C.-E.; Atanase, L.I.; Jérôme, C.; Sol, V.; Martin, P.; Popa, M.; Ochiuz, L. Polysaccharides-based complex particles' protective role on the stability and bioactivity of immobilized curcumin. *Int. J. Mol. Sci.* **2021**, *22*, 3075. [CrossRef] [PubMed]
30. McCubrey, J.A.; Lertpiriyapong, K.; Steelman, L.S.; Abrams, S.L.; Cocco, L.; Ratti, S.; Martelli, A.M.; Candido, S.; Libra, M.; Montalto, G.; et al. Regulation of gsk-3 activity by curcumin, berberine and resveratrol: Potential effects on multiple diseases. *Adv. Biol. Regul.* **2017**, *65*, 77–88. [CrossRef] [PubMed]
31. Urbanska, M.; Gozdz, A.; Macias, M.; Cymerman, I.A.; Liszewska, E.; Kondratiuk, I.; Devijver, H.; Lechat, B.; Van Leuven, F.; Jaworski, J. Gsk3β controls mtor and prosurvival signaling in neurons. *Mol. Neurobiol.* **2018**, *55*, 6050–6062. [CrossRef] [PubMed]
32. Gómez-Sintes, R.; Hernández, F.; Lucas, J.J.; Avila, J. Gsk-3 mouse models to study neuronal apoptosis and neurodegeneration. *Front. Mol. Neurosci.* **2011**, *4*, 45. [CrossRef]
33. Song, B.; Lai, B.; Zheng, Z.; Zhang, Y.; Luo, J.; Wang, C.; Chen, Y.; Woodgett, J.R.; Li, M. Inhibitory phosphorylation of gsk-3 by camkii couples depolarization to neuronal survival. *J. Biol. Chem.* **2010**, *285*, 41122–41134. [CrossRef] [PubMed]
34. Grama, C.N.; Suryanarayana, P.; Patil, M.A.; Raghu, G.; Balakrishna, N.; Kumar, M.N.; Reddy, G.B. Efficacy of biodegradable curcumin nanoparticles in delaying cataract in diabetic rat model. *PloS ONE* **2013**, *8*, e78217.
35. Szerdahelyi, P.; Kása, P. Histochemical demonstration of copper in normal rat brain and spinal cord. *Histochemistry* **1986**, *85*, 341–347. [CrossRef]
36. Gunther, M.R.; Hanna, P.M.; Mason, R.P.; Cohen, M.S. Hydroxyl radical formation from cuprous ion and hydrogen peroxide: A spin-trapping study. *Arch. Biochem. Biophys.* **1995**, *316*, 515–522. [CrossRef]
37. Liu, J.; Chakraborty, S.; Hosseinzadeh, P.; Yu, Y.; Tian, S.; Petrik, I.; Bhagi, A.; Lu, Y. Metalloproteins containing cytochrome, iron-sulfur, or copper redox centers. *Chem. Rev.* **2014**, *114*, 4366–4469. [CrossRef]
38. Sheline, C.T.; Choi, D.W. Cu2+ toxicity inhibition of mitochondrial dehydrogenases in vitro and in vivo. *Ann. Neurol.* **2004**, *55*, 645–653. [CrossRef] [PubMed]
39. Gaetke, L.M.; Chow-Johnson, H.S.; Chow, C.K. Copper: Toxicological relevance and mechanisms. *Arch. Toxicol.* **2014**, *88*, 1929–1938. [CrossRef] [PubMed]
40. Halliwell, B. Oxidative stress and neurodegeneration: Where are we now? *J. Neurochem.* **2006**, *97*, 1634–1658. [CrossRef]
41. Farkhondeh, T.; Samarghandian, S.; Samini, F. Antidotal effects of curcumin against neurotoxic agents: An updated review. *Asian Pac. J. Trop. Med.* **2016**, *9*, 947–953. [CrossRef]
42. Satta, S.; Mahmoud, A.M.; Wilkinson, F.L.; Yvonne Alexander, M.; White, S.J. The role of nrf2 in cardiovascular function and disease. *Oxidative Med. Cell. Longev.* **2017**, *2017*, 9237263. [CrossRef] [PubMed]
43. González-Reyes, S.; Guzmán-Beltrán, S.; Medina-Campos, O.N.; Pedraza-Chaverri, J. Curcumin pretreatment induces nrf2 and an antioxidant response and prevents hemin-induced toxicity in primary cultures of cerebellar granule neurons of rats. *Oxidative Med. Cell. Longev.* **2013**, *2013*, 801418. [CrossRef]
44. Santana-Martínez, R.A.; Silva-Islas, C.A.; Fernández-Orihuela, Y.Y.; Barrera-Oviedo, D.; Pedraza-Chaverri, J.; Hernández-Pando, R.; Maldonado, P.D. The therapeutic effect of curcumin in quinolinic acid-induced neurotoxicity in rats is associated with bdnf, erk1/2, nrf2, and antioxidant enzymes. *Antioxidants* **2019**, *8*, 388. [CrossRef] [PubMed]
45. Soulé, J.; Messaoudi, E.; Bramham, C.R. Brain-derived neurotrophic factor and control of synaptic consolidation in the adult brain. *Biochem. Soc. Trans.* **2006**, *34*, 600–604. [CrossRef]
46. Ishii, T.; Warabi, E.; Mann, G.E. Circadian control of p75 neurotrophin receptor leads to alternate activation of nrf2 and c-rel to reset energy metabolism in astrocytes via brain-derived neurotrophic factor. *Free Radic. Biol. Med.* **2018**, *119*, 34–44. [CrossRef]
47. Chen, T.; Wu, Y.; Wang, Y.; Zhu, J.; Chu, H.; Kong, L.; Yin, L.; Ma, H. Brain-derived neurotrophic factor increases synaptic protein levels via the mapk/erk signaling pathway and nrf2/trx axis following the transplantation of neural stem cells in a rat model of traumatic brain injury. *Neurochem. Res.* **2017**, *42*, 3073–3083. [CrossRef] [PubMed]
48. Bonizzi, G.; Karin, M. The two nf-kappab activation pathways and their role in innate and adaptive immunity. *Trends Immunol.* **2004**, *25*, 280–288. [CrossRef]
49. Guo, J.; Cao, X.; Hu, X.; Li, S.; Wang, J. The anti-apoptotic, antioxidant and anti-inflammatory effects of curcumin on acrylamide-induced neurotoxicity in rats. *Bmc. Pharm. Toxicol.* **2020**, *21*, 62. [CrossRef]
50. Tangpong, J. 227—neuroprotective efficacy of curcumin in lead (pb) induced inflammation and cholinergic dysfunction in mice. *Free Radic. Biol. Med.* **2018**, *128*, S99. [CrossRef]
51. Reddy, P.V.; Rao, K.V.; Norenberg, M.D. The mitochondrial permeability transition, and oxidative and nitrosative stress in the mechanism of copper toxicity in cultured neurons and astrocytes. *Lab. Investig. A J. Tech. Methods Pathol.* **2008**, *88*, 816–830. [CrossRef] [PubMed]
52. Roy, D.N.; Mandal, S.; Sen, G.; Biswas, T. Superoxide anion mediated mitochondrial dysfunction leads to hepatocyte apoptosis preferentially in the periportal region during copper toxicity in rats. *Chem. Biol. Interact.* **2009**, *182*, 136–147. [CrossRef]
53. Shi, Y.; Chen, J.; Weng, C.; Chen, R.; Zheng, Y.; Chen, Q.; Tang, H. Identification of the protein-protein contact site and interaction mode of human vdac1 with bcl-2 family proteins. *Biochem. Biophys. Res. Commun.* **2003**, *305*, 989–996. [CrossRef]
54. Almog, N.; Rotter, V. Involvement of p53 in cell differentiation and development. *Biochim. Et Biophys. Acta* **1997**, *1333*, F1–F27. [CrossRef]

55. Schuler, M.; Bossy-Wetzel, E.; Goldstein, J.C.; Fitzgerald, P.; Green, D.R. P53 induces apoptosis by caspase activation through mitochondrial cytochrome c release. *J. Biol. Chem.* **2000**, *275*, 7337–7342. [CrossRef]
56. Herrera, B.; Fernández, M.; Alvarez, A.M.; Roncero, C.; Benito, M.; Gil, J.; Fabregat, I. Activation of caspases occurs downstream from radical oxygen species production, bcl-xl down-regulation, and early cytochrome c release in apoptosis induced by transforming growth factor β in rat fetal hepatocytes. *Hepatology* **2001**, *34*, 548–556. [CrossRef]
57. Chongtham, A.; Agrawal, N. Curcumin modulates cell death and is protective in huntington's disease model. *Sci. Rep.* **2016**, *6*, 18736. [CrossRef] [PubMed]
58. Risso, G.; Blaustein, M.; Pozzi, B.; Mammi, P.; Srebrow, A. Akt/pkb: One kinase, many modifications. *Biochem. J.* **2015**, *468*, 203–214. [CrossRef]
59. Kaidanovich-Beilin, O.; Woodgett, J.R. Gsk-3: Functional insights from cell biology and animal models. *Front. Mol. Neurosci.* **2011**, *4*, 40. [CrossRef]
60. Ren, F.; Zhang, L.; Zhang, X.; Shi, H.; Wen, T.; Bai, L.; Zheng, S.; Chen, Y.; Chen, D.; Li, L.; et al. Inhibition of glycogen synthase kinase 3β promotes autophagy to protect mice from acute liver failure mediated by peroxisome proliferator-activated receptor α. *Cell Death Dis.* **2016**, *7*, e2151. [CrossRef] [PubMed]
61. Bhushan, B.; Poudel, S.; Manley, M.W., Jr.; Roy, N.; Apte, U. Inhibition of glycogen synthase kinase 3 accelerated liver regeneration after acetaminophen-induced hepatotoxicity in mice. *Am. J. Pathol* **2017**, *187*, 543–552. [CrossRef]
62. Alhusaini, A.; Fadda, L.; Hasan, I.H.; Ali, H.M.; El Orabi, N.F.; Badr, A.M.; Zakaria, E.; Alenazi, A.M.; Mahmoud, A.M. Arctium lappa root extract prevents lead-induced liver injury by attenuating oxidative stress and inflammation, and activating akt/gsk-3β signaling. *Antioxidants* **2019**, *8*, 582. [CrossRef]
63. Pap, M.; Cooper, G.M. Role of glycogen synthase kinase-3 in the phosphatidylinositol 3-kinase/akt cell survival pathway. *J. Biol Chem* **1998**, *273*, 19929–19932. [CrossRef] [PubMed]
64. Linseman, D.A.; Butts, B.D.; Precht, T.A.; Phelps, R.A.; Le, S.S.; Laessig, T.A.; Bouchard, R.J.; Florez-McClure, M.L.; Heidenreich, K.A. Glycogen synthase kinase-3beta phosphorylates bax and promotes its mitochondrial localization during neuronal apoptosis. *J. Neurosci.* **2004**, *24*, 9993–10002. [CrossRef]
65. Hongisto, V.; Smeds, N.; Brecht, S.; Herdegen, T.; Courtney, M.J.; Coffey, E.T. Lithium blocks the c-jun stress response and protects neurons via its action on glycogen synthase kinase 3. *Mol. Cell Biol.* **2003**, *23*, 6027–6036. [CrossRef] [PubMed]
66. Bustanji, Y.; Taha, M.O.; Almasri, I.M.; Al-Ghussein, M.A.; Mohammad, M.K.; Alkhatib, H.S. Inhibition of glycogen synthase kinase by curcumin: Investigation by simulated molecular docking and subsequent in vitro/in vivo evaluation. *J. Enzym. Inhib. Med. Chem.* **2009**, *24*, 771–778. [CrossRef]
67. Mishra, H.; Kesharwani, R.K.; Singh, D.B.; Tripathi, S.; Dubey, S.K.; Misra, K. Computational simulation of inhibitory effects of curcumin, retinoic acid and their conjugates on gsk-3 beta. *Netw. Modeling Anal. Health Inf. Bioinform.* **2019**, *8*, 3. [CrossRef]
68. Balasubramanian, K. Quantum chemical insights into alzheimer's disease: Curcumin's chelation with Cu(II), Zn(II), and Pd(II) as a mechanism for its prevention. *Int. J. Quantum Chem.* **2016**, *116*, 1107–1119. [CrossRef]
69. Balasubramanian, K. Molecular orbital basis for yellow curry spice curcumin's prevention of alzheimer's disease. *J. Agric. Food Chem.* **2006**, *54*, 3512–3520. [CrossRef]
70. Patil, V.M.; Das, S.; Balasubramanian, K. Quantum chemical and docking insights into bioavailability enhancement of curcumin by piperine in pepper. *J. Phys. Chem. A* **2016**, *120*, 3643–3653. [CrossRef]
71. Singh, S.; Jamwal, S.; Kumar, P. Piperine enhances the protective effect of curcumin against 3-np induced neurotoxicity: Possible neurotransmitters modulation mechanism. *Neurochem. Res.* **2015**, *40*, 1758–1766. [CrossRef] [PubMed]
72. Alhusaini, A.; Fadda, L.; Hassan, I.; Ali, H.M.; Alsaadan, N.; Aldowsari, N.; Aldosari, A.; Alharbi, B. Liposomal curcumin attenuates the incidence of oxidative stress, inflammation, and DNA damage induced by copper sulfate in rat liver. *Dose-Response A Publ. Int. Hormesis Soc.* **2018**, *16*, 1559325818790869. [CrossRef] [PubMed]
73. Mihara, M.; Uchiyama, M. Determination of malonaldehyde precursor in tissues by thiobarbituric acid test. *Anal. Biochem.* **1978**, *86*, 271–278. [PubMed]
74. Ellman, G.L. Tissue sulfhydryl groups. *Arch. Biochem. Biophys.* **1959**, *82*, 70–77. [CrossRef]
75. Marklund, S.L. Superoxide dismutase isoenzymes in tissues and plasma from new zealand black mice, nude mice and normal balb/c mice. *Mutat. Res.* **1985**, *148*, 129–134. [CrossRef]
76. Cohen, G.; Dembiec, D.; Marcus, J. Measurement of catalase activity in tissue extracts. *Anal. Biochem.* **1970**, *34*, 30–38. [CrossRef]
77. Hickey, E.J.; Raje, R.R.; Reid, V.E.; Gross, S.M.; Ray, S.D. Diclofenac induced in vivo nephrotoxicity may involve oxidative stress-mediated massive genomic DNA fragmentation and apoptotic cell death. *Free Radic. Biol. Med.* **2001**, *31*, 139–152. [CrossRef]
78. Mahmoud, A.M. Hematological alterations in diabetic rats - role of adipocytokines and effect of citrus flavonoids. *Excli J.* **2013**, *12*, 647–657. [PubMed]

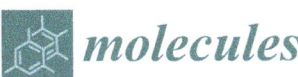

Review

Caffeic Acid on Metabolic Syndrome: A Review

Nellysha Namela Muhammad Abdul Kadar [1,2], Fairus Ahmad [1], Seong Lin Teoh [1] and Mohamad Fairuz Yahaya [1,*]

[1] Department of Anatomy, Faculty of Medicine, Universiti Kebangsaan Malaysia Medical Centre, Cheras, Kuala Lumpur 56000, Malaysia; nellysha.namela@ums.edu.my (N.N.M.A.K.); fairusahmad@ukm.edu.my (F.A.); teohseonglin@ukm.edu.my (S.L.T.)
[2] Department of Biomedical Sciences and Therapeutics, Faculty of Medicine and Health Sciences, Universiti Malaysia Sabah, Kota Kinabalu 88400, Malaysia
* Correspondence: mfairuzy@ukm.edu.my

Abstract: Metabolic syndrome (MetS) is a constellation of risk factors that may lead to a more sinister disease. Raised blood pressure, dyslipidemia in the form of elevated triglycerides and lowered high-density lipoprotein cholesterol, raised fasting glucose, and central obesity are the risk factors that could lead to full-blown diabetes, heart disease, and many others. With increasing sedentary lifestyles, coupled with the current COVID-19 pandemic, the numbers of people affected with MetS will be expected to grow in the coming years. While keeping these factors checked with the polypharmacy available currently, there is no single strategy that can halt or minimize the effect of MetS to patients. This opens the door for a more natural way of controlling the disease. Caffeic acid (CA) is a phytonutrient belonging to the flavonoids that can be found in abundance in plants, fruits, and vegetables. CA possesses a wide range of beneficial properties from antioxidant, immunomodulatory, antimicrobial, neuroprotective, antianxiolytic, antiproliferative, and anti-inflammatory activities. This review discusses the current discovery of the effect of CA against MetS.

Keywords: caffeic acid; metabolic syndrome; phenolic compound; obesity; dyslipidemia; hyperglycemia; hypertension

1. Introduction

Metabolic syndrome (MetS) has affected almost one fifth of the adult population and increases the risk of cardiovascular disease, type-2 diabetes, and all-cause mortality compared to a healthy person [1]. In Asia, Malaysia is recognized as one of the countries that has a high MetS prevalence [2]. MetS is a complication of the modern lifestyle that includes overeating and underactivity [3]. With the current COVID-19 pandemic situation and increasing state of sedentary lifestyle, the numbers are bound to be more than the expected figures in the coming years [4].

The current definition of MetS still uses the Harmonized Criteria that state that abnormal findings of 3 out of 5 of the following risk factors would qualify a person of having MetS: raised blood pressure, dyslipidemia (raised triglycerides (TG) and lowered high-density lipoprotein cholesterol), raised fasting glucose, and central obesity [5,6]. These components have the ability to precede into cardiac dysfunction, but together, they can also cause an additional risk to morbidity and mortality [7]. Although MetS has been collectively accepted as an alarming condition, the clinical world has yet to mutually agree on a uniform terminology and diagnostic criteria. This is mainly due to the adversity of genetic predisposition, diet history, and physical, geographical, and endocrinal attributes that together take part in forming this intricate syndrome [8]. One of the causes of MetS is the increase in oxidative stress and chronic inflammation. In many instances, it has been shown that an antioxidant imbalance may play a role in its development where there is an overproduction of reactive oxygen species (ROS) and nitrogen (RNS) species that can react

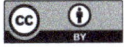

with virtually all biomolecules, causing oxidative damage [9,10]. Similarly, human studies have also shown that MetS is associated with oxidative stress and a proinflammatory state that comes with a high antioxidant defense in the peripheral blood mononuclear cells assumed to be derived from a pre-activation state of human cells [11].

Although obesity and insulin resistance remain at the root of MetS pathogenesis, other factors such as chronic stress and dysregulation of the hypothalamic–pituitary–adrenal axis and autonomic nervous system, increased cellular oxidative stress, renin–angiotensin–aldosterone activity, and intrinsic tissue glucocorticoid reaction, as well as the newly discovered miRNAs, have been identified to play roles in this condition [12,13].

At the core of many pathological diseases, including MetS, an increase in ROS has played a crucial element that can be tipped over with the aid of a longstanding diet comprising antioxidants [14]. Reactive species are essential signaling molecules that are involved in nearly every physiological activity, from cell division to metabolic regulation. They modulate the activity of biomolecules, and redox-sensitive transcription factors activate a cell's adaptive endogenous response, including antioxidant defense. The degree of reactive species production and neutralization that are tightly associated with oxidative metabolism determines the redox homeostasis of cells and their surroundings. Setting the redox states of cells is critical in both health and disorders such as MetS [15]. The question is, which antioxidant and at what aliquot would be the optimum elixir to shorten the period in combating the specific diseases.

The research world has, for many years, focused on a more natural approach toward combatting human diseases. Synthetic medications have slowly proven its downside over years of pharmacological use. Polypharmacy in the treatment of MetS has become a substantial healthcare burden due to adverse drug reactions, morbidity, and cost [16]. One of the phytonutrient compounds that caught the attention of researchers were the flavonoids. These are a very diverse group of polyphenolic compounds that consists of a benzo-γ-pyrone and can be found in several parts of a plant. They are classified as plant secondary metabolites having a polyphenolic structure [17,18]. These compounds, which can be found in abundance in the Mediterranean diet, has increasingly shown a beneficial effect in maintaining cardiometabolic and cardiovascular health, which, in turn, reduces the risks of MetS development. This positive impression may be due to the diets that are high in polyphenolic antioxidant content derived from vegetables, grapes, and olive oils [19]. Similarly, treatment with naringin, a type of glycoside flavonoid, has been reported to reverse MetS by reducing visceral obesity, blood glucose, blood pressure, and lipid profile [20].

In this review, we discuss a phenolic compound found in many herbs, caffeic acid (CA), or its chemical name 3,4-dihydroxycinnamic acid, which belongs to a group called phenolic compounds, which are a naturally occurring chemical structure found abundantly in fruits and vegetables [21,22].

2. Caffeic Acid as a Phenolic Compound

Phenolic compounds provide protection against noncommunicable diseases not only by their means of antioxidant activity but also by regulating a variety of cellular processes at different levels, including enzyme inhibition, modification of gene expression, and protein phosphorylation [23]. An increase in phenolic compounds can alter their health benefits [24]. There are over 8000 phenolic compounds that can be classified into two main groups: flavonoids and nonflavonoids. Flavonoids contain a phenyl benzopyran skeleton: two phenyl rings joined through a heterocyclic pyran ring. Nonflavonoids, on the other hand, are mostly smaller and simpler in comparison to flavonoids [17].

Phenolic acids (PAs) are a group of nonflavonoid phenolic compounds that contain a single phenyl group substituted by a carboxylic group and one or more hydroxyl (OH) groups [25]. PAs are further divided according to the length of the chain that contains the carboxylic group into: hydroxybenzoic acids, hydroxycinnamic acids, and hydroxyphenyl acids. The group hydroxycinnamic acid has a C6-C3 (phenylpropanoid) basic skeleton.

Hydroxy derivatives of cinnamic acid are more effective as an antioxidant than the hydroxyl derivatives of benzoic acid as the presence of a $CH_2 = CH\text{-}COOH$ group in the cinnamic acids ensures a greater antioxidant capacity than the COOH group in benzoic acid (Figure 1). One of the major hydroxycinnamic acids is CA [26–28].

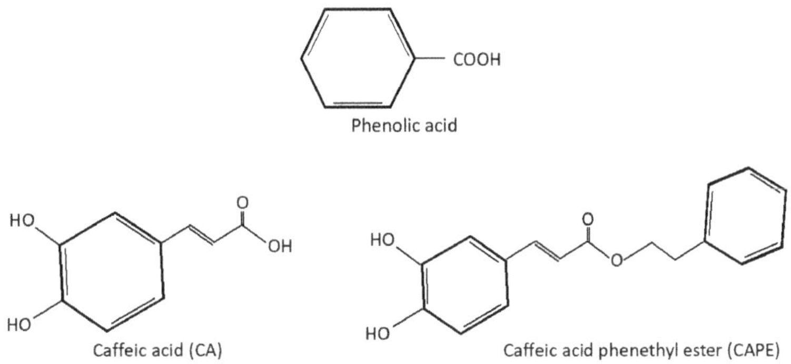

Figure 1. Chemical structure of PA, CA, and CAPE.

CA is found in coffee, honey, potatoes, berries, herbs, and vegetables such as olives, Swiss chard, and carrot [29]. In vitro and in vivo studies have shown that CA not only possesses antioxidant capacity but also has immunomodulatory [30], antimicrobial [31], neuroprotective, antianxiolytic [32], antiproliferative, and anti-inflammatory activities [33], and has shown to improve inflammation and oxidative stress in chronic metabolic diseases. Besides the therapeutic potentials of CA, studies have also shown that the pure form of CA has the availability to be absorbed in the intestines and form subsequent interactions with the target tissue [34]. This solidifies the potential of using CA as an oral route of administration as an appealing choice for a phytonutrient.

CA has also been found in Gelam honey and stingless bee honey through HPLC analysis [35,36]. The antioxidant capability of CA is due to its ability to scavenge ROS, including $O2-$, $OH-$, and H_2O_2 [37]. CA has shown to be an effective ABTS, DPPH, and superoxide anion radical scavenger, with a total reducing power and metal chelates on ferrous ion activities, in comparison to other standard antioxidant compounds such as BHA, BHT, alpha-tocopherol, and trolox in different in vitro antioxidant assays [38]. Multiple factors influence PA efficacy in vivo, including the amount of consumed chemical, whether it is absorbed or metabolized, its plasma or tissue concentrations, PA type and dosage, and synergistic effects [39].

Besides pure CA, its derivatives in the form of caffeic acid phenyl ester (CAPE) and caffeic acid phenylethyl amide (CAPA) have also been found to have a therapeutic effect against MetS. However, CAPA and CAPE are less stable in its form compared to CA [40]. CAPE is an active component of the propolis substance and has been known for its anti-inflammatory, antioxidant, and anti-cancer effects [41]. The following section discusses the effects of CA and its derivatives on different components of MetS.

3. CA vs. Obesity

Obesity is a condition where excess body fat accumulates either due to the enlargement of lipids in existing adipocytes (hypertrophy), or through an increase in the number of adipocytes (hyperplasia) [42]. Adipose tissue in the human body functions as an energy storage system, an endocrine gland, and a heat producer (nonshivering thermogenesis) [43]. In healthy slender individuals, adipocytes are smaller, more insulin-sensitive, and secretes anti-inflammatory mediators such as adiponectin, IL-10, IL-4, IL-13, IL-1 receptor agonist (IL-1Ra), apelin, and transforming growth factor beta (TGFβ). In contrast, the adipocytes of an obese individual are enlarged and infiltrated by a large number of pro-inflammatory M1 macrophages that secrete pro-inflammatory cytokines such as TNFα, IL-6, visfatin, leptin, MCP-1, Ang-II, and plasminogen activator inhibitor-1 [44]. With the surplus of these pro-inflammatory compounds within the obese adipocyte, they are often referred to be in a state of inflammation. This state of chronic low-grade activation of the innate immune system is critical in the pathophysiology of obesity and MetS [45].

Visceral fat is localized within the abdomen and is metabolically active with the constant release of free fatty acids into the portal circulation [46]. In a state of caloric excess, the hypertrophied adipocytes will secrete adipokines that result in the increment of additional pre-adipocytes that will later mature. However, this compensatory act reaches its threshold and causes fat accumulation in the visceral depots. The accumulation and distribution of the fat depots play a key role in forming metabolic complications. A metabolically healthy obese individual that remains insulin-sensitive and displays a normal metabolic and hormonal profile and is physically different compares to a metabolically unhealthy obese person through their higher abdominal circumference measurement [47].

Metabolic changes in obesity are associated with a persistent low-grade inflammatory state that impairs energy homeostasis and glucose metabolism [44,48]. The c-Jun N-terminal kinase (JNK) and the nuclear factor-kappa B (NF-κB) signaling pathways contribute to inflammation and play a key role in obesity, insulin-resistance, and in regulating the expression of proinflammatory molecules [49]. Zhang and colleagues found that CA was able to exert anti-inflammatory effects in dextran sulfate sodium-induced colitis mice, showing a significantly suppressed secretion of IL-6 and TNFα and colonic infiltration of CD3+ T cells, CD177+ neutrophils, and F4/80+ macrophages through the activation of the NF-κB signaling pathway. Their study concluded that CA was able to amend the colonic pathology and inflammation, indirectly contributing toward reducing obesity [50].

Obesity may also be associated with adipocyte necrosis, which could be the start of a pro-inflammatory response. Adipocytes grow hypertrophic when their caloric intake and energy expenditure increase, which has been linked to cell hypoxia and death. These hypertrophic adipocytes will subsequently start secreting TNFα in small amounts, resulting in a chemotactic response that draws macrophages [48]. An in vitro study using adipose stem cells (ASCs) showed that CAPE had the ability to inverse the effects of high glucose and lipopolysaccharide exposure. Through this study, they found that CAPE treatment was able to restore the functions of adipocytes by increasing the adiponectin and peroxisome proliferator-activated receptor gamma (PPARγ), resulting in the reduction in pro-inflammatory factors [51]. CA also acts on adipogenesis by reducing intracellular lipid accumulation in an in vitro model [52].

Increasing evidence has shown that gut microbiota plays a role in the development of obesity and MetS through the modulation of energy absorption, and subsequently influences glucose and lipid metabolism [53,54]. It was recently postulated that gut microbiota producing t10,c12-conjugated linoleic acid induced lipogenesis [8]. Dietary polyphenols have been found to promote the growth of beneficial bacteria while inhibiting pathogenic bacteria [55]. In an in vivo study to determine the anti-obesity effect of CA, high-fat-diet (HFD)-induced mice were seen to have a positive effect after being given a daily dose of 50 mg/kg CA for a span of 12 weeks. The researchers noted a significant reduction in body weight and fat accumulation, increases in energy expenditure and beneficial gut bacteria (i.e., Muribaculaceae), and a decrease in pathogenic bacteriae (i.e., Lachnospiraceae) [56].

In another study, HFDs in nonalcoholic fatty liver disease (NAFLD)-induced mice were used to demonstrate the effectiveness of CA treatment and its effects toward the gut microbiota. CA was able to significantly reduce the body weight of the HFD-fed mice and attenuated the expression of lipogenesis-related protein expression (Srebp1, Fas, Acc, and Scd1) in the liver. It was concluded that CA exerted protective effects on the NAFLD mice by inhibiting gut dysbiosis, pro-inflammatory LPS release, and subsequent lipid synthesis [57].

4. CA vs. Hyperglycemia and Insulin Resistance

One of the primary causes of metabolic and endocrine abnormalities, as well as cellular damage in afflicted tissue, is hyperglycemia-related oxidative stress [15]. Nutrient-induced toxicity due to overnutrition may lead to insulin-resistance in tissues such as the heart and the skeletal muscle, which normally responds to insulin for glucose uptake [58]. Insulin resistance is a condition where the tissues use their adaptive mechanism to avoid toxic nutrient overload [59]. Over time, insulin resistance will cause an increase in fasting glucose and reduced insulin-mediated glucose clearance. Eventually, hyperinsulinemia will occur as a negative feedback from the target cells, signaling inadequate insulin response, and, in turn, the pancreatic β-cells will produce more insulin. The prolonged inability to correct the state of insulin resistance will eventually give rise to hyperglycemia and type 2 diabetes [60].

CA is found to increase insulin sensitivity through the reduction in proinflammatory cytokines and increase in adiponectins under the hyperglycemic state [51]. In a study that used MetS diet-induced rats, where it caused increases in BMI and abdominal circumference, blood glucose, triglycerides, and LDLc, and lowered the HDLc, the group that received a dose of 40 mg/kg oral gavage of CA daily for 6 weeks showcased a significant reduction in serum leptin, adiponectin, insulin, TNF-a, IL-6, and IL-8. The study showed that CA had the highest superoxide dismutase (SOD), catalase, and glutathione peroxidase antioxidant enzymes in the liver after 4 weeks of CA administration in comparison to ferulic acid, gallic acid, and protocatechuic acid under the same doses [61]. This suggests that the scavenging activity as a result of CA administration shows the most promising effectivity amongst the listed phenolic acids that protect against hyperglycemic damages.

Nasry et al. investigated the role of pioglitazone (a synthetic PPARγ agonist that causes a decrease in insulin resistance) on HFD-induced-MetS rats, and CA was able to show promising results. There was a significant reduction in insulin resistance, fasting blood glucose, and fasting serum insulin with an increase of insulin sensitivity and β cell function. CA also reduces the nitric oxide (NO) liver contents to almost half of those of the HFD-induced MetS rats [62]. This shows the efficacy of CA as scavenging activity toward correcting the insulin resistance through the reduction in oxidative stress caused by the HFD.

CA also suppresses the hepatic glucose output by enhancing its utilization and inhibiting overproduction [63]. This can be seen by the increase in glucokinase activity through an increase in its mRNA expression and glycogen content. It was also found to simultaneously lower the G6Pase and phosphoenolpyruvate carboxykinase activities together with their respective mRNA expressions, along with a decline in the GLUT2 expression in the liver [63].

CA methyl and ethyl esters exert antidiabetic activities in insulin-responsive cells through insulin-independent mechanisms involving AMPK and adipogenic factors [64]. A 2-week treatment of CAPA toward streptozotocin and diet-induced diabetic mice were able to protect them against hepatic inflammation and glucose intolerance associated with the NF-κB-mediated induction of inflammatory cytokines and the increase in the expression of antioxidant protein. HepG2 cell models were then used to further investigate CAPA's ability. They were able to show that CAPA was able to ameliorate TNFα-induced pIKKα/β expression and prevent TG accumulation in H_2O_2-treated HepG2 cells [40]. These findings strengthen the belief that chronic oral administration of CAPA is able to protect against MetS.

Stress-induced inflammation may cause the development of insulin resistance [65–67]. Stress activates the hypothalamic–pituitary–adrenal axis, renin–angiotensin system pathway, and sympathoadrenal system, all of which are involved in the production of pro-inflammatory cytokines, resulting in the negative downregulation of insulin signaling by either phosphorylating insulin resistance serine residues or inhibiting Akt, resulting in insulin resistance. CA given to chronic restraint stress-induced insulin-resistance mice showed to reduce fasting blood sugar, systemic inflammation, and oxidative stress, and improve insulin sensitivity [68].

5. CA vs. Dyslipidemia

Dyslipidemia is described as an abnormal level of circulating lipids. It has been acknowledged that dyslipidaemia increases the risk of cardiovascular disease development [69]. This condition may be of primary cause (genetic) or secondary (diet, drugs, chronic diseases, and metabolic disorders, including MetS). Dyslipidemia is detected through a biochemical analysis of fasting lipid profile, which consists of TG, total cholesterol (TC), high-density lipoprotein cholesterol (HDL-c), low-density lipoprotein cholesterol (LDL-c), and non-HDL-c. Dyslipidemia is diagnosed when there is an increased concentration of TG, TC, LDL-c, and non-HDL-c, along with a decreased level of HDL-c [70].

Free fatty acids (FFA) are abundantly released in an obese body due to the increase in the adipose tissue mass. FFA causes an increase in the synthesis of glucose and TG in the liver, as well as an increase in VLDL secretion. This occurs together with the reduction in HDL-C and increased density of LDL [71]. CA has shown improvement in the serum lipid profile, serum liver biomarker enzymes, and hepatic tissue architecture to normal in HFD-induced hyperlipidemic rat models by showing antihyperlipidemic and hepatoprotective activities. CA was found able to reduce the levels of endoplasmic reticulum stress markers in the liver after a HFD obese induction [72]. Besides CA's ability to revert dyslipidemia by reducing TG and TC, studies have shown that CA was able to revert hepatic steatosis in the long run [49,73–75]. In a recent in vivo study, a 12 week CA supplementation on HFD obese mice revealed that CA was able to reduce body weight and fat accumulation together with readings of improved lipid profile with an increased HDL [56]. This suggests that CA's ability to impair the formation of bad white fat tissue could subsequently reduce FFA production, thereby showing its hepatoprotective ability.

CA is capable of providing a TG-lowering, anticoagulatory, antioxidative, and anti-inflammatory protection for the cardiac tissue and also downregulating the TNF-α and monocyte chemoattractant protein-1 mRNA expression in the kidney of diet-induced diabetic rats [76]. Studies on diet-induced hypercholesterolemic rats by Agunloye and Oboh compared the modulatory properties of CA and chlorogenic acid, proving that CA was a better candidate in ameliorating the pathological condition. They also tested two different dosages of the drug (10 mg/kg and 15 mg/kg of CA) and concluded the lipid-lowering effects were more effective at larger doses [77].

It is possible that an excessive amount of oxidative stress and/or inflammation can convert circulating LDL and HDL particles into oxidized LDL (oxLDL) and oxidized HDL particles (oxHDL). OxLDL and oxHDL both stay longer in the bloodstream due to their impaired interaction with their specific receptors. Their diminished clearance and imbalance of lipid profile ultimately contributes to the onset of atherosclerosis [19]. CA is thought to prevent atherosclerosis by lowering the functional and structural changes in the arteries [78]. This has been demonstrated by its ability to inhibit thrombogenic thromboxane A2 (TXA2) production together with other platelet-aggregating molecules [79,80]. CA also downregulated platelet-activating molecules such as COX-1, calcium ions, and P-selectin and upregulated platelet-inhibiting molecules such as cAMP and cGMP, resulting in an inhibition toward thrombogenic processes [81].

6. CA vs. Hypertension

Almost 80% of the individuals with MetS suffer from hypertension. Evidence concurred that 65–75% of the risk factor for primary hypertension is contributed by obesity and excess weight gain [82]. Besides, insulin resistance has also been linked to hypertension as insulin is able to cross the blood–brain barrier and subsequently activate the systemic nervous system, in addition to its ability to upregulate the angiotensin II (AT-II) receptor and reduce NO [60]. NO is one of the most important ROS in the cardiovascular system. ROS are produced by NO synthase enzymatically, and they act as a prototype endothelial-derived vasodilator [83].

Nω-Nitro-L-arginine-methyl ester (L-NAME) is a well-known active inhibitor of NO production in the nerves and the endothelial cell. A study using L-NAME-induced hypertensive rats showed that a combination of caffeine and CA was able to reduce the systolic BP. A decrease in ACE and arginase activity coupled with high NO and low MDA levels might be associated with their antihypertensive effects [84,85]. In another study using CAPE against the high-fructose corn syrup diet-induced vascular damage in rats, blood pressure values were significantly reduced after a two-week intraperitoneal injection with CA derivative. This study also noted that CAPE has the ability to correct the reduced levels of endothelial NO synthase levels caused by the high-fructose corn syrup diet [73].

According to a more recent study, CA has a favorable effect on the vascular function and blood pressure stabilization. In this study, male SERCA2a knockout mice and its wild-type were surgically implanted with mini osmotic pumps filled with AT-II solutions and fed with a normal diet of 0.05% CA in drinking water. CA significantly attenuated the AT-II-induced increase in blood pressure reading in the wildtype mice but showed no hypotensive effect to the SERCA2a knockout mice. This suggests that the CA might act by activating the SERCA2a on the primary vascular smooth muscle cells [86].

CA has also been reported to be a potent antihypertensive agent and has been confirmed to have a nontoxic manifestation [87,88]. Agunloye and Oboh's in vitro study revealed that CA was capable of inhibiting key enzymes associated with hypertension that includes E-NTPDase, 5'-ectonucleotidase, ADA, ACE, arginase, and AChE. This study suggested that CA targets specific enzymes associated with hypertension [89]. Decreased ACE and arginase activity, as well as high NO and low MDA levels, might be associated with their antihypertensive effects [77]. The summary for MetS studies related to CA can be found in Table 1, whereas the proposed pathway for CA against MetS can be found in Figure 2.

Table 1. MetS studies related to CA.

Pathological Induction/State	Dose of CA or Its Derivates and Administration Route	Duration of Treatment	Observations	Reference
Diet-induced MetS with HFD in male Wistar rats	40 mg/kg via oral gavage	6 weeks	Reduced: —Insulin —HOMA-IR —Leptin —TNFα —IL-6 —IL-8 —Total cholesterol, TG, VLDLc, LDLc, HDLc Increased: —Adiponectin	[61]
Diet-induced hypercholesterolemic rats	10 and 15 mg/kg	21 days	Reduced: —Total cholesterol —TG —LDL —HDL (With dose 15 mg/kg showing better results) Increased: —Plasma and heart SOD activity	[77]
Nω-Nitro-L-argininge-methylester (L-NAME)-induced hypertensive in male Wistar rats	5 mg/kg and 25 mg/kg via oral gavage	20 days	Reduced: —SBP —MDA Increased: —ACE activity —NOx level	[85]

Table 1. Cont.

Pathological Induction/State	Dose of CA or Its Derivates and Administration Route	Duration of Treatment	Observations	Reference
Surgically implanted mini osmotic pumps filled with Ang II solution in wild type mice and SERCA2a knockout mice	0.05% CA in drinking water	8 weeks	CA was able to: —Relax mesenteric artery —Smooth norepinephrine-induced vasoconstriction —Reduced intracellular Ca^{2+} ions —Bind to SERCA forming strong hydrogen bonds —Significantly attenuated AngII-induced hypertension. However, CA failed to do so in SERCA2a knockout mice	[86]
HFD obesity-induced C57BL/6J mice	50 mg/kg via oral gavage	12 weeks	Reduced serum insulin	[56]
Alloxan-induced type-1 diabetic in Swiss albino mice	50 mg/kg intraperitoneal injection	7 days	Protective effects on liver and kidneys Hypoglycemic and hypolipidemic properties.	[75]
STZ-induced diabetic male Wistar rats	10 and 50 mg/kg via oral gavage (diluted in canola oil)	30 days	Reduced —FBS —oxidative stress parameters (lipid peroxidation, reactive species production, protein oxidation, and MPO activity).	[90]
STZ-induced diabetic rats	orally	5 weeks	Increased: —serum insulin level —GSH, CAT, and SOD levels Reduced: —Blood glucose level Histologically seen normal islet morphology in CA administered diabetic rats.	[91]
STZ and high-fat high-fructose-diet-induced CD1 (ICR) mice	10 mg/kg/day of CAPA orally	2 weeks	Reduced —Body weight increase —Plasma retinol binding protein 4 (RBP4) —Adiponectin level —TNFα in liver Preserved glucose tolerance Prevented glucose intolerance Preserved basal coronary flow	[40]
Insulin-resistant adipocytes ASCs exposed to high glucose levels			Decreased lipid droplets and radical oxygen species formation. Increased insulin sensitivity (showed reduction in pro-inflammatory cytokines level and increased adiponectins).	[51]
HFD inducing NAFLD in C57BL/6J mice	0.08% or 0.16% CA added to pellet diet	8 weeks	Reduced body weight in both concentrations. Positively altered the community compositional structure of gut microbiota.	[57]

Table 1. Cont.

Pathological Induction/State	Dose of CA or Its Derivates and Administration Route	Duration of Treatment	Observations	Reference
Non-insulin-dependent DM (NIDDM) and insulin-resistant (IR) mice models	15 and 30 mg/kg CAPE dissolved in PEG-400 given via oral gavage.	5 weeks	Improved: —Insulin sensitivity —Hyperlipidemia —Peroxisome-proliferator-activated receptor-α (PPAR-α) —TNFα —Glucose consumption —Glucose uptake —Glycogen content —Oxidative stress level —Decreased level of glucose-6-phosphotase expression (G6Pase).	[49]
HFD-induced obesity in mice	50 mg/kg/day orally	10 weeks	Reduced: —Body weight —Liver weight —Liver lipid accumulation —Levels of ER stress markers in the liver Improved glucose intolerance and insulin sensitivity.	[72]
High fructose corn syrup-induced vascular dysfunction in Sprague Dawley rats	50 mmol/kg intraperitoneal injection	2 weeks	Reduced SBP Increased NO synthase production. Significant reduction in TC and LDL. No significant change to HDL nor TG.	[73]
Chronic restraint stress-induced insulin resistance in LACA mice	5 and 10 mg/kg intraperitoneal injections	30 days	Reduces: —Fasting blood sugar —Systemic inflammation —Oxidative stress —Improved insulin sensitivity	[68]
HFD-induced MetS in C57 mice	A combination of ferulic acid (50 mg/kg/day) with CA 0.9 mg/kg/day via subcutaneous injection	40 days	Prevents obesity. Reverts hyperglycemia. Reverts dyslipidemia. Reverts hepatic steatosis.	[74]
High-fat-diet and STZ-induced diabetic male Wistar rats	40 mg/kg via oral gavage	8 weeks	Improved albumin excretion by kidneys. Improved blood glucose Reduced renal mesangial matrix extension. CA results were seen better in reversing the diabetic nephropathy in comparison to prevention.	[92]
L-NAME-induced Sprague Dawley rats	50 µmol/kg/day intraperitoneally	14 days	Kidney tissue analysis shows that CA was: —Unable to preserve PON1 activity —Unable to reduce NF-κB significantly	[93]
Hyperlipidemic Wistar Albino	20 mg/kg/day	30 days	Significantly reduced: —Total cholesterol —TG —HDL-c	[94]

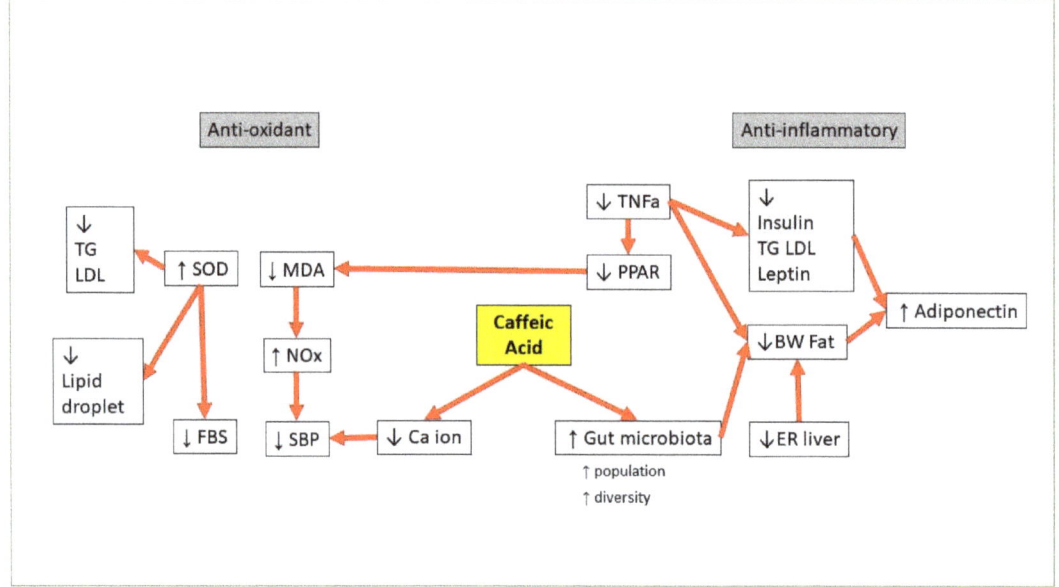

Figure 2. Proposed CA pathways against MetS.

7. Conclusions

There has been enormous progress in understanding the effect of CA through retrospective research. Strong evidence of the ability of CA to reverse the MetS effects through the reduction in inflammatory markers such as TNFα coupled with reduced oxidative stress parameters have guided researchers to a more proteomic and metabolomic approach. Besides the singular usage of CA, studies of using CA as an enhancer together with more commonly used drugs have surfaced. Through this review, we can conclude that CA holds strong potential to be used as MetS management by its anti-obesity, antidiabetic, hypolipidemic, and hypotensive activities. During the course of drafting this manuscript, we identified a substantial gap in which the wealth of knowledge about CA is limited to findings in animal models or cell lines. Further studies in the form of a clinical trial or a population cohort study would further strengthen the beneficial effect of CA on MetS.

Author Contributions: Conceptualization, N.N.M.A.K. and M.F.Y.; writing—original draft preparation, N.N.M.A.K.; writing—review and editing, M.F.Y., F.A. and S.L.T.; supervision, M.F.Y., F.A. and S.L.T.; project administration, M.F.Y.; funding acquisition, M.F.Y. All authors have read and agreed to the published version of the manuscript.

Funding: This research was funded by PPUKM Fundamental Grant, grant number FF-2019-014.

Conflicts of Interest: The authors declare no conflict of interest.

References

1. Ranasinghe, P.; Mathangasinghe, Y.; Jayawardena, R.; Hills, A.; Misra, A. Prevalence and trends of metabolic syndrome among adults in the asia-pacific region: A systematic review. *BMC Public Health* **2017**, *17*, 107. [CrossRef]
2. Manaf, M.R.A.; Nawi, A.M.; Tauhid, N.M.; Othman, H.; Rahman, M.R.A.; Yusoff, H.M.; Safian, N.; Ng, P.Y.; Manaf, Z.A.; Kadir, N.B.A.; et al. Prevalence of metabolic syndrome and its associated risk factors among staffs in a Malaysian public university. *Sci. Rep.* **2021**, *11*, 1–11. [CrossRef]
3. Ando, K.; Fujita, T. Metabolic syndrome and oxidative stress. *Free Radic. Biol. Med.* **2009**, *47*, 213–218. [CrossRef]
4. Martinez-Ferran, M.; De La Guía-Galipienso, F.; Sanchis-Gomar, F.; Pareja-Galeano, H. Metabolic Impacts of Confinement during the COVID-19 Pandemic due to Modified Diet and Physical Activity Habits. *Nutrients* **2020**, *12*, 1549. [CrossRef]

5. Alberti, K.G.M.M.; Eckel, R.H.; Grundy, S.M.; Zimmet, P.; Cleeman, J.I.; Donato, K.A.; Fruchart, J.-C.; James, W.P.T.; Loria, C.M.; Smith, S.C., Jr. Harmonizing the Metabolic Syndrome. *Circulation* **2009**, *120*, 1640–1645. [CrossRef]
6. EEckel, R.H.; Alberti, K.G.M.M.; Grundy, S.M.; Zimmet, P.Z. The metabolic syndrome. *Lancet* **2010**, *375*, 181–183. [CrossRef]
7. Li, A.; Zheng, N.; Ding, X. Mitochondrial abnormalities: A hub in metabolic syndrome-related cardiac dysfunction caused by oxidative stress. *Heart Fail. Rev.* **2021**, 1–8. [CrossRef]
8. Etchegoyen, M.; Nobile, M.H.; Baez, F.; Posesorski, B.; González, J.; Lago, N.; Milei, J.; Otero-Losada, M. Metabolic Syndrome and Neuroprotection. *Front. Neurosci.* **2018**, *12*, 196. [CrossRef]
9. Li, S.; Tan, H.-Y.; Wang, N.; Zhang, Z.-J.; Lao, L.; Wong, C.-W.; Feng, Y. The Role of Oxidative Stress and Antioxidants in Liver Diseases. *Int. J. Mol. Sci.* **2015**, *16*, 26087–26124. [CrossRef] [PubMed]
10. Maritim, A.C.; Sanders, R.A.; Watkins, J.B. Diabetes, oxidative stress, and antioxidants: A review. *J. Biochem. Mol. Toxicol.* **2003**, *17*, 24–38. [CrossRef]
11. Monserrat-Mesquida, M.; Quetglas-Llabrés, M.; Capó, X.; Bouzas, C.; Mateos, D.; Pons, A.; Tur, J.A.; Sureda, A. Metabolic Syndrome Is Associated with Oxidative Stress and Proinflammatory State. *Antioxidants* **2020**, *9*, 236. [CrossRef] [PubMed]
12. Hanson, R.L.; Imperatore, G.; Bennett, P.H.; Knowler, W.C. Components of the "metabolic syndrome" and incidence of type 2 diabetes. *Diabetes* **2002**, *51*, 3120–3127. [CrossRef]
13. Kassi, E.; Pervanidou, P.; Kaltsas, G.; Chrousos, G. Metabolic syndrome: Definitions and controversies. *BMC Med.* **2011**, *9*, 48. [CrossRef] [PubMed]
14. Sies, H.; Jones, D.P. Reactive oxygen species (ROS) as pleiotropic physiological signalling agents. *Nat. Rev. Mol. Cell Biol.* **2020**, *21*, 363–383. [CrossRef] [PubMed]
15. Korac, B.; Kalezic, A.; Pekovic-Vaughan, V.; Korac, A.; Jankovic, A. Redox changes in obesity, metabolic syndrome, and diabetes. *Redox Biol.* **2021**, *42*, 101887. [CrossRef]
16. Quinn, K.J.; Shah, N.H. A dataset quantifying polypharmacy in the United States. *Sci. Data* **2017**, *4*, 170167. [CrossRef] [PubMed]
17. Kumar, S.; Pandey, A.K. Chemistry and Biological Activities of Flavonoids: An Overview. *Sci. World J.* **2013**, *2013*, e162750. [CrossRef] [PubMed]
18. Panche, A.N.; Diwan, A.D.; Chandra, S.R. Flavonoids: An overview. *J. Nutr. Sci.* **2016**, *5*, e47. [CrossRef]
19. Feldman, F.; Koudoufio, M.; Desjardins, Y.; Spahis, S.; Delvin, E.; Levy, E. Efficacy of Polyphenols in the Management of Dyslipidemia: A Focus on Clinical Studies. *Nutrients* **2021**, *13*, 672. [CrossRef]
20. Kumar, S.R.; Ramli, E.S.M.; Nasir, N.A.A.; Ismail, N.H.M.; Fahami, N.A.M. Preventive Effect of Naringin on Metabolic Syndrome and Its Mechanism of Action: A Systematic Review. *Altern. Med.* **2019**, *2019*, e9752826. [CrossRef]
21. Azuma, K.; Ippoushi, K.; Nakayama, M.; Ito, H.; Higashio, H.; Terao, J. Absorption of chlorogenic acid and caffeic acid in rats after oral administration. *J. Agric. Food Chem.* **2000**, *48*, 5496–5500. [CrossRef] [PubMed]
22. Manish, P.; Wei Ling, L.; Seong Lin, T.; Mohamad Fairuz, Y. Flavonoids and its Neuroprotective Effects on Brain Ischemia and Neurodegenerative Diseases. *Curr. Drug Targets* **2018**, *19*, 1710–1720. [CrossRef]
23. Kasprzak-Drozd, K.; Oniszczuk, T.; Stasiak, M.; Oniszczuk, A. Beneficial Effects of Phenolic Compounds on Gut Microbiota and Metabolic Syndrome. *Int. J. Mol. Sci.* **2021**, *22*, 3715. [CrossRef] [PubMed]
24. Saibabu, V.; Fatima, Z.; Khan, L.A.; Hameed, S. Therapeutic Potential of Dietary Phenolic Acids. *Adv. Pharmacol. Sci.* **2015**, *2015*, 823539. [CrossRef] [PubMed]
25. Leonard, W.; Zhang, P.; Ying, D.; Fang, Z. Hydroxycinnamic acids on gut microbiota and health. *Compr. Rev. Food Sci. Food Saf.* **2021**, *20*, 710–737. [CrossRef]
26. Göçer, H.; Gülçin, I. Caffeic acid phenethyl ester (CAPE): Correlation of structure and antioxidant properties. *Int. J. Food Sci. Nutr.* **2011**, *62*, 821–825. [CrossRef] [PubMed]
27. Filipe, H.; Sousa, C.; Marquês, J.T.; Vila-Viçosa, D.; de Granada-Flor, A.; Viana, A.; Santos, M.; Machuqueiro, M.; de Almeida, R.F. Differential targeting of membrane lipid domains by caffeic acid and its ester derivatives. *Free Radic. Biol. Med.* **2018**, *115*, 232–245. [CrossRef]
28. Vinayagam, R.; Jayachandran, M.; Xu, B. Antidiabetic Effects of Simple Phenolic Acids: A Comprehensive Review. *Phytother. Res.* **2016**, *30*, 184–199. [CrossRef]
29. Armutcu, F.; Akyol, S.; Ustunsoy, S.; Turan, F.F. Therapeutic potential of caffeic acid phenethyl ester and its anti-inflammatory and immunomodulatory effects (Review). *Exp. Ther. Med.* **2015**, *9*, 1582–1588. [CrossRef] [PubMed]
30. KKępa, M.; Miklasińska-Majdanik, M.; Wojtyczka, R.D.; Idzik, D.; Korzeniowski, K.; Smoleń-Dzirba, J.; Wąsik, T.J. Antimicrobial Potential of Caffeic Acid against Staphylococcus aureus Clinical Strains. *BioMed Res. Int.* **2018**, *2018*, e7413504. [CrossRef]
31. Kim, Y.H.; Sung, Y.-H.; Lee, H.-H.; Ko, I.-G.; Kim, S.-E.; Shin, M.-S.; Kim, B.-K. Postnatal treadmill exercise alleviates short-term memory impairment by enhancing cell proliferation and suppressing apoptosis in the hippocampus of rat pups born to diabetic rats. *J. Exerc. Rehabil.* **2014**, *10*, 209–217. [CrossRef]
32. Koga, M.; Nakagawa, S.; Kato, A.; Kusumi, I. Caffeic acid reduces oxidative stress and microglial activation in the mouse hippocampus. *Tissue Cell* **2019**, *60*, 14–20. [CrossRef]
33. Pereira, P.; De Oliveira, P.A.; Ardenghi, P.; Rotta, L.; Henriques, J.A.P.; Picada, J.N. Neuropharmacological analysis of caffeic acid in rats. *Basic Clin. Pharmacol. Toxicol.* **2006**, *99*, 374–378. [CrossRef]
34. Sato, Y.; Itagaki, S.; Kurokawa, T.; Ogura, J.; Kobayashi, M.; Hirano, T.; Sugawara, M.; Iseki, K. In vitro and in vivo antioxidant properties of chlorogenic acid and caffeic acid. *Int. J. Pharm.* **2011**, *403*, 136–138. [CrossRef] [PubMed]

35. Kassim, M.; Achoui, M.; Mustafa, M.R.; Mohd, M.A.; Yusoff, K.M. Ellagic acid, phenolic acids, and flavonoids in Malaysian honey extracts demonstrate in vitro anti-inflammatory activity. *Nutr. Res.* **2010**, *30*, 650–659. [CrossRef]
36. Ramli, N.Z.; Chin, K.-Y.; Zarkasi, K.A.; Ahmad, F. The Beneficial Effects of Stingless Bee Honey from Heterotrigona itama against Metabolic Changes in Rats Fed with High-Carbohydrate and High-Fat Diet. *Environ. Res. Public Health* **2019**, *16*, 4987. [CrossRef] [PubMed]
37. Kolgazi, M.; Cilingir, S.; Yilmaz, O.; Gemici, M.; Yazar, H.; Ozer, S.; Acikel-Elmas, M.; Arbak, S.; Suyen, G.G. Caffeic acid attenuates gastric mucosal damage induced by ethanol in rats via nitric oxide modulation. *Chem.-Biol. Interact.* **2021**, *334*, 109351. [CrossRef]
38. Gülçin, İ. Antioxidant activity of caffeic acid (3,4-dihydroxycinnamic acid). *Toxicology* **2006**, *217*, 213–220. [CrossRef] [PubMed]
39. Piazzon, A.; Vrhovsek, U.; Masuero, D.; Mattivi, F.; Mandoj, F.; Nardini, M. Antioxidant activity of phenolic acids and their metabolites: Synthesis and antioxidant properties of the sulfate derivatives of ferulic and caffeic acids and of the acyl glucuronide of ferulic acid. *J. Agric. Food Chem.* **2012**, *60*, 12312–12323. [CrossRef] [PubMed]
40. Weng, Y.-C.; Chuang, S.-T.; Lin, Y.-C.; Chuang, C.-F.; Chi, T.-C.; Chiu, H.-L.; Kuo, Y.-H.; Su, M.-J. Caffeic Acid Phenylethyl Amide Protects against the Metabolic Consequences in Diabetes Mellitus Induced by Diet and Streptozocin. *Evid.-Based Complement. Altern. Med.* **2012**, *2012*, e984780. [CrossRef]
41. Shin, E.J.; Jo, S.; Choi, H.-K.; Choi, S.; Byun, S.; Lim, T.-G. Caffeic Acid Phenethyl Ester Inhibits UV-Induced MMP-1 Expression by Targeting Histone Acetyltransferases in Human Skin. *Int. J. Mol. Sci.* **2019**, *20*, 3055. [CrossRef]
42. Honecker, J.; Weidlich, D.; Heisz, S.; Lindgren, C.M.; Karampinos, D.C.; Claussnitzer, M.; Hauner, H. A distribution-centered approach for analyzing human adipocyte size estimates and their association with obesity-related traits and mitochondrial function. *Int. J. Obes.* **2021**, *45*, 2108–2117. [CrossRef] [PubMed]
43. Cannon, B.; Nedergaard, J. Brown adipose tissue: Function and physiological significance. *Physiol. Rev.* **2004**, *84*, 277–359. [CrossRef]
44. Jayarathne, S.; Koboziev, I.; Park, O.-H.; Oldewage-Theron, W.; Shen, C.-L.; Moustaid-Moussa, N. Anti-Inflammatory and Anti-Obesity Properties of Food Bioactive Components: Effects on Adipose Tissue. *Prev. Nutr. Food Sci.* **2017**, *22*, 251–262. [CrossRef] [PubMed]
45. Engin, A.B. Adipocyte-Macrophage Cross-Talk in Obesity. In *Obesity and Lipotoxicity*; Engin, A.B., Engin, A., Eds.; Springer International Publishing: Cham, Switzerland, 2017; pp. 327–343. [CrossRef]
46. Jensen, M.D. Visceral Fat: Culprit or Canary? *Endocrinol. Metab. Clin. N. Am.* **2020**, *49*, 229–237. [CrossRef] [PubMed]
47. Chait, A.; den Hartigh, L.J. Adipose Tissue Distribution, Inflammation and Its Metabolic Consequences, Including Diabetes and Cardiovascular Disease. *Front. Cardiovasc. Med.* **2020**, *7*, 22. [CrossRef] [PubMed]
48. Parekh, P.J.; Arusi, E.; Vinik, A.I.; Johnson, D.A. The Role and Influence of Gut Microbiota in Pathogenesis and Management of Obesity and Metabolic Syndrome. *Front. Endocrinol.* **2014**, *5*, 47. [CrossRef]
49. Nie, J.; Chang, Y.; Li, Y.; Zhou, Y.; Qin, J.; Sun, Z.; Li, H. Caffeic Acid Phenethyl Ester (Propolis Extract) Ameliorates Insulin Resistance by Inhibiting JNK and NF-κB Inflammatory Pathways in Diabetic Mice and HepG2 Cell Models. *J. Agric. Food Chem.* **2017**, *65*, 9041–9053. [CrossRef]
50. Zhang, Z.; Wu, X.; Cao, S.; Wang, L.; Wang, D.; Yang, H.; Feng, Y.; Wang, S.; Shoulin, W. Caffeic acid ameliorates colitis in association with increased Akkermansia population in the gut microbiota of mice. *Oncotarget* **2016**, *7*, 31790–31799. [CrossRef]
51. Vanella, L.; Tibullo, D.; Godos, J.; Pluchinotta, F.R.; Di Giacomo, C.; Sorrenti, V.; Acquaviva, R.; Russo, A.; Volti, G.L.; Barbagallo, I. Caffeic Acid Phenethyl Ester Regulates PPAR's Levels in Stem Cells-Derived Adipocytes. *PPAR Res.* **2016**, *2016*, e7359521. [CrossRef] [PubMed]
52. Mariana, B.D.; Tiago, L.S.; Ramon, R.P.P.B.D.M.; Jamile, M.F.; Tiago, S.M.; Richard, R.C.M.; Hector, G.R.; Dânya, B.L.; Alice, M.C.M.; Maria, G.R.D.Q. Caffeic acid reduces lipid accumulation and reactive oxygen species production in adipocytes. *Afr. J. Pharm. Pharmacol.* **2018**, *12*, 263–268. [CrossRef]
53. Boulangé, C.L.; Neves, A.L.; Chilloux, J.; Nicholson, J.K.; Dumas, M.-E. Impact of the gut microbiota on inflammation, obesity, and metabolic disease. *Genome Med.* **2016**, *8*, 42. [CrossRef]
54. Ridaura, V.K.; Faith, J.J.; Rey, F.E.; Cheng, J.; Duncan, A.E.; Kau, A.; Griffin, N.W.; Lombard, V.; Henrissat, B.; Bain, J.R.; et al. Gut Microbiota from Twins Discordant for Obesity Modulate Metabolism in Mice. *Science* **2013**, *341*, 1241214. [CrossRef]
55. Dueñas, M.; Muñoz-Gonzalez, I.; Cueva, C.; Jiménez-Girón, A.; Sánchez-Patán, F.; Santos-Buelga, C.; Moreno-Arribas, M.; Bartolomé, B. A Survey of Modulation of Gut Microbiota by Dietary Polyphenols. *BioMed Res. Int.* **2015**, *2015*, e850902. [CrossRef] [PubMed]
56. Xu, J.; Ge, J.; He, X.; Sheng, Y.; Zheng, S.; Zhang, C.; Xu, W.; Huang, K. Caffeic acid reduces body weight by regulating gut microbiota in diet-induced-obese mice. *J. Funct. Foods* **2020**, *74*, 104061. [CrossRef]
57. Mu, H.-N.; Zhou, Q.; Yang, R.-Y.; Tang, W.-Q.; Li, H.-X.; Wang, S.-M.; Li, J.; Chen, W.-X.; Dong, J. Caffeic acid prevents non-alcoholic fatty liver disease induced by a high-fat diet through gut microbiota modulation in mice. *Food Res. Int.* **2021**, *143*, 110240. [CrossRef]
58. Freeman, A.M.; Pennings, N. Insulin Resistance. In *StatPearls*; StatPearls Publishing: Treasure Island, FL, USA, 2021. Available online: http://www.ncbi.nlm.nih.gov/books/NBK507839/ (accessed on 12 August 2021).
59. Nolan, C.J.; Ruderman, N.B.; Kahn, S.E.; Pedersen, O.; Prentki, M. Insulin Resistance as a Physiological Defense Against Metabolic Stress: Implications for the Management of Subsets of Type 2 Diabetes. *Diabetes* **2015**, *64*, 673–686. [CrossRef]

60. Hashim, K.-N.; Chin, K.-Y.; Ahmad, F. The Mechanism of Honey in Reversing Metabolic Syndrome. *Molecules* **2021**, *26*, 808. [CrossRef]
61. Ibitoye, O.B.; Ajiboye, T.O. Dietary phenolic acids reverse insulin resistance, hyperglycaemia, dyslipidaemia, inflammation and oxidative stress in high-fructose diet-induced metabolic syndrome rats. *Arch. Physiol. Biochem.* **2018**, *124*, 410–417. [CrossRef]
62. Nasry, M.R.; Abo-Youssef, A.M.; Zaki, H.F.; El-Denshary, E.-E.-D.S. Effect of caffeic acid and pioglitazone in an experimental model of metabolic syndrome. *Int. J.Sci. Res. Publ.* **2015**, *5*, 1–9.
63. JJung, U.J.; Lee, M.-K.; Park, Y.B.; Jeon, S.-M.; Choi, M.-S. Antihyperglycemic and Antioxidant Properties of Caffeic Acid in db/db Mice. *J. Pharmacol. Exp. Ther.* **2006**, *318*, 476–483. [CrossRef]
64. Eid, H.M.; Thong, F.; Nachar, A.; Haddad, P.S. Caffeic acid methyl and ethyl esters exert potential antidiabetic effects on glucose and lipid metabolism in cultured murine insulin-sensitive cells through mechanisms implicating activation of AMPK. *Pharm. Biol.* **2017**, *55*, 2026–2034. [CrossRef] [PubMed]
65. Feng, Y.; Feng, Q.; Qu, H.; Song, X.; Hu, J.; Xu, X.; Zhang, L.; Yin, S. Stress adaptation is associated with insulin resistance in women with gestational diabetes mellitus. *Nutr. Diabetes* **2020**, *10*, 4. [CrossRef] [PubMed]
66. Jimenez, V.; Sanchez, N.; Clark, E.L.M.; Miller, R.L.; Casamassima, M.; Verros, M.; Conte, I.; Ruiz-Jaquez, M.; Gulley, L.D.; Johnson, S.A.; et al. Associations of adverse childhood experiences with stress physiology and insulin resistance in adolescents at risk for adult obesity. *Dev. Psychobiol.* **2021**, *63*, 1–10. [CrossRef] [PubMed]
67. Poplawski, J.; Radmilovic, A.; Montina, T.D.; Metz, G.A.S. Cardiorenal metabolic biomarkers link early life stress to risk of non-communicable diseases and adverse mental health outcomes. *Sci. Rep.* **2020**, *10*, 13295. [CrossRef]
68. Choudhary, S.; Mourya, A.; Ahuja, S.; Sah, S.P.; Kumar, A. Plausible anti-inflammatory mechanism of resveratrol and caffeic acid against chronic stress-induced insulin resistance in mice. *Inflammopharmacology* **2016**, *24*, 347–361. [CrossRef]
69. Gonna, H.; Ray, K.K. The importance of dyslipidaemia in the pathogenesis of cardiovascular disease in people with diabetes. *Diabetes Obes. Metab.* **2019**, *21*, 6–16. [CrossRef]
70. Pappan, N.; Rehman, A. Dyslipidemia. In *StatPearls*; StatPearls Publishing: Treasure Island, FL, USA, 2021. Available online: http://www.ncbi.nlm.nih.gov/books/NBK560891/ (accessed on 12 August 2021).
71. Cornier, M.-A.; Dabelea, D.; Hernandez, T.L.; Lindstrom, R.C.; Steig, A.J.; Stob, N.R.; Van Pelt, R.E.; Wang, H.; Eckel, R.H. The Metabolic Syndrome. *Endocr. Rev.* **2008**, *29*, 777–822. [CrossRef] [PubMed]
72. Kim, H.; Kim, Y.; Lee, E.S.; Huh, J.H.; Chung, C.H. Caffeic acid ameliorates hepatic steatosis and reduces ER stress in high fat diet–induced obese mice by regulating autophagy. *Nutrition* **2018**, *55–56*, 63–70. [CrossRef] [PubMed]
73. Gun, A.; Ozer, M.K.; Bilgiç, S.; Kocaman, N.; Ozan, G. Effect of Caffeic Acid Phenethyl Ester on Vascular Damage Caused by Consumption of High Fructose Corn Syrup in Rats. *Oxidative Med. Cell. Longev.* **2016**, *2016*, e3419479. [CrossRef] [PubMed]
74. Bocco, B.M.L.D.C.; Fernandes, G.W.; Lorena, F.; Cysneiros, R.; Christoffolete, M.; Grecco, S.; Lancellotti, C.; Romoff, P.; Lago, J.H.G.; Bianco, A.; et al. Combined treatment with caffeic and ferulic acid from *Baccharis uncinella* C. DC. (Asteraceae) protects against metabolic syndrome in mice. *Braz. J. Med Biol. Res.* **2016**, *49*, e5003. [CrossRef] [PubMed]
75. Oršolić, N.; Sirovina, D.; Odeh, D.; Gajski, G.; Balta, V.; Šver, L.; Jembrek, M.J. Efficacy of Caffeic Acid on Diabetes and Its Complications in the Mouse. *Molecules* **2021**, *26*, 3262. [CrossRef]
76. Chao, C.-Y.; Mong, M.-C.; Chan, K.-C.; Yin, M.-C. Anti-glycative and anti-inflammatory effects of caffeic acid and ellagic acid in kidney of diabetic mice. *Mol. Nutr. Food Res.* **2010**, *54*, 388–395. [CrossRef]
77. Agunloye, O.M.; Oboh, G. Hypercholesterolemia, angiotensin converting enzyme and ecto-enzymes of purinergic system: Ameliorative properties of caffeic and chlorogenic acid in hypercholesterolemic rats. *J. Food Biochem.* **2018**, *42*, e12604. [CrossRef]
78. Hassan, N.A.; El-Bassossy, H.M.; Mahmoud, M.; Fahmy, A. Caffeic acid phenethyl ester, a 5-lipoxygenase enzyme inhibitor, alleviates diabetic atherosclerotic manifestations: Effect on vascular reactivity and stiffness. *Chem.-Biol. Interact.* **2014**, *213*, 28–36. [CrossRef] [PubMed]
79. Lee, D.-H.; Kim, H.-H.; Cho, H.-J.; Bae, J.-S.; Yu, Y.-B.; Park, H.-J. Antiplatelet effects of caffeic acid due to Ca^{2+} mobilization-inhibition via cAMP-dependent inositol-1, 4, 5-trisphosphate receptor phosphorylation. *J. Atheroscler. Thromb.* **2014**, *21*, 23–37. [CrossRef]
80. Lu, Y.; Li, Q.; Liu, Y.-Y.; Sun, K.; Fan, J.-Y.; Wang, C.-S.; Han, J.-Y. Inhibitory effect of caffeic acid on ADP-induced thrombus formation and platelet activation involves mitogen-activated protein kinases. *Sci. Rep.* **2015**, *5*, 13824. [CrossRef]
81. Nam, G.S.; Nam, K.-S.; Park, H.-J. Caffeic Acid Diminishes the Production and Release of Thrombogenic Molecules in Human Platelets. *Biotechnol. Bioprocess Eng.* **2018**, *23*, 641–648. [CrossRef]
82. Mendoza, M.F.; Kachur, S.M.; Lavie, C.J. Hypertension in obesity. *Curr. Opin. Cardiol.* **2020**, *35*, 389–396. [CrossRef]
83. Touyz, R.M.; Rios, F.J.; Alves-Lopes, R.; Neves, K.B.; Camargo, L.D.L.; Montezano, A.C. Oxidative Stress: A Unifying Paradigm in Hypertension. *Can. J. Cardiol.* **2020**, *36*, 659–670. [CrossRef]
84. Surikow, S.; Nguyen, T.; Stafford, I.; Horowitz, J. Inhibition of Nitric Oxide Synthase: Impact on Cardiovascular Injury and Mortality in a Model of Takotsubo Syndrome. *Heart Lung Circ.* **2019**, *28*, S132. [CrossRef]
85. Oboh, G.; Ojueromi, O.O.; Ademosun, A.O.; Omayone, T.P.; Oyagbemi, A.A.; Ajibade, T.O.; Adedapo, A.A. Effects of caffeine and caffeic acid on selected biochemical parameters in L-NAME-induced hypertensive rats. *J. Food Biochem.* **2021**, *45*, 13384. [CrossRef] [PubMed]
86. Wu, H.; Zhang, L.; Gao, P.; Liu, D.; Zhu, Z. Caffeic Acid Ameliorates Angiotensin II-induced Increase In Blood Pressure by Activating Vascular Sarco-/Endoplasmic Reticulum CA-ATPASE2A. *J. Hypertens.* **2021**, *39*, e248. [CrossRef]

87. Li, P.-G.; Xu, J.-W.; Ikeda, K.; Kobayakawa, A.; Kayano, Y.; Mitani, T.; Ikami, T.; Yamori, Y. Caffeic Acid Inhibits Vascular Smooth Muscle Cell Proliferation Induced by Angiotensin II in Stroke-Prone Spontaneously Hypertensive Rats. *Hypertens. Res.* **2005**, *28*, 369–377. [CrossRef]
88. Bhullar, K.S.; Lassalle-Claux, G.; Touaibia, M.; Rupasinghe, H.V. Antihypertensive effect of caffeic acid and its analogs through dual renin–angiotensin–aldosterone system inhibition. *Eur. J. Pharmacol.* **2014**, *730*, 125–132. [CrossRef]
89. Agunloye, O.M.; Oboh, G. Caffeic acid and chlorogenic acid: Evaluation of antioxidant effect and inhibition of key enzymes linked with hypertension. *J. Food Biochem.* **2018**, *42*, e12541. [CrossRef]
90. Castro, M.F.V.; Stefanello, N.; Assmann, C.E.; Baldissarelli, J.; Bagatini, M.D.; da Silva, A.D.; da Costa, P.; Borba, L.; da Cruz, I.B.M.; Morsch, V.M.; et al. Modulatory effects of caffeic acid on purinergic and cholinergic systems and oxi-inflammatory parameters of streptozotocin-induced diabetic rats. *Life Sci.* **2021**, *277*, 119421. [CrossRef]
91. Xu, W.; Luo, Q.; Wen, X.; Xiao, M.; Mei, Q. Antioxidant and anti-diabetic effects of caffeic acid in a rat model of diabetes. *Trop. J. Pharm. Res.* **2020**, *19*, 1227–1232. [CrossRef]
92. Matboli, M.; Eissa, S.; Ibrahim, D.; Hegazy, M.; Imam, S.S.; Habib, E.K. Caffeic Acid Attenuates Diabetic Kidney Disease via Modulation of Autophagy in a High-Fat Diet/Streptozotocin- Induced Diabetic Rat. *Sci. Rep.* **2017**, *7*, 2263. [CrossRef]
93. Salmas, R.E.; Gulhan, M.F.; Durdagi, S.; Sahna, E.; Abdullah, H.I.; Selamoglu, Z. Effects of propolis, caffeic acid phenethyl ester, and pollen on renal injury in hypertensive rat: An experimental and theoretical approach. *Cell Biochem. Funct.* **2017**, *35*, 304–314. [CrossRef]
94. Taher, M.A.; Hussain, D.A.A.; Hasan, H.F.; Fahmi, Z.M.; Luaibi, O.K.; Ali, M.G. Hypolipidemic Effect of Caffeic Acid Isolated From Arctium Lappa Cultivated In Iraq, in Hyperlipidemic Rat Model. *Iraqi J. Pharm. Sci.* **2015**, *24*, 18–24.

MDPI
St. Alban-Anlage 66
4052 Basel
Switzerland
Tel. +41 61 683 77 34
Fax +41 61 302 89 18
www.mdpi.com

Molecules Editorial Office
E-mail: molecules@mdpi.com
www.mdpi.com/journal/molecules

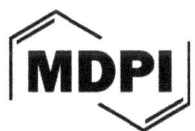

www.ingramcontent.com/pod-product-compliance
Lightning Source LLC
LaVergne TN
LVHW070428100526
838202LV00014B/1548